Treasures of Healthy Living

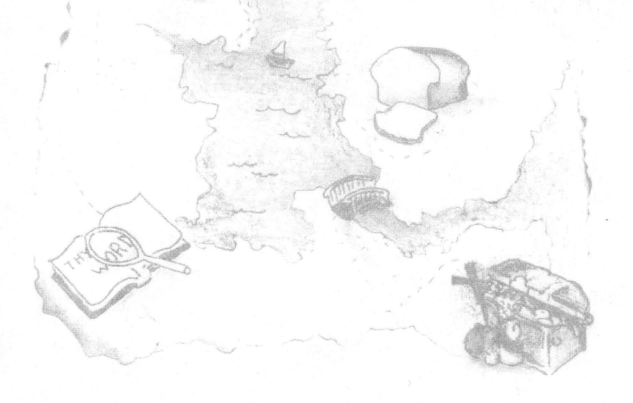

Treasures of Healthy Living

A treasure hunt unveiling God's ultimate plan for health

Annette Reeder and Dr. Richard Couey

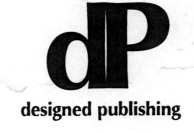

designed publishing

Photo: Dennis Waterman
watermanphoto@yahoo.com
GlimpsesofHisCanvas.blogspot.com

ISBN 13: 978-8-9853969-0-9

Library of Congress Catalog Card Number: 2009908023

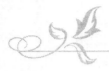

Contents

    Are You Ready to Make a Discovery?

    Why We Need the Treasure

    What Is Keeping Us from the Treasure?

    Tools for the Journey

PART I: FEASTING IN THE TREASURE OF GOD'S DESIGN

    Treasure from the Well

    Got Milk?

    The Joy of Juice

    Beverages Good and Not So Good

    Bread of Life Adds Value to the Treasure

    Wholesome Benefits

    Types of Whole Grains

    Fill Your Basket with Grains, Seeds, and Nuts

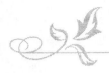

What others are saying....

"This well organized book is full of good scriptural tips and sweet stories. I know God will use this book in a mighty way. Rex would have been thrilled with this Bible study and would have enjoyed being friends."

—Judy Russell, wife of the late Dr. Rex Russell;
author of *What the Bible Says About Healthy Living*

"Based on a passion to bring glory to God alone, Annette Reeder and Dr. Couey present sound scriptural truths, coupled with extensive research data. This journey will teach the readers the joy and benefits of living healthy. Information is given in a unified way that is intriguing to follow and easy to understand. Look forward to being rewarded with life-changing application and treasures you will eagerly want to embrace and share with others!"

—Jerry and Bobbye Rankin, International Mission Board, SBC

"Our bodies were made by God and for God. We are to honor Him through living a healthy lifestyle. In *Treasures of Healthy Living* Annette Reeder and Dr. Richard Couey equip us to maximize our bodies for God. This Bible Study is packed with helpful information. Read and apply to live!"

—Steve Reynolds, Pastor, Capital Baptist Church,
Annandale, Virginia, and author of *Bod4God*

"This book provides a map showing the way to a nutritious lifestyle. These daily teachings serve as a 'GPS' on the journey toward health and wellness in the midst of so many confusing choices. Annette and Dr. Couey's passion to share the treasures and lasting benefits of healthy living, to the glory of God, leaps off these pages."

—Rhonda Sutton, RN, MSN, CHCR

"Annette and Dr. Couey present a practical, biblical, and natural guide for improving health while making it interesting and relevant."

—Kim P. Davis, author of *My Life His Mission*,
compiler of *Voices of the Faithful* books

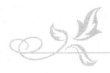

Tribute

Greatest Tribute: The greatest tribute goes to Dr. Rex Russell, who wrote a book, *What the Bible Says about Healthy Living*, that changed my life. His application of the Three Principles made going healthy not only practical but easy to verify in scripture. Along with Dr. Russell is Kim Davis, missionary to Africa, who started me on the search for a foundation to my health and the health of my family. Kim introduced me to Dr. Russell's book and has been a cherished mentor all along the journey.

My partner, co-author, and content advisor: Dr. Couey has a heart for missions and missionaries. His desire to see them stay healthy and continue going forth made writing this book with his expertise a delight.

My foodie friends: Thanks to all participants of the healthy living classes who were persuasive to get this completed book out to more churches and individuals. You can never have enough foodie friends. They are responsible for many of the ideas presented in this book.

My writing team: Without the help of Jessica Buckalew, Dr. Couey, and Carol McLaren (www.uniquelifestories.com), this book would never have been in your hands. They spent endless hours editing and encouraging every step of the way.

My writing group: Tom and Pat Lacy saw in me more than I saw myself. They gave me confidence each step of the way as they do with all members of Richmond Christians Who Write.

My contributing authors: Joel Sutton, with his years of counseling experience, helped tremendously on the forgiveness chapter; Pastor Jeff Brauer, who contributed his personal journey in the exercise chapter; and to Hunter Stoner, who compiled and wrote most of the exercise chapter.

My family: Their support and prayer never ended. I love each one of them dearly: Steve, Stacey, Brent, Mollie, Chris, Lillie, and our newest grandchild, Stella, who was born just in time to get her name in print.

The work of this book is not one or two people but a collection of gifts God has given to each of these people plus many more. Everyone listed here has the same goal: to reach the world with the treasure of God's health through His Word one person at a time.

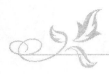

About the Authors

Annette Reeder is a national speaker and author changing lives one meal and a prayer at a time. She is the founder of Designed Healthy Living, author of 5 popular health and cooking books, and encourager to women, men, families and students nationwide through her tasteful cooking classes and life-changing seminars. Annette obtained her B.H.S. Nutrition from Huntington College and diploma in Biblical Studies from Liberty University and is certified in nutrition consulting, but her greatest training came from being a wife, mother, and caretaker for more than twenty-five years. Her career as a biblical nutrition consultant allows her the blessings of seeing lives changed as people apply Scripture to their physical, emotional, and spiritual health. Annette loves the Lord and continually thanks God for the treasures that come from His Word. She eagerly and generously shares her personal journey into God's truths and treasures.

Dr. Richard (Dick) Couey is professor emeritus of health sciences at Baylor University in Waco, Texas. His areas of specialty are human physiology, human anatomy, sports medicine, and nutrition. He is a former member of the President's Commission on Physical Fitness and Sports, and served as exercise physiology consultant for the U.S. Olympic team. Prior to coming to Baylor he was a pitcher in the Chicago Cubs organization. Dr. Couey was educated at Baylor (B.A), Sam Houston State University (M.A.), and Texas A&M University (PhD). He has written and published more than twenty books on subjects ranging from nutrition, physical fitness, wellness, and enzymes. He has spoken in more than three hundred churches throughout the U.S. and internationally on "Why Christians Should Care For Their Temple (body)." His hobbies include working out, serving as a deacon at his church, and golf.

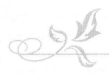

Introduction

A word from Annette Reeder

Have you ever tried to get your kids to eat healthy? One day, years ago, I thought it was time for my kids to try spinach…from the can, of course. My six-year-old son had chosen to be a picky eater, and he did not trust my choice of vegetables for the evening meal. I told him the spinach was smashed green beans, because that was a vegetable he would eat! My son was required to try everything I served, so he obediently took several bites. The problem was that he was not enjoying it. After several bites his face became distorted, his cheeks grew larger, and he threw up the spinach across the table…right at his younger sister. Then I had two kids who no longer enjoyed spinach. Needless to say, we never had canned spinach again.

Have you had similar experiences at the dinner table? Has God been tugging at your heart to make some diet changes but you don't know how? Change can be confusing. Did you know that what you feed your family can contribute to your kids suffering from common illnesses or even tragic health problems? Are you ready to look to the Scriptures and unveil the health plan God has designed just for you?

Several years ago I was in your seat. We were a family battling many health challenges such as cancer, severe PMS, depression, Osgood Slater's disease, multiple cavities, lethargy, muscle complaints, high cholesterol, acid reflux, weight issues, and other more serious health problems. It tires me out just thinking about all the problems we had and yet we were considered "normal." On the outside we appeared as a normal healthy family but inside we were sick and needed answers.

God was tugging at my heart and mind to prepare better meals for my family and therefore improve our health. But I didn't know how. I looked into some health food stores only to feel like I was abandoning my faith and going into New Age. Some of the food looked weird. If I served sprouts for dinner my family would be fighting for the phone to order a pizza.

Praise the Lord, that all changed. Through the next several years God placed strategic people into my life. I was mentored and taught how to search the Scriptures with a focus on health. These new answers matched what I had studied in college. Once the Bible became my foundation, the food and nutrition fell right into place. I started making changes in my family's diet, which surprisingly tasted great! Health and vitality started returning. Truly, the treasure chest was opened! The foods God gifted us to bring hope and an energized life came flowing forth, and the blessings continue to this day.

A word from Dr. Couey

I was introduced to the gospel by a professional hall of fame baseball player who challenged me "to serve God as long and as best that I can." My biology teacher in high school told me that if I could learn everything in one human cell I could change the health of mankind. As my education progressed I realized that I could use my knowledge of the human cell to help Christians live longer, free of health problems, and serve God better. Since those high school and college years I have dedicated my life to helping Christians become better servants. I believe the ideas presented in this book will definitely enhance the health of every Christian, not only in the physical sense but also in the mental, emotional, and spiritual. To be the best Christians possible we need to develop equally in each of these areas in our lives. Annette and I have written this book with this philosophy in mind so that you can find and experience the treasures that God has in store for you.

A word for you to join us

This is a fun and rewarding hunt, and even though Dr. Couey and I have found the treasure chest we continue to search the Scriptures for more blessings to keep it full and guarded. God has promised us His mercies are new every morning.

This Bible study is for those of you who are looking for the answers found in Scripture. Your heart's desire is to provide the very best that God has to offer.

This Bible study is intended to be helpful, but it does not make claims for dramatic healing. It is meant to encourage you to search the Old and New Testaments as you seek God's design for your life and discover a healthier lifestyle.

This study will lead you to God's answers so that He can show you how He designed your body to glorify Him. You will find scriptures and scientific studies that will encourage you to make better choices that lead to becoming a healthier person. As God transforms your life, you will witness His marvelous works.

We will learn which foods to purchase and how to prepare them. The food and tasting may become your favorite part. As we begin our study together, take a moment to read this verse from Proverbs as a prayer to the God who made you and moves with a redeeming love.

Trust in the Lord with all your heart and do not lean on your own understanding. In all your ways acknowledge Him, and He will make your paths straight. Do not be wise in your own eyes; fear the Lord and turn away from evil. It will be healing to your body and refreshment to your bones.
—Prov. 3:5-8 NASB

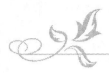

Starting the Treasure Hunt

The *Treasures of Healthy Living Bible Study, Treasures of Health Nutrition Manual,* and *Healthy Treasures Cookbook* are designed to guide you to a balanced approach to improve your health and understand God's provision. The balance comes from understanding God's Word, applying modern scientific studies, and preparing satisfying meals. If we separate the equation we will be unbalanced; all three are needed to balance the body, mind, and spirit. This balance will be presented throughout the next twelve weeks to achieve the highest level of health God has in store for us. The Designed Healthy Living website (www.designedhealthyliving.com) will be updated with new studies, class notes / suggestions, DVDs, CDs, and recipes to help you in this transition and to share with others. Keep watching for new updates.

The *Healthy Treasures Cookbook* is a great accompaniment and is a collection of recipes that incorporates better ingredients. These are designed for enjoyment with all that God has given us to please our taste. If you do not have this book already you can get one from the website.

This study is designed to be completed with a church group or in a home setting. You will be asked to look up verses from the Bible, primarily the New American Standard Bible (NASB) and the New King James (NKJV). If you do not have these translations then you can find these verses on the internet at www.biblegateway.com. To fully benefit from this course, complete all the reading assignments each week and attend the classes or listen to the recorded sessions online. The entertaining and sometimes humorous videos and recorded teachings from Annette Reeder and Dr. Couey will complement your reading and give practical tips to implementing changes. The teachings will also include many pertinent talks on understanding your health and making wise shopping choices. The topics included in the Bible study and *Nutrition Manual* will not all be covered during class time and vice-versa; topics covered in classes are not fully discussed in the Bible study. So don't miss out on any part of the equation.

Getting started:

- **Sample Day in Treasures of Healthy Living—** Read "A Sample Day in Treasures of Healthy Living" in the *Nutrition Manual* to get an idea of how a person can have a healthy lifestyle.

- **Health Assessment**—In the appendix you will find a Health Assessment form. This will assist you in tracking the changes in your life as you begin to apply the principles learned. Fill this out now so that you will have a reference to see the physical, mental, and emotional changes you will experience by personally applying God's treasure.
- **Action Plan**—Weekly you will be given a chance to implement the truths you learned by making one commitment on the Action Plan located in the Appendix of this book. The Action Plan page will give you the opportunity to check off the items as you complete them. The growing list of changes will reflect improvements in your health and life. Both Dr. Couey and I encourage you to not overlook this simple task—it is a rewarding experience.
- **Foodie Friend**—With whom would you like to cook or share cooking ideas? Who would you enjoy as a fun partner in the kitchen? This person or group of people—whether it is your spouse, children, good friend, or group of friends—will be your foodie friends. Foodie friends are great for accountability, sharing spices, and being a cooking partner. They are also people with whom you can share what God is teaching you. Fabulous Foodie Friday will give you ideas each week to make health fun and easy to accomplish. Remember to pray for your foodie friend daily.

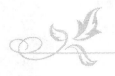

Treasure of Health

DAY ONE—ARE YOU READY TO MAKE A DISCOVERY?

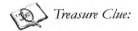 *Treasure Clue:*

My son, if you will receive my words and treasure my commandments
within you…then you will…discover the knowledge of God.

—Prov. 2:1, 5 NIV

Imagine yourself standing in awe as you gaze at an unbelievably huge room full of gold coins and priceless artifacts glistening on the floor, draping the walls, and hanging from the ceiling. The farther you step into the room and feast your eyes on the treasure, the more details stand out of the intricate jade jewelry and breathtaking diamonds. Such a marvelous discovery is beyond anything you ever have imagined, yet you realize that without a map with the clues to the real treasure, it would still be a mystery.

We have all seen movies or read books where encrypted clues on a frail weathered map lead the hero or heroine on a suspenseful trek to a promised fortune. Perils and tragedy lurk around every corner as the clues begin to unveil themselves. Some who follow the leader begin to quit for fear of the unknown, but with each turn more clues emerge, and the treasure is just around the next bend. Those that keep on have renewed energy to keep going, and they don't give up until they reach their reward.

This sounds like the typical, wonderful, incredible discovery of many movies and books, but in our lives is there a treasure we should be looking for? Money and gems are wonderful, but they are not typically what we want most in life. What if you replaced the gold and diamonds for a rewarding adventure to discover vibrant health, healthy relationships, and a grateful heart? Would such rewards be worth getting your hands on the treasure map? Would these rewards be worth following the clues?

Imagine another scene. Imagine you, your family, and your friends are enjoying a picnic on a beautiful day. Your kids are breathing in the crisp, clean air, running after the dog, and laughing contagiously. The adults are enjoying a game of volleyball in the warm sand. Everyone is enjoying the time together. It is time for lunch; everyone is hungry. It takes you and two other people to lift up the picnic chest and share with everyone. As the lid opens, oohs and aahs come from everyone as the tempting aromas and vivid colors of the inviting food fill their senses. Someone gives a prayer of thanks, and the plates are filled. Contentment, health, freedom, and gratitude mark this second scene and are parts of the far greater treasure that God has given us.

Years ago, my family and I were following the wrong map regarding our health. It led us to challenges beyond our ability to handle. The more we continued down the wrong perilous path, the more problems we endured. High blood pressure, pre-diabetes, obesity, joint problems, high cholesterol, allergies, and other severe health challenges seemed to be our destiny. It seemed there were no other choices.

Then I was shown an old encrypted map, and inside was the answer to our health problems. This map is older than any other on the planet. It has been proven for centuries to be the truth. That map is the Bible, and all I had to do was unroll or open the pages. I was very skeptical at first. How could the Bible answer our health dilemmas? I knew the Bible to be true. Yes, it was a treasure, but I never saw answers to my family's health in it. Now it was time to prove it true for health. With a new vigor, I began poring over Scripture to see what God had to say regarding health. Suddenly the words began jumping off the pages! From the very first day of this new search on my heart, God began revealing His Word in a new and refreshing way. Every verse I read, every sermon I listened to, every song I sang began to speak to my heart. I began to delight myself in the Lord! (See Ps. 37:4.) After much study, I began to apply what God teaches in His Word. My family became much healthier, and the persistent health problems began to disappear. Psalm 119:92-93 says, "If Your law had not been my delight, then I would have perished in my affliction. I will never forget Your precepts, for by them you have revived me!" (NASB). This is what I call a praise tickle (my version of "tickled pink")! I was praising God for the joy of discovery He brings.

You may have searched for answers to your health problems. If you were like me you searched everywhere and asked for advice from everyone—expert or not. Did you encounter the pirates of counterfeits and substitutes that did not bring you good health? Since you are still looking for answers, join Dr. Couey and me on this new adventure. Let's be intentional with our search. Our map will be the Bible, our guide will be the Holy Spirit, and the angels will be cheering us on as we discover praise tickles!

The revelation of Your words brings light and gives understanding to the inexperienced.
—Ps. 119:130 HCSB

Great health is in God's plan. Good health is more than food choices. It includes our attitudes, relationships, and outlook on life. This study will take us deep into the eye-opening trails on our map. At different junctions we will compare our directions with various health experts. This hunt is an opportunity for God to reveal His abundant blessings through deeper fellowship, refreshed fulfillment, fabulous food, harmonious families, and endearing friends. Are you ready? Remember, those who quit too early never get to see the full reward.

Fellowship

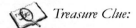 *Treasure Clue:*

My son, if you will receive my words and treasure my commandments within you...then you will...discover the knowledge of God.

—Prov. 2:1, 5 NIV

The first clue on our map is found in our Treasure Clue, Proverbs 2:1-6. Read all the verses in your Bible. Identify the imperative verbs in these verses, and fill in the blanks.

R _____ my words.

T_____ my commandments.

D_____ the knowledge.

In verse 6, what three things does God say He will give us?

_____

God invites us to "receive [His] words" with an open heart and mind. Even more than that, He tells us to treasure His words so we can discover His knowledge and wisdom. The clue of receiving His words will help unlock the door to ultimate health. God's most important words have to do with our fellowship with Him through a relationship with Jesus Christ.

Fellowship is defined as shared interest or companionship. The fellowship with our friends and family is a shared interest when we listen to them and treasure that relationship. By listening and treasuring the other person, we are able to discover more about him or her and deepen our friendship. It is the same with our relationship with Christ. If we want health, if we want freedom, then we need to develop fellowship with Him. We are designed for fellowship with God, according to 1 Corinthians 1:9, "God, who has called you into fellowship with his Son Jesus Christ our Lord, is faithful" (NIV). It may seem strange to consider fellowship a part of health, but it all fits together. Health is more than just food.

Read Psalm 139:13-16. At what time in our life did God desire a fellowship with us?

_____

It is refreshing to understand that God desired fellowship before we were even born.

Throughout this study you will be asked to paraphrase scriptures. This gives you an opportunity to personalize and remember them. It is a way to turn a verse into a prayer. Paraphrase the verses in Psalm 139:13-16 as a prayer of thanksgiving.

_____

_____

_____

God works amazingly in people's lives as they start looking to Scripture for health. Not only do they get great health results, but fellowship with God also keeps increasing. Since my family has been using the Bible as our map to greater health, the physical changes have increased our faith and fellowship. I want you to realize that in order to have true health, you must understand that God wants to have continual fellowship with you.

Leviticus 26:12 says, "I will also walk among you and be your God, and you shall be My people" (NASB). That is fellowship. God wants to walk with us as we learn about health. What better companion could we have?

Can you see how your walk with the Lord (fellowship) may affect your view of God's design for health? Write a prayer of commitment to treasure God's Word as you continue this study.

_____

_____

_____

For further reading about fellowship, read 1 John 1:1-7.

Food

Everyone loves food. Chances are, you have already had some tasty morsel today, but the question is, "Was it truly healthy?" Much of this study is devoted to criteria needed to answer this question. Let's go from loving all food to loving the One who gave us food that builds health. Food is a gift for both necessity and pleasure.

I love trying out new foods and seeing the reaction on the faces of my family or friends when they bite into an innovation from my kitchen. As you partner with your foodie friend, you will have fun making new discoveries also.

The foods God gave us will please even the pickiest eater. As your family members begin to sample new foods, they will each discover at least one new favorite and hopefully many more. Our bodies are not born with a favorite foods gene; favorite foods develop from culture and personal habits. So if we change our habits, our taste preferences change. Many of us have been on diets of cheeseburgers and french fries or fried chicken with lots of gravy. Through this type of eating, our natural taste for nutritious foods has probably become somewhat dulled. Let's awaken those innate sensitivities and broaden our food horizon.

What does Psalm 132:15 say about how God uses food in our lives?

_____

Is that how you have viewed food? God-designed food is a treasure to regain much of our health and return the glory to Him. This will lead to great fulfillment.

Fulfillment

Fulfillment is a sense of achieving something expected, desired, or promised. As we learn to trust God in the area of eating and health, we will discover fulfillment. We will be everything that God intended for us to be and this fulfillment brings gratification and satisfaction in who we are and whose we are.

Write out John 10:10.

_____

_____

How would fulfillment feel to you?

_____

_____

Have you ever considered how your health can bring fulfillment?

_____

_____

In order to completely open the treasure chest and allow absolute health to penetrate our body, mind, and spirit, our twelve-week journey will show us the mudslides of stress and bitterness while giving us an oasis as we camp out on exercise, fasting, and gratitude. As we personally address these issues and make changes under God's leadership, the feelings of fulfillment and satisfaction will fill our daily lives.

Family

> My grandmother had a special cedar box that she kept all of her prized possessions in. I used to sit with her at the kitchen table as she would unwrap her treasures. There were old pictures, coins, gems, a lock of hair, a ribbon from a long passed contest, a pair of old glasses, a hand carved spinning top and a dozen other knick-knacks. My grandmother would tell the story of each and every one, and the love and affection she shared with those memories will stay with me all of my life.[1]

God continues to work in families through generations. This is an asset that can give meaning in the present and guidance for the future. As you receive the valuable riches of God's Word, you will have an opportunity to share with your family how God's treasures have impacted your life. Like the grandmother who has a story to share about each prized possession, you also will have a story to share about how you allowed God to work in your life regarding healing. My husband, Steve, and I can share with our grandchildren that God brought us to a point where we had to go back and rediscover the Old and New Testament for answers to health questions. Those answers have brought us years of health, and prayerfully many more years to come. Psalm 78:4 says, "We will not hide them from their children; we will tell the next generation the praiseworthy deeds of the Lord, his power, and the wonders he has done" (NIV).

No matter what our family situation, we can receive counsel, guidance, and leadership through our Lord and the Scriptures. Your family's spiritual heritage begins with you as you learn from the lives of Abraham, Esther, Ruth, Paul, and Timothy. From them we can understand how God works and apply those ancient lessons to our lives today.

As you make this paradigm change and develop an attitude of looking to God for all your provision, get ready for an impact in your relationships. It continues to amaze me how being physically out of balance transferred to every area of my life, especially family relationships. Family members were easy targets for negative attitudes, and I would treat strangers with kindness. As my family began to realize the benefits of total health, our home became more peaceful, and problems could be solved quickly and with grace. This new attitude that comes with health brings cooperation and well-being into our relationships with others.

We know that family members can either help or hinder our walk with the Lord. List the family members who can assist you in making positive food and health changes. This week let them know of your commitment to a new action plan.

_____

_____

What areas in your life would you like to commit to the Lord and give up your hold on so that He can do marvelous things?

_____

_____

List a few ways God could be glorified by following through with these commitments.

_____

_____

Family Meals a Priority

Which one is better, to grab meals on the go or eat at the kitchen table? According to the British Columbia Medical Association, children who eat at least one meal a day with their families in the home develop more nutritious eating habits, since mealtimes give parents a chance to lead by example and demonstrate healthy food choices. Further research has shown that kids who eat meals at home are more likely to have higher grades, better vocabulary, and improved communication skills.[2] This is good reason to be intentional about family meals. In addition, families usually save money by eating food prepared at home.

Sharing mealtimes together helps to instill a sense of belonging in children and provides a way to transmit Christian family values and traditions. Think of the opportunities you will have to help develop character in your kids as you spend time enjoying a home-cooked meal together. The longer it takes to prepare, serve, and enjoy a meal, the more opportunity there will be for sharing conversations. Consider involving every family member in shopping, cutting, preparing, cooking, and setting the table.

Take a moment to set a goal for how often your family will eat meals together at home this week. We will eat _____ meals per week at home at the kitchen table.

Friends

"A friend is someone who knows all about you and likes you just the same," according to Ralph Waldo Emerson. Friends help us when we are down, they pray with us, and they are the ones we can go to when we're excited. God has put many friends in my life, and they were the ones who helped me get started on this biblical health scavenger hunt.

In 2004, my husband was dealing with many health issues, and we were getting tired of problems, prescriptions, and side effects. When he visited the doctor, he was given three new prescriptions and was informed that he would need all of them for the rest of his life. I began to understand what Matthew 9:36 means, "When he saw the crowds, he had compassion on them, because they were harassed and helpless, like sheep without a shepherd" (NIV).

We felt harassed and helpless like sheep without a shepherd. We wanted a different answer. The previous year, God had moved us from St. Louis, Missouri, to Richmond, Virginia. Being new to the area, I had only made a few friends. I went to my new friend Kim when we couldn't figure out what to do about Steve's health. She showed me the shepherd's plan for eating and health. I affectionately refer to her as Dr. Kim; she is not a doctor, but a missionary who found God's treasure for her family's health.

After Kim, God sent other people who have encouraged me to continue to follow God's plan for health and healing. These friends became instrumental in our health and the birth of the Designed Healthy Living classes. We can follow God's plan successfully on our own with only a Bible, but it's more fun to have friends joining us on the journey.

Here are some suggestions as to how can you be a friend along this valuable hunt:

- Share scriptures that mean the most to you.
- Encourage friends to join you.
- Pray for your friends.
- Share healthy recipes and herbs, but never the spice of gossip.
- Invite friends to dinner and have an "Everything Goes on Pizza Night."
- Find foodie friends. A foodist can never find enough fabulous foodie friends!

Read Proverbs 18:24. How must we act if we want friends?

_____

What friends are joining you in this treasure hunt? Star the ones that are foodie friends.

_____

Finally

There are several great authors who have written about health. Those who have looked to Scripture and applied it have come to the same conclusion: God's laws (commandments) are a blessing to His people. This blessing was not just a spiritual blessing; it was a holistic blessing. Specifically, the laws God gave His people were both a method God used to teach His people obedience and a way to spare them from many easily preventable illnesses and problems. Fellowship, food, fulfillment, family, and friends are all clues to this holistic blessing. Can you just imagine that treasure chest overflowing with all these blessings you are learning to experience? What a great opportunity to see God in a new way! Hang on; the joy of discovery is just beginning.

Day Two—Why We Need the Treasure

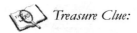 *Treasure Clue:*

*My son, do not forget my teaching, but let your heart keep my command-
ments; for length of days and years of life and peace they will add to you.*
—Prov. 3:1-2 NASB

Read Proverbs 3:1-6. How is God speaking to you in these verses?

_____

_____

Take a moment to say a prayer of thanks for these words. Commit this truth to memory, saying it several times throughout the day.

Some people ask, "Why do we need to look at Scripture for our health?" The answer is so we can be balanced, wise, and healthy. There are many lopsided Christians who are not reaching their potential because they do not look at Scripture in regard to their health.

Be Balanced

These verses in Proverbs help us see that keeping our body (vs. 2), mind (vs. 6), and spirit (vs. 5) in balance is necessary for total health. Scripture tells us many times to treasure His Word in our heart, to never forget it, and to keep telling it to our children and grandchildren. God knows how easy it is for us to forget His teachings when we are faced with the barrage of information coming at us from all directions. He wants us to always remember His words so that we can keep His commandments. By following His commandments, we may be given many more years here on this earth to rejoice in the Lord, and peace will be added to those years.

This peace is not something the world can give us. We can follow all the guidelines for eating a healthy diet, and we can even gain health, but peace will only come from following the God of peace. The apostle Paul speaks of the God of peace and how He wants to sanctify us.

Read 1 Thessalonians 5:23-24. This is another very important clue in our treasure hunt, so read it carefully.

In the book *Praying God's Word,* Beth Moore discusses this verse in view of a triangle. Our God is a God of peace and that peace comes when our body, soul, and spirit are properly surrendered to His wise, loving, and liberating authority. She says, "God deeply desires for us to grant Him total access, to set apart every single part of our lives-body, soul and spirit-to His glorious work."[3] Look at the triangle below, and imagine that the point at the top represents what is in control of our lives. When the body is on top of the triangle, we are controlled by our appetites, physical drives, and bad habits. When the soul (mind) is on top we are controlled by our feelings and personality types. We do not always act the best toward ourselves or others when we are controlled momentarily by either body or soul. As you know, our feelings can drive our physical appetites just as our physical appetites can drive our feelings. Instead, we need to be controlled by the spirit—it should be at the top of the triangle. As Moore says, "The spirit represents that part of us that was created in the image of God to know and enjoy His fellowship. Our bodies, our feelings, and personalities are wonderful components sanctified by God when the Holy Spirit is in control."[4]

Label each triangle below using the words *body, soul,* and *spirit.*

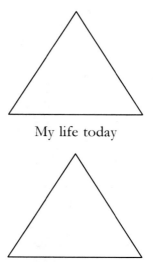

My life today

My commitment to how I want my daily life to be

Take a moment to ask God to lead you to a balanced life. Allow God to sanctify your whole spirit, soul, and body.

Be Wise

In order to be wise, we need to take the teachings that we receive from man and measure them against God's Word. If they match, then the teachings are sound advice. Steve Reynolds, pastor of Capital Baptist Church in Annandale Virginia, learned the wisdom of listening to God.

I weighed 104 pounds in first grade. I still have a report card that says, "Your son is thirty-six pounds overweight." I started playing football when I was eight years old, and played all the way through until I was twenty-two. Then, when I finished, I made myself a promise: "Nobody's ever going to make me run again in my life."

Unfortunately, I kept that promise from age twenty-two to forty-eight. Here I was, not exercising and eating whatever I wanted. I grew and grew to 340 pounds. I had terrible health: high blood pressure, high cholesterol, and diabetes. I was literally digging my grave with a knife, fork, and, of course, an ice cream spoon. At that point God was working and telling me I needed to do something about my overeating and lack of exercise.

God is faithful and He is able. From Colossians 1:16 I learned everything that exists was created for Him and by Him. That included me. If He was in control of all things, then He was in control of my life, and if I'd let Him, He could be in control of my weight issues too.

God gave me a prescription for making a huge change in my life. Once I began to follow it, I began to see results. My faith increased with each change I made and each pound I shed. Today, I am proud to announce that I'm a loser. I've lost more than one hundred pounds. God has helped me get to this point and I intend to stay on track."[5]

Pastor Reynolds applied the treasure map to his health. He is no longer limited with physical aliments, and he is able to reach more people with the gospel of Christ.

Because of a lack of wisdom, disease fills our daily lives. We experience everything from the common cold to cancer to high blood pressure. Genesis starts with a perfect world that God called good. In Genesis 3 everything changed. Sin came into the world and with it came harmful influences that were not a part of God's original grand design.

The Bible gives another clue about how we can avoid some of these problems and be wise. Look up Exodus 15:26 and write it here. Then underline all the verbs and verb phrases.

_____

_____

_____

Let's look at this verse in depth, using Hebrew definitions.

- The term "listen carefully" in Hebrew is *shema*—to be earnest, heed, hear intelligently, consider, be content, or obey.

When you are about to tell your kids something that is very important, you want them to really listen to you. You want your kids to listen carefully so that you can avoid repeating yourself and so they will learn the importance of immediate obedience. This usually happens when you get down on their level and look them straight in the eye.

- The term "do" in Hebrew is *asah*—to accomplish, advance, be busy, execute, finish, fulfill, sacrifice, maintain, or bring to pass.

We all know what *sacrifice* means, but now God is applying it to this verse, asking for us to listen intelligently and to sacrificially do whatever it takes.

- The term "pay attention" in Hebrew is *azon*—to give ear, expand, or listen.
- The term "keep" in Hebrew is *shamar*—to keep, hedge about, guard, protect, take heed, beware, or observe.

We protect what is important. Typically parents pray for a hedge of protection around their children. This continues to show the intensity of this verse.

God is calling to us in these verbs. You will sacrifice your time and risk having your family looked upon as being different as you start changing your eating habits. To help with this, you should realize that you are called to put a "hedge about" your family, which carries a heavy responsibility. These verbs tell us a lot about this passage. If we do these things, *then* He will not bring certain things upon us. God gives us steps and responsibilities to follow in order to take care of our bodies.

John Jay, a Christian statesman in the late 1700s, also knew what it meant to be wise. Consider his words:

> In order to become wise, [we] have much to unlearn as well as to learn—much to undo as well as to do. The Israelites had little comfort in Egypt, and yet they were not very anxious to go to the promised land. Figuratively speaking, we are all at this Day in Egypt, and a Prince worse than Pharaoh reigns in it, although the prophet "like unto Moses" offers to deliver from Bondage, and invites us to prepare and be ready to go with him, under divine guidance and Protection, to the promised land; yet great is the number who prefer remaining in slavery and dying in Egypt.[6]

Write down what you have learned and what you need to unlearn. What wise and sacrificial choices might you need to make for your own health and that of your family?

_____

_____

Be Healthy

Read Deuteronomy 4:39-40, and consider what God is telling you.

_____

_____

The Bible is God's owner's manual. Everything we need to know is in this manual, including how to help our bodies. In Deuteronomy, God confirms that He has the authority to guide us and has given us His statutes and commandments. Keeping His commandments are the means by which we will do well, including with our health. Obey God; do well.

Being healthy or being well does not mean being perfect. We still live in a sin-cursed earth. We live in a toxic environment. We will grow older. Even though we cannot achieve perfection in our health, we should take care of ourselves.

Read 3 John 2 and write it here:

_____

_____

Consider the advantages of being healthy:

- It's easier to be cheerful and vibrant.
- It helps us represent our Lord.
- It helps us not feel tired and run down.
- There is less time for discouragement.

However, we also need to realize that there are exceptions to healing. God does use sickness in the following ways:

- God uses sickness for testing and to bring glory to Him, as in the case of Job and the blind man in John 9. "My grace is sufficient for thee: for my strength is made perfect in weakness," God said in 2 Corinthians 12:9 (KJV).
- Sickness can be a result of disobedience or ignorance. Hosea 4:6 says, "My people are destroyed for lack of knowledge" (KJV). And Isaiah 1:19-20 says, "If ye be willing and obedient, ye shall eat the good of the land: But if ye refuse and rebel, ye shall be devoured with the sword" (KJV).
- The purpose of sickness may also be for death. It is one way we get to heaven! "It is appointed unto men once to die, but after this the judgment" (Heb. 9:27 KJV).

Taking this treasure to heart: Being balanced, wise, and healthy requires an understanding that the biblical stewardship of our whole life, body, mind, and spirit—they all belong to God. We are custodians of what He has given us. If He is our Lord and we are His servants, then shouldn't we take care of what He has given us?

Look back at the triangles you labeled a few pages ago. What steps can you take to begin to improve the care of your body, mind, and spirit today?

_____

_____

_____

Applying this treasure at home: Fill out the Health Assessment in the Appendix if you have not done so already.

DAY THREE—WHAT IS KEEPING US FROM THE TREASURE?

Knowledge is love, life, and vision.

—Helen Keller

"The cat spit first!" My daughter and I heard this defensive remark as we arrived at Sarah's home. She was trying to discipline her two rambunctious boys after the neighbor had complained that the boys were spitting at her cat. Their response—which made perfect sense to them—was to defend themselves against a spitting cat by spitting back.

How many times do we as parents have to hide our snickers when our kids do something as comical as spitting at a cat, especially when discipline is necessary? Sometimes I believe God is wondering and often laughing at the mistakes I make. But there are other times when I know God is disappointed with my decisions, when He had clearly given me the knowledge and directions I should follow.

Look up Hosea 4:6 and write it down.

_____

_____

Rewrite the verse in your own words or as a prayer request.

_____

_____

Hosea, the ancient prophet to the kingdom of Judah, expressed this mournful cry as his generation broke their covenant with God and shamelessly disobeyed God's commandments. Even the priests had exchanged the glory of God for something disgraceful. Hosea understood and communicated the consequences of ignoring God's law—destruction and death. As we look at this principle regarding our health, we will see it still holds true today. If we pay attention to God's design, health and blessing will follow, and God will be glorified in our lives. If we ignore God's design, the consequences can be dire indeed.

Lack of Knowledge

National Treasure was a treasure-seeking movie in which the hero followed a map found on the back of the Declaration of Independence. The encrypted clues led to a discovery of precious treasures worth billions of dollars sitting in the middle of a city. These treasures were hidden, yet within the reach of thousands of people.

Similarly, our health is within reach when we open up God's Word. The truth has been there for thousands of years. You may have heard the saying "ignorance is bliss," but when it comes to our health that is not true. Ignorance is costing us everything.

Debbie Grice, an RN in a prestigious hospital in Richmond, Virginia, knew about health care, but she wishes she had known about God's foods earlier in life.

For forty-nine years I was so energetic, vibrant, and enthusiastic. I thought I was living a healthy life. I thought nothing would happen to me, simply because I didn't feel sick.

Suddenly, in 2007, I suffered a seizure and was diagnosed with malignant brain cancer—*glioblastoma multiforme*. All I could say was that I was suffering due to a lack of knowledge and to disobedience, because I was too busy to learn to eat according to God's instruction.

My mistake was that I followed the culture—it was an easy and more convenient way to eat. But deep down inside me, I had a secret longing to learn. I just didn't know where and how to start learning. I didn't know who to approach.

Wasted years, oh how foolish! Since 2007, pharmaceutical drugs have been my food. I have missed summer vacations and Christmas celebrations with my family and kids. Wrong eating has even brought on heart disease in my husband.[7]

Throughout history, men have thought they could improve or replace God's teachings. Many other times people, including Christians, forgot God's teachings. Look at Moses and the example he left for us.

Moses Gained Knowledge

Moses was raised in Pharaoh's royal court and was educated in all the wisdom of the Egyptians (Acts 7:22). Doubtless, he knew Egyptian remedies and all the latest medical breakthroughs. Who would expect Moses to make breakthroughs in epidemic prevention? Yet in the Pentateuch (the first five books in the Old Testament), Moses recorded important prescripts on how to live a healthy lifestyle. And he attached a blessing and a promise of freedom from disease. Take a moment to refer back to Exodus 15:26 and continue to ask God how to apply it to your life.

Throughout the centuries, as people have not followed God's Law in the writings of Moses, they suffered and died. When scientific breakthroughs have discovered these same truths, doctors have saved lives and prevented the spread of epidemics. Thus, Moses could be called the father of modern infection control. Even today we are still benefiting from God's 3,500-year-old prescription for health.

Lack of Knowledge Leads to Spread of Leprosy

When we lack adequate knowledge about health matters, diseases can spread. For instance, there was a time when doctors thought spicy foods, spoiled fish, or diseased pork caused leprosy. Therefore, they would allow the sick to continue living among others, not realizing that this would cause an epidemic. Since the physicians had nothing to offer, the church took over. When the church began separating the sick from the healthy and building communities for them, the epidemic stopped. "As long as he has [leprosy]…he must live alone…outside the camp" (Lev. 13:46 NIV). Today we call that a quarantine.

Like the ancient Hebrews, we can experience this promise: "If you will give earnest heed to the voice of the Lord your God…I will put none of these diseases upon you" (Ex. 15:26 NASB).

Lack of Knowledge Leads to Unnecessary Death

Numbers 19:11 says, "The one who touches the corpse of any person shall be unclean for seven days" (NASB). And Leviticus 12:2 reads, "When a woman gives birth…she shall be unclean for seven days, as in the days of her menstruation she shall be unclean" (NASB).

In Vienna, Austria, in 1847, one out of every six women who had just given birth was dying. During those times, the physicians and interns routinely alternated between delivering babies and examining bodies in the morgue. Then one physician, Dr. Semmelweiss, requested every physician to wash his hands between the morgue and the delivery room. The death rate dropped to one in eighty-four women—a life-saving difference. But Dr. Semmelweiss, who discovered this link between hand washing and infection, was ridiculed and forced out of practice. Dr. Semmelweiss did not believe truth was a democracy. The majority could just as easily agree on error as truth, especially if they refused to look at the truth.[8]

Lack of Knowledge Leads to Cholera Epidemic

"Designate a place outside the camp where you can go to relieve yourself. As part of your equipment have something to dig with, and when you relieve yourself, dig a hole and cover up your excrement" (Deut. 23:12-13 NIV).

There was an epidemic of cholera in England during the 1800s. As a result, Dr. Chadwick tried to convince Parliament to bring sanitation to the poor villages. Again, people did not follow the laws God gave us in his Word, and more than 72,000 people died.

Knowledge Saves the Camp

Compare the previous events to the leadership of George Washington, who ordered the army to follow these rules for hygiene and to police the camps.

> In the History of these People, the soldiers must admire the singular attention that was paid to the Rules of Cleanliness. They were obliged to wash their Hands two or three Times a Day. Foul garments were counted abominable: every Thing that was polluted or dirty was absolutely Forbidden: and such Persons as had Sores or Diseases in their skin were turned out of the Camp. They were commanded to have a place without the Camp, whither they should go, and have a paddle with which they should dig so that when they went abroad to ease themselves they might turn back and cover that which came from them.[9]

Lack of Knowledge in Christians Today

These examples mentioned happened long before any of us were born, but what about today? Apply these principles to our culture today. What teachings are you hearing that may go against Scripture?

_____

_____

_____

For years I had read the Old Testament laws and had been taught that they were no longer necessary for our lives today. They said the New Testament was the end to the laws or that Jesus fulfilled the Law. But is that the whole truth?

Read Joshua 1:7-8. In verse 7, how much of the law was Joshua commanded to do?

_____

_____

According to verse 8, what was the command regarding God's laws?

_____

_____

Read Matthew 5:17-19. What do we learn about the law in these verses?

_____

_____

Read 2 Timothy 3:16-17. Which scriptures are inspired by God?

_____

_____

Does that include the Old Testament, New Testament, or both?

_____

_____

What are the directions regarding the verses in the Old Testament?

_____

_____

Verse 17 gives us a promise. Write it here.

_____

_____

The laws in Scripture are for our good. We will go over many of them in detail throughout our journey. For now it is important to understand that the laws were written for our good from a God who loves us and knows what is best for us.

Has your physical condition ever stopped you from doing something that would have brought glory to God?

_____

Do you know of Christians who are unable to physically help others when called upon?

_____

_____

Have you or anyone you know been unable to go on missions due to a health problem?

_____

God designed our bodies in His image, and He cares enough to give us a plan to follow. For years I was too ignorant of this. My latest job was working in the medical office of a mission organization. The more I learned about *biblical* health, the more my heart broke for the missionaries who were returning home from overseas due to health problems. Many of these health problems were from following man's altered diet—a diet void of God's whole foods. Stacks of applications represented people who dreamed of serving God in missions, but who would never see the soil they felt called to serve because of health problems. I knew if my husband and I were serving overseas we, too, would have been brought home because of health problems.

However, the tide is turning and the answers are becoming clear. There will be a day when our health testimony will be one of the tools God uses to draw all men unto Him. Do you want to be the one holding that tool? I know I do.

Day Four—Tools for the Journey

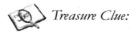 *Treasure Clue:*

But if from there you seek the LORD your God, you will find him if you look for him with all your heart and with all your soul.

—Deut. 4:29 NIV

The Lord wants us to find Him, and He wants us to search for Him as if we are searching for silver and gold with all our heart and all our soul. We are to leave nothing out of this search. Our treasure hunt is better than any fictional plot written. Those heroes had to wait to see their rewards. In contrast, we get to fill our treasure chest with each new or relearned discovery. Today we'll learn about the tools that are needed for this adventure.

Tool #1—Delight Yourself in the Law

From Genesis to Revelation, scriptures instruct us to live a fulfilled life. Just as God was intentional to place these specific scriptures, we should be intentional to understand them.

Read Psalm 19:7-11. How does David describe the law of the Lord? List all the examples given.

_____

_____

_____

Psalm 119 is a deep ocean of verses where the author is in absolute devotion to the Lord. He truly delights in the law. But what is the law? In the complete chapter, the psalmist uses eight different words for God's law.

- Law (or *torah*)—This refers to the instruction given to Moses as the basis for life and action.
- Word—This includes any word that proceeds from the mouth of the Lord.
- Laws—God is a great judge; this word pertains to the legal system.

- Statutes—This word means "testimony" and is synonymous with *covenant*. The observance of the statutes of the Lord signifies loyalty to the terms of the covenant between God and Israel.
- Commands—This refers to anything that the Lord has ordered.
- Decrees—This means "engraved" or "inscribe." God reveals his royal sovereignty by establishing his divine will in nature and in the covenant community.
- Precepts—This is synonymous with covenant and revelation of God.
- Word or Promise—This is anything God has spoken, commanded, or promised.

Read or skim through this chapter, and count how many times the author declares his delight in the law. _____

What spiritual, physical, and emotional benefits did you discover from this chapter about following the Law?

_____

_____

_____

_____

LOOK AT THE TEN COMMANDMENTS

Exodus 20 begins with the words of God. "And God spoke all these words, saying: 'I am the Lord your God, who brought you out of the land of Egypt, out of the house of bondage'" (Ex. 20:1-2 NKJV). The Ten Commandments are part of the laws God gave us to protect us, give us direction, and keep us from bondage. All of the Mosaic Laws are designed to be a tutor to lead us to Christ. There is no way we can fulfill all the laws given on our own. But that does not mean we are to ignore them. God gave us those laws to bring Him glory.

Today if I speed on the highway I will probably get a ticket. That is a law of our culture. Speed laws were designed to keep the driver in control of the vehicle and to prevent accidents. As a citizen I am free to either drive the speed limit or to speed. It is my choice. It is the same with God's laws. They were given to protect us, but we can choose whether or not to follow them. God instructed Moses to write ten commandments on stone for the Israelites to carry with them. Today many Christians encourage their children to memorize these commandments and follow them.

Take a moment now to write as many of the 10 commandments as you can remember.

_____

_____

_____

_____

_____

_____

_____

Which commandments might adversely affect our health if we broke them? Write them down, and then write what the ill effect might be.

_____

_____

_____

LEARN THE MOSIAC LAW

Can you recall a situation where reading the directions would have saved you a lot of headaches or mishaps? We have a book with lots of laws, commandments, and guidelines. Unless we read the whole book, we may not be familiar with the reason for many of God's directives. It helps to understand that God is thoroughly interested and involved in every single part of our life: body, mind, and spirit.

It is important to understand that we need to read God's Word for ourselves and not just accept another person's interpretation. Remember, God created us individually and wrote His "letter" to us personally.

Read Ecclesiastes 12:13-14 and fill in the blanks. "Now _____ has been heard; here is the conclusion of the matter: Fear God and _____ his commandments, for this is the _____ duty of man" (NIV).

Who should keep the commandments?

_____

For a deeper study, read Isaiah 8:20 and Proverbs 28:9.

We are going to look at the dietary law, but first I want us to basically understand the three types of laws God gave us.

- The moral law, which is summed up in the Ten Commandments—Exodus 20.
- The dietary law—Leviticus 11 and Deuteronomy 14:3-21.
- The ceremonial law—Exodus 25–40 and the book of Leviticus.

There are many views on Old Testament law. Some people would say that Old Testament dietary laws were only for the nation of Israel or for ceremonial purposes. Some people speak of "legalism" to those who obediently respect the Law. Others are enslaved to the Law, believing its perfect obedience is essential to eternal salvation (Rom. 3:19-28, 4:5; Gal. 2:16). Some people believe we should obey parts of the Law such as the Ten Commandments. Some claim if it is not written in the New Testament, it should be rejected. What do you think?

_____

_____

_____

God is perfect and righteous; therefore, His laws are also. Man is imperfect and unrighteous and cannot keep the law perfectly, and therefore he falls under the total penalty of the law: death. God did not allow this to be the end of humanity, though (John 3:16). He sent His Son to be the fulfillment of the law and allowed Jesus' blood to be the payment for our sins.

There is therefore now no condemnation to those who are in Christ Jesus, who do not walk according to the flesh, but according to the Spirit. For the law of the Spirit of life in Christ Jesus has made me free from the law of sin and death. For what the law could not do in that it was weak through the flesh, God did by sending His own Son in the likeness of sinful flesh, on account of sin: He condemned sin in the flesh, that the righteous requirement of the law might be fulfilled in us who do not walk according to the flesh but according to the Spirit.

—Romans 8:1-4 NKJV

Now what should be our attitude toward the Law?

_____

Because we are dead to sin and alive in Christ, the Holy Spirit lives in us and gives us direction and strength to live a righteous life. He not only puts the desire within us to want to keep God's Law, but His Spirit actually helps us succeed as we surrender to Him. We rejoice because God wants us to be healthy, but we cannot lose our salvation due to not following dietary laws.

Tool #2—The Three Principles

Through his writings, Dr. Rex Russell has been a significant influence in my understanding of how Scripture and science fit together. Here is his testimony.

I was diagnosed with juvenile diabetes when I was thirteen years old. At that time I was told I could expect to live about twenty more years before serious complications would shorten my life. I immediately had two thoughts. The first was, "Why me?" The next was, "God, use this to help people come to know You."

Then at the predicted age of thirty-three the two big D's—Diabetes and Death—contributed to my kidneys, arteries, and eyesight deteriorating.

Desperate, I searched for anything that might alleviate my health crisis. One evening, I was sprawled out on the couch in a funk—but still with a Bible in my hand. I read Psalm 139:4. The psalmist, in praise, lifted his voice to God and said, "I am fearfully and wonderfully made." Uncomforted and angry I said, "God, if I am so wonderfully made, why am I so sick? Why didn't You give us a way to be healthy?" And then, like a feather making a gentle descent, The Question dropped into my mind: "Have you read my Instruction Book?" No longer the one asking the questions, I felt compelled to answer the one God posed to me. I began a journey to discover what the Bible says about healthy living.

The first thing that caught my attention was that God wanted his people to be healthy. Exodus 15:26 and other verses cemented the idea that there was a relationship between God's ordinances and the health of His people. I began to learn that God had laws and commands relating to health.

But I was a scientist. Would science speak to the adverse effects of eating pork or shellfish?

God's health plan slowly began to fit together. Each time, I looked at what the Bible said and then found confirmation in science. I would shake my head in amusement and smile with a grateful heart. We are fearfully and wonderfully made.

I faithfully lived out what I learned and I experienced enormous positive health changes from applying the Three Principles to my life.

One might say at age sixty-seven, I have lived on borrowed time. I would not put it that way. I live each day as a gift—a gift wrapped in the wisdom of God's Instruction Book.[10]

Foodie Test: In five minutes or less, walk into a grocery store and see if you can find ice cream with five or less ingredients. Can you do it? How many packages will you need to pick up to read the back label? Do you look for a short name on the front, such as "vanilla"?

There are 320,000 edible items for sale on a typical day in the United States. Most subu grocery stores carry as many as 40,000 of these items. Do you have a plan for finding food that will build health? Do you have a measuring stick to use for making good choices? How do you decide between low-fat and heart-healthy foods?

Dr. Rex Russell's book, *What the Bible Says About Healthy Living*, led me to one of the best discoveries to help simplify shopping choices: The Three Principles. These principles form the foundation for making choices in regard to all areas of our health.

Principle I—Eat only substances God created for food. Avoid what is not designed for food.

Principle II—As much as possible, eat foods as they were created—before they are changed or converted into something humans think might be better.

Principle III—Avoid food addictions. Don't let any food or drink become your god.[11]

PRINCIPLE I: EAT ONLY SUBSTANCES GOD CREATED FOR FOOD

The story of Adam and Eve begins with God giving them food to eat. Read Genesis 1:29-30. List the foods given to eat.

_____

_____

Some Christian health plans preclude and conclude with Genesis 1:29. It is true that Genesis 1:29 is loaded with lots of nutrition, as it includes fruits, vegetables, grains, and nuts. Even Daniel and his friends followed this diet and appeared "better...than all the youths who had been eating the king's choice food" (Dan. 1:15 NASB).

But after Adam and Eve sinned, everything changed. What foods were added to their diet in Genesis 3? What foods do you think this includes?

_____

_____

This was the food previously designated for animals. Many think that these were the herbs without seed in them, such as lettuce, cabbage, broccoli, cauliflower, spinach, and asparagus, as well as tubers, which include yams, potatoes, carrots, beets, and so on.

Then along comes a worldwide flood that wipes out everything, including the vegetation. So God gave Noah a new food group to add to his food pyramid.

Read Genesis 9:3-4. List the foods that were given in these verses and the restriction that came along with them.

_____

_____

_____

Many people like to think—or want to think—that Noah was allowed to have a barbeque at this point and start pigging out. Let's take a closer look.

Were there any rules? In the Garden, God gave Adam and Eve seeds to eat. He wanted them to be disciplined—to not eat from the Tree of Knowledge of Good and Evil. Then later He added herbs without seeds and told them to cultivate the ground.

Now take a look at God's instructions to Noah in Genesis 7:2. How many of each animal was Noah instructed to take on the ark?

_____

Up to this point in Scripture, there is no instruction about which animals are clean and unclean. So who told Noah?

Recently I was with my two-year-old granddaughter, Lillie, and we were walking to the boat dock for a fun day on the lake. The evening before, we had experienced a downpour of rain, and as we walked along hand-in-hand, Lillie's little shoe landed in some mud. She immediately lifted her foot and said, "Yucky!" Now, some grandchildren would step into the mud and say, "Cool!" To one child mud equals a dirty shoe, but to another child mud is a chance for fun. Who taught them the difference? Did they just know it? Some parents would disagree with me, but most of the time it is learned. Obviously Noah had learned which animals were unclean for human consumption. Noah knew which animals should be brought on the ark in groups of seven and which ones in groups of two. We also see that in Genesis 6:21, Noah was instructed to gather up some of all edible food to take on the ark, which tells us that he had also learned which types of plant foods were edible. Then after the flood, in Genesis 8:20, we read, "Noah built an altar to the Lord and took of every clean animal and of every clean bird and offered burnt offerings on the altar" (N.ASB). Again, Noah knew what was clean and unclean.

I have talked with people from different parts of the US in regard to following Principle I. Those who have followed it for more than ten years report few doctor visits and illnesses. Their learned discipline in diet carries over to other areas of the Christian life. What a treasure to pass on to our children and grandchildren!

To apply Principle I, when you question a food you are about to eat, ask yourself, "Is this something God called food?" Make a list of the top five foods you enjoy that God gave us to eat.

_____

_____

PRINCIPLE II – EAT THE FOODS CLOSE TO THE WAY GOD DESIGNED, WITH VERY LITTLE ALTERATION

Write Proverbs 14:12 here.

_____

_____

The spiritual truth stated in this proverb is that our attempts to be good, to do things our own way, or to earn righteousness by good deeds all lead to spiritual death. The verse has a practical secondary truth important for our study here—a warning against our incessant presumption that we can somehow improve on God's design.

In our compulsive and pleasure-seeking culture, we often formulate additives, chemicals, and processed foods that take us away from our Creator's perfect design for nutrition. Altering foods has caused an alarming rate of obesity and diabetes, and many now believe today's children will live shorter lives than their parents. "The report, published in *The New England Journal of Medicine*, says the prevalence and severity of obesity is so great, especially in children, that the associated diseases and complications—Type 2 diabetes, heart disease, kidney failure, and cancer—are likely to strike people at younger and younger ages."[12]

To follow Principle II, eat vegetables raw, steamed, or lightly cooked. Eat bread that you have made yourself by self-milling the flour. Otherwise, eat bread that says "stone-ground" on the label. Eat an apple instead of an apple-flavored cereal, which is an altered food.

List some altered foods that you typically eat that are not healthy, such as potato chips, marshmallows, and candy.

_____

_____

PRINCIPLE III: DON'T LET ANY FOOD BECOME YOUR GOD

Exodus 20:3 says, "You shall have no other gods before Me" (NASB). Your treasure chest is full of foods beyond what science can explain. But even foods given to us by the hand of God can become a god themselves by our misuse or by allowing them to consume our primary attention—a place God reserves for Himself.

We often use the word *addiction* to describe this difficulty. Our society commonly talks of addictions to drugs, tobacco, alcohol, and work, and there are support groups for each of these categories. However, even food can become an addiction. The foods commonly referred to an addiction would be chocolate, sugar, caffeine, and possibly salt.

Even good food can become an addiction. One of the doctors with whom I worked in an emergency room had been away for several weeks. When he returned to work, it was apparent that he had lost weight and looked much healthier, except for one thing—his skin was orange. His coloring caused quite a reaction, and finally one brave person asked how he acquired such an unusual look. He replied that he was trying to lose weight and he constantly carried carrots with him to eat as a snack. Obviously, from his skin color, he got hungry often.

When food consumes our thoughts and actions, the best way to gain control is to fast. Fasting is a very effective way of freeing ourselves from a preoccupation with our physical wants and desires so that we can concentrate on our relationship with God. Are there any foods you think you might be addicted to?

_____

Take a moment to write a prayer about this addiction, asking God to reveal His plan for you to place Him—not the food—back on the throne.

_____

_____

_____

The greatest truth to be learned for health is that we have a loving Creator who has left us a map that wonderfully matches the design of His creation. In 2 Timothy, Paul wrote, "All Scripture is inspired by God and is useful for teaching, for showing people what is wrong in their lives, for correcting faults, and for teaching how to live right. Using the Scriptures, the person who serves God will be capable, having all that is needed to do every good work" (2 Tim. 3:16-17 NCV).

The laws of science are the thoughts of God.

—Florence Nightingale

Tool #3—The Healthy Treasures Mediterranean Pyramid

What would Jesus eat? Would you like a tool to use as a guide to the foods Jesus ate and declared for our good? Then look at the Healthy Treasures Mediterranean Pyramid.

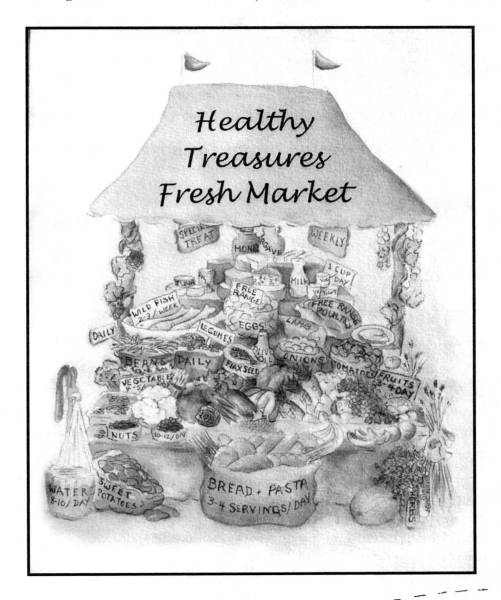

Dieticians and physicians have given us several food pyramids, but the one with the most solid foundation—with extensive research going back fifty years—is the Mediterranean Pyramid. According to the Mayo Clinic, this pyramid has demonstrated the highest average life expectancy and the lowest rates of chronic diseases among adults.[13]

This pyramid maximizes natural, whole foods and minimizes highly processed ones. Dr. Steven Parker summarizes the Mediterranean Diet Pyramid in his book *The Advanced Mediterranean Diet*. "Clinical studies have clearly shown that a Mediterranean style diet is associated with overall greater health and longevity, lower incidence of cancers, and lower incidence of cardiovascular disease. Furthermore, recent studies suggest that such a diet may reduce dementia of both Alzheimer's and vascular types. Expert consensus is that the health benefits are due to diet composition coupled with a physically active lifestyle."[14,15]

People have taken notice, and now restaurants, cooking shows, and cookbooks have embraced this way of meal planning. You and your foodie friend can join in on the culinary delight.

For the Healthy Treasures Mediterranean Pyramid, we have designed a useful tool with the unclean foods eliminated and the categories such as herbs, grains, and vegetables easy to measure.

Which of your food habits need to change in order for your eating lifestyle to match this food pyramid? What about your family?

_____

_____

_____

Understanding Our Fears

As we end this first week, our treasure hunt may have brought to light some concerns about how you are going to deal with the information you learn. This information can mean changes, and those changes might be a challenge. You may be thinking:

- What if I don't like what I learn?
- Doesn't eating organic cost too much for my budget?
- What will my family and friends think?
- What if it means eating differently from everyone with whom we spend time?
- Will my family like the new foods?

- How will I learn to cook new foods and still have time for my other obligations?
- What if following Scripture doesn't work?

Over and over, many people who have taken this course and followed this approach to their health had some fears to work through. What are some of the challenges you face when thinking about looking to Scripture for answers for your health?

_____

_____

Write out Proverbs 3:13 and Proverbs 4:7.

_____

_____

_____

_____

How can you apply these verses to your fears?

_____

_____

Take a moment to pray for wisdom and discernment as you study God's Word.

Finally, while health is important and should be treasured, we must remember that there is a greater human blessing: "The free gift of God is eternal life in Christ Jesus our Lord" (Rom. 6:23 NASB).

Taking this treasure to heart: What is one nugget that you have gained from this week's lesson?

_____

_____

Applying this treasure at home: What commitment are you going to make regarding at least one of the treasures you learned this week? Add it to your Action Plan.

FABULOUS FOODIE FRIDAY

A wife invited some people to dinner. At the table, she turned to her six-year-old daughter and said, "Would you like to say the blessing?"

"I wouldn't know what to say," the girl replied.

"Just say what you hear Mommy say," the wife answered.

The daughter bowed her head and said, "Lord, why on earth did I invite all these people to dinner?"

Obviously this mom hasn't opened the treasure chest yet. She might not even be able to find the treasure chest. Do you feel as if your kitchen has a treasure chest waiting to be opened? The *Treasures of Healthy Living* will help you have fun as a foodie while gaining new health.

Anyone Can Be a Foodie

To be a foodie is not only to like food, but to be interested in it. Just as a good student will have a thirst for knowledge, a foodie wants to learn about food. A foodie will never answer the question, "What are you eating?" with "I don't know." There are some basic traits of being a foodie, as there are basic traits that come with all labels. Generally, you have to know what you like, why you like it, recognize why some foods are better than others, and want to have good tasting food all or most of the time. This doesn't mean that you can't eat Cheetos every now and again, but it does mean that you don't fool yourself into thinking that it's a nutritionally-balanced meal. Do you have to know the difference between a beefsteak tomato and an heirloom tomato? No, but you might be interested to find out what it is. Do you have to only shop at farmer's markets? No, but you still look for good, fresh produce. Are there some foods you just don't like or weird foods you like? That's OK; it doesn't make you any less of a foodie. Just like food, learn about food, and, most importantly, eat food.

Foodie Time

For your first Fabulous Foodie Friday adventure, we will take a look at your eating plan and your kitchen.

PERSONAL

This week, keep a journal of the food you eat. Record everything you do that will affect your health. This includes food, exercise, thoughts, stress level, and prayer time. Pay special attention to how many fruits and vegetables you eat and what colors they are.

FAMILY

Try a recipe from the *Healthy Treasures Cookbook*. Send a note to the Designed Healthy Living staff and let them know how your family liked or was challenged by this new dish.
Email us at yourfriends@designedhealthyliving.com.

KITCHEN SUPPLIES

Take an inventory of your kitchen supplies:
- Cutting Utensils—What do you use to cut or peel food? Make sure your knives don't have rust or places where mold or mildew can grow. Discard all damaged utensils.
- Pots and pans—If you use pots and pans with non-stick coating…good news, it's time for new cookware. Don't even wait for them to peel, just chuck them in the trash. Look at other pot and pan options, and consider using stainless steel. Waterless stainless steel is by far the healthiest type of cookware, but it will cost you an investment. But you can will it to your kids! I have had my set for more than twenty-five years and it still outperforms any cookware on the market. Use glass for casseroles and other baking. Stoneware is also a good choice for baking.
- Cooking and Serving Utensils—Just as you should think about stainless steel for your pots and pans, also consider it for your cooking utensils. You do not want plastic spatulas melting in your organic spaghetti sauce.

- Food Storage—Try to avoid plastic. As your food sits in the container, plastic leaches into the food and all the toxins that it holds may be ingested with the food. Use glass as much as possible. If you need to cover food with plastic wrap, make sure the wrap does not touch the food. Save your plastic containers for seeds, grains, and powdered ingredients.

It would be hard to make a lot of changes in the kitchen at once, so don't get frustrated. Start small and work a little at a time. Look for deals at store sales and garage sales; you can get a lot of glassware this way. This is what Fabulous Foodie Fridays are all about. Now think about what you are going to commit to first. Tell your foodie friend, and get it done by next week!

PART I

FEASTING IN THE TREASURE OF GOD'S DESIGN

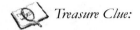 *Treasure Clue:*

My son, give attention to my words; incline your ear to my sayings. Do not let them depart from your sight; keep them in the midst of your heart. For they are life to those who find them and health to all their body.

—Prov. 4:20-22 N.ASB

New adventures can be exciting. We now have our bags packed with the tools we need, we have checked our compass and it is pointed heavenward, so we are on our way.

Because this journey results in a total transformation in our life, it is best approached in two parts. Part I is the opportunity to fill the treasure chest with the richest of foods gifted to us. This will benefit our bodies and in turn glorify God. Then in Part II, we will learn the secrets to keeping our treasure chest full and not letting any pirates steal from our bounty. The discoveries found in both parts will be reflected in our total health: body, mind, and spirit. We will have total balance in our walk with the Lord.

Check out our Treasure Clue above. This verse gives us a very valuable hint to acquire life and health. In fact, it has even given us the steps to follow. Isn't that just like God to make it simple for us?

"Give attention to my words," He says. We are giving attention to His words by using them as our map. Those of us who are parents want our kids to listen when we speak. We want them to hear us so they can do what is right. God wants us to do the same—to give attention to the words that may change your health.

"Incline your ear to my sayings," He continues. This may sound strange, but the simplest way to do this is to speak His words out loud. Practice this now with today's clue; read Proverbs 4:20-22 out loud. The more we hear the Scriptures out loud, the better our retention is. We will need these words later when situations come and we lack direction.

"Do not let them depart from your sight." We are embarking on an incredible journey with a biblical itinerary, so don't hide the map in a drawer and forget about it. Scripture will stay as our focus so that we will be prepared for whatever God has in store for us. As you find scriptures on your map that are useful to restore your health, write them down on a card. Keep God's words in sight so you can stay focused.

"Keep them in the midst of your heart," the Lord says. Spiritually, we can move mountains by keeping God's Word in our hearts. Physically, our lives can take on a whole new look. The key to this is not letting Satan take away the value of the promises laid out for us. Guard your heart; keep the words as a treasure. Give God the glory as your healing comes.

We have looked at the four steps to God's plan. Now where will this clue take us? "They are life to those who find them and health to all their body." Wow, what a treasure: life and health to the whole body. Does that excite you? That is another praise tickle!

Before we go any farther, read Deuteronomy 23:5 and learn why God is offering this for us. Fill in the blanks, "Because the _____ you" (NASB). God's love will carry us on this journey.

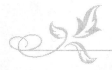

Beverages

DAY ONE—TREASURE FROM THE WELL

Let's reflect on this verse. "The Lord will guide you always; he will satisfy your needs in a sun-scorched land and will strengthen your frame. You will be like a well-watered garden, like a spring whose waters never fail" (Isa. 58:11 NIV). Underline the words that describe what the Lord wants to do for you. Then rewrite the verse as a prayer of thanksgiving to God for this spring of water.

_____

_____

_____

I Baptized a Priest

"Water, please."

"With bubbles or without?" That was the question following my request from the Swedish flight attendant as we traveled from New York to Amsterdam. But what was the correct answer? I had no idea, so I choose to play it safe and requested water without bubbles. After the stewardess gave me my drink, I placed it on the modest tray in my cramped seat that would be home for the next ten hours. I was seated between two people I had never met, one of whom was a priest. I started to sip on my water when I overheard my husband and son ordering bubbly water in the row behind me. I wanted to see their expressions as they drank this new water, so I turned to watch through the opening between the seats. No sooner had I twisted my body than I heard the priest exclaim, "Miss, your water!" As I turned back around I realized what had happened. The water on my tray had baptized the priest!

Water, Water Everywhere

If we were to fill up our treasure chest with water, you might fear that it would overflow or slosh out. Would that be bad if it did? Should we keep the water in our chest at a level that will never spill out? Let's see what you think after we study the spiritual application of water. I hope you will discover better uses for water other than baptizing people on an airplane. In case you were wondering, during the long flight his attire did dry out, but he only spoke a foreign language the remainder of the flight. It is probably good I did not understand.

Water is used throughout Scripture. See if these verses begin to quench your thirst.

Read Proverbs 18:4. What is the symbol of water in this verse?

_____

How can you apply that to learning about health biblically?

_____

Words and knowledge are all around us. It has been said that the more we know, the more we know we don't know. This is very true when it comes to health. When we take the knowledge we have been given by man and measure it against God's Word, we can see if it leaks or holds truth. Wisdom comes from looking to God's Word first and then measuring man's teaching against it. If man's teaching doesn't hold water, then let it spill onto the ground. Wisdom, in the sense of our treasure hunt, is to take what we learn from Scripture and apply it to our health. As we gain wisdom, it will be like a flowing brook—one that never ends.

Read Isaiah 12:2-3. What is the symbol of water in this verse?

_____

Don't you love the connection of "joy" and "salvation"? How can you apply this verse to learning about health biblically?

_____

_____

Read Isaiah 44:3. What is the reference to water in this verse? What truths can you gather?

_____

_____

The Lord promises that He is going to give water to the person who is thirsty and He is going to give us His Holy Spirit. Can you see this in the view of the treasure chest being filled with the Holy Spirit and God's promises? Just as a drink of water satisfies our thirst, the promises from God also bring satisfaction.

Read Isaiah 55:1. What do you need to bring to purchase salvation?

_____

If you had all the money in the world could it purchase salvation? No. This water is not available for money; it is free. If you are willing, you can have it. The poorest person in the world who does not have anything else can have this water. The Lord essentially says, "Come and get all you need. You are going to be satisfied, and you do not need to have any money. I am not going to charge you a price."

Read John 7:37-39. Compare these verses in John to the ones you read in Isaiah 44:3 and 55:1. What is required for anyone to receive from God?

_____

Remember, He is not talking about physical water. He is talking about spiritual water, and He makes an appeal to people who are thirsty. They are the ones that are invited. He says, "If you come, I will give you water." What makes someone a thirsty person?

_____

A thirsty person is one who is dissatisfied. When you are thirsty, you are dissatisfied with your condition, and you are never going to be satisfied again until you can get some water. Why did Jesus appeal to people who were thirsty? It's simple. Have you ever tried to give a drink to someone who was not thirsty or, as we will learn in our study, one who does not know he or she is thirsty? It is not easy.

Many people are dissatisfied or thirsty and don't even realize it. They fill the void with other beverages to quench the physical aspect and they fill their lives with things, power, or knowledge to fill the spiritual portion. Jesus knew those things would not satisfy us. So He said to the people of His day, "If you are still thirsty, if you are still dissatisfied, come to Me and you will be satisfied." He invites the rich, poor, high, and low and He says, "If you come to me, I will relieve your burdened mind. I will comfort your sorrowing heart. I will refresh your bones. I will give you back hope." The good news is that this spiritual water is available to us now; we don't even have to wait till we get to heaven.

Let's see how this teaching applies to the physical side of water. Does water really quench our thirst, strengthen our bones, and satisfy our body?

God's Fingerprints in the Design

On many mission trips with the youth group at First Baptist Church in Arnold, Missouri, we taught the children a fun song called the Hippo Song.[16]

> In the beginning God made the seas,
> Made the forest full of trees,
> Stacked the mountains way up high,
> And right in the middle he placed the sky.
>
> God's fingerprints are everywhere,
> Showing us how much he cares
> And right in the middle he made some fun;
> He made a hippo that weighed a ton!

If you ever want to see God's fingerprints, look not only at the hippo but at the ice crystals frozen on your window or the snowflake that lands on your jacket. These are what I consider God's fingerprints. Water is a design of God's fingerprints.

What happens if you get a drop of water on the counter in your kitchen? Does it appear to be flat or bubbled up? The perfect hexagon alignment of the hydrogen and oxygen in the molecule of water gives it the surface tension that causes it to bubble up. That also explains why ice crystals take up more space than liquid water, making it denser than water so it floats. If it did not expand—as all other molecules do during their transitions from liquid to solid—it would sink. The earth would soon be lifeless, frozen tundra. All bodies of water would freeze from the bottom up, destroying all life in the water. That also explains why water can dissolve other molecules, such as salt. Do you see why I call water and snowflakes God's fingerprints?

Without water, nothing lives. Water is an essential nutrient, more important than any other. It has two primary properties in the body: life-sustaining and life-giving functions. You can survive only a few days without water, whereas a deficiency of the other nutrients may take weeks, months, or even years to develop.

In the previous paragraph, what similarities do you find between water and Jesus?

_____

_____

The role of water has not changed since the beginning of creation, and neither has the role of God in our life.

Adult bodies are made up of 67 percent water, and it's an even higher percentage in children. In the body, water becomes the fluid in which all life processes occur. Water makes up 80 percent of your muscle mass, 60 percent of your red blood cells, and more than 90 percent of your blood plasma. Take a look at the important role water plays in your body and the spiritual application:

- Water helps with digestion. It carries nutrients and waste products throughout the body. Similarly, studying God's Word helps us to get nutrition into our mind and remove the waste from our world.
- Water serves as the solvent for minerals, vitamins, amino acids, glucose, and many other small molecules so that they can participate in metabolic activities. Likewise, God takes every part of our innermost being and acts as our solvent.
- Water acts as a lubricant and cushion around joints and inside eyes, the spinal cord, and, in pregnancy, the amniotic sac surrounding the fetus in the womb. Jesus is a cushion around us in our daily life, protecting us from harm and keeping us moving freely.
- Water aids in regulation of normal body temperature. Evaporation of sweat from the skin removes excess heat from the body; dehydrated people don't sweat. When we let God handle our battles we can remain calm, not over-heated.
- Water maintains blood volume and is the major component in blood and body fluids. Every day our body replaces trillions of cells, including our blood. Every day we think thousands of thoughts; keeping our focus on God and His will keeps us balanced.

All of these physical functions require an adequate daily water balance. All of these spiritual functions require an adequate daily intake from prayer, Bible study, and worship. We don't want to be prune-faced in our walk with the Lord.

Are You Thirsty?

If you were to take a nice juicy plum and place it next to a dried prune, which one has more water? That's easy: the plum. Now if you were to apply the same logic to a person, imagine someone who is well hydrated and has been for more than ten years. She has great looking skin and no wrinkles.

When I worked at Missouri Baptist Hospital, elderly people would commonly be admitted with dehydration. Their skin was paper thin and wrinkled. Their veins were so dehydrated IVs were hard to start. Many had mental confusion. Immediately they would be hooked up to an IV for fluid replacement. After a couple hours on this therapy, often their mental ability would improve along with their ability to function. Their faces would even show more expression.

Dehydration affects all areas of our body. This is why it is important to understand the signs. Just as not everyone recognizes a thirst for God's Word, some people do not recognize the thirst for water.

The research of F. Batmanghelidj, M.D., author of *Your Body's Many Cries for Water*, points out that many people are dehydrated in part because our natural thirst mechanism is turned off by drinking beverages such as soda, juice, and tea. These drinks actually dehydrate us because they draw water from the body's reserves so the body can digest them. He also noted in his research that most pain and sickness we experience is actually the result of chronic dehydration.

Exercise, sweating, diarrhea, temperature, or altitude can significantly increase the amount of water we lose each day. The most common cause of dehydration is exercise and sweating. Even though we are all at risk of water loss, the people most vulnerable are infants, elderly adults, and athletes. They are either not able to adequately express their thirst sensation or they aren't able to detect it and do something in time. Early signs of dehydration include the following:

- Blood pressure changes
- Fatigue
- Flushed skin
- Headache
- Infrequent urination and dark yellow urine
- Light-headedness, dizziness, and decreased coordination
- Loss of appetite
- Muscle cramping

Have you ever had symptoms like these? Was your first thought to reach for a glass of water or an aspirin?

Stress, headache, back pain, allergies, asthma, high blood pressure, and many serious degenerative health problems are the result of chronic dehydration. When chronic dehydration continues, it can lead to constipation, Type 2 diabetes, and autoimmune disease. According to Dr. Batmanghelidj, all of these ailments can be easily corrected with water.

How Do You Know If You're Dehydrated?

A man went to his doctor and told him that he wasn't feeling well. The doctor examined him, left the room, and came back with three bottles of pills. He told his patient, "Take the green pill with a big glass of water when you get up. Take the blue pill with a big glass of water after lunch. Just before going to bed, take the red pill with another big glass of water."

Startled at being put on so much medicine, the man stammered, "My goodness, Doc, exactly what's my problem?"

The doctor replied, "You're not drinking enough water."[17]

If you are thirsty, it means your cells are already dehydrated. A dry mouth should be regarded as the last outward sign of dehydration. That's because thirst does not develop until body fluids are depleted well below levels required for optimal functioning.[18]

We should prevent dehydration rather than wait to correct it.

DIGGING DEEPER: Read the 10 Commandments of Good Hydration in the *Treasures of Health Nutrition Manual.* Then calculate the number of ounces you need to drink each day. (Weight _____ divided by 2 equals _____.)

Treasure of Pure Water

Read Deuteronomy 33:28. What will Israel receive from heaven?

Dew is pure water; it is the equivalent of distilled water. A reverse osmosis filter also gives water that would compare to the dew from heaven.

Many people assume tap water is clean. This is not always true. Some bottled waters even come from city tap water supplies. There are more than 3,800 chemicals in daily use, many of which make their way into our drinking water. What is in our water? Agricultural pollutants, including pesticides and chemicals from fertilizer and manure; contaminants from polluted urban runoff and wastewater treatment plants; industrial chemicals from factory waste and consumer products; and pollutants that are byproducts of the water treatment process or that leach from pipes and storage tanks. In short, more than half of the contaminants found in treated drinking water are not regulated by the EPA (Environmental Protection Agency).[19] To read more about this you will need to dig deeper into the well.

DIGGING DEEPER: In the *Treasures of Health Nutrition Handbook,* read about fluoride and water. This will give you tips on choosing the best water source for your health.

Taking this treasure to heart: Are you satisfied? Are you dehydrated? The water Jesus offers us will never allow dehydration or dissatisfaction. The water we have here on this earth will also keep us hydrated and satisfied. What affirmation can you write to reaffirm this gift to fill your treasure chest? Example: As I drink pure water I am reminded of this gift given to me from a loving God. This water will keep my body balanced in health.

_____

_____

How would you apply the Three Principles to water?

Principle I _____

Principle II _____

Principle III _____

Applying this treasure at home: Water is in all natural foods, fruits, vegetables, meat, dairy, bread, etc. Look at a box of cereal or crackers. How much water content is in it? Maybe that is why you need something to help rinse it down. When you learn to drink more water, fruits and vegetables will count toward your daily water supply along with green and herbal teas. Fresh squeezed juice also counts toward part of your water supply. Eventually you will want to get in all the ounces with just pure water.

How many ounces of water did you drink today? _____

Keep track of how many you drink each day this week. If you don't remember how many ounces are needed look back in today's lesson.

Day Two _____ Day Three _____ Day Four _____

Day Five _____ Day Six _____ Day Seven _____

It may be helpful to post a marker board on the refrigerator to help your kids keep track of their water intake also. Make it fun by rewarding them with an activity they enjoy.

Day Two—Got Milk?

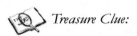 *Treasure Clue:*

*Be glad then, you children of Zion, and rejoice in the Lord, your God; for He gives
you the former or early rain in just measure and in righteousness, and He causes to
come down for you the rain, the former rain and the latter rain, as before.*

—Joel 2:23 AMP

Affirmation: As God's child, I will rejoice and be glad continually, for He has given me a teacher and a guide. He rains blessings down upon me like an autumn rain and causes me to gather a harvest even as I am sowing my seed.

Affirmations are a way of taking words or truth and writing them in a positive way. Write an affirmation of your own using the verse from Joel.

_____

_____

_____

Read Genesis 18:8. List the food Abraham fed the three men (or angels) representing God himself.

_____

_____

Read Deuteronomy 32:12-14. List the food God brought to Jacob.

_____

_____

Read Exodus 3:8. What is in the Promised Land?

_____

The American Dairy Association says we need several glasses of pasteurized, homogenized milk every day. Still others say we should consume goat's milk only. Clean cow's milk and clean goat's milk are some of the most complete health-giving foods on earth.[20]

Read Proverbs 27:27. How much goat's milk will they have?

_____

Read 1 Corinthians 3:1-2, Hebrews 5:12, and 1 Peter 2:2. What conclusion can you draw from the use of milk in these verses?

_____

_____

Is milk only for babies, or do people of all ages need nourishment for growth? Since they did not have pasteurization and homogenization in those days, was the milk safe to drink? How do we know?

_____

_____

It is obvious clean milk is an excellent beverage given to us by the Creator. God provides the best for our physical needs and gives us what we need spiritually to grow.

Few people are aware that clean, raw milk from grass-fed cows was actually used as a medicine in the early part of the last century.[21] That's right. Milk straight from the udder belongs in the treasure chest and was used as medicine to treat some serious chronic diseases.[22] From the earliest recordings to just after World War II, this "white blood" nourished and healed uncounted millions.

Milk as a New Food Group

Clean raw milk from pastured cows is a complete and properly balanced food. You could live on it exclusively if you had to. Indeed, published accounts exist of people who have done just that.[23] What's in it that makes it so great? Let's look at the ingredients to see what makes it such a powerful food.[24]

PROTEINS

Raw cow's milk has all nine essential amino acids. Amino acids are the building blocks of every cell in your body. There are very few foods that make it so easy to live.

LACTOFERRIN

This nutrient has numerous beneficial properties, including improved absorption and assimilation of iron, anti-cancer properties, and anti-microbial action against several species of bacteria responsible for dental cavities.[25] Studies have shown a significant loss of these important disease fighters when milk is heated in pasteurization.[26,27]

CARBOHYDRATES

Lactose, or milk sugar, is the primary carbohydrate in cow's milk. People with lactose intolerance no longer make the enzyme lactase and so can't digest milk sugar. Raw milk has lactose-digesting bacteria and may allow people who have an intolerance to give it another try.

FATS

Approximately two-thirds of the fat in milk is saturated. So is it good or bad for you? Saturated fats play a number of key roles in our body, from construction of cell membranes and important hormones, to providing energy storage and padding for delicate organs, to serving as a vehicle for important fat-soluble vitamins. We will study this in more detail later, but the good news is that fats from foods God designed will not cause heart disease. Keep in mind the Three Principles.

VITAMINS

Volumes have been written about the two groups of vitamins, water and fat-soluble, and their contribution to health. Whole raw milk has them all, and they're completely available for your body to use. Whether regulating your metabolism or helping the biochemical reactions that free energy from the food you eat, they're all present and ready to go to work for you.[28]

MINERALS

Raw milk contains a broad selection of completely available minerals ranging from the familiar calcium and phosphorus on down to trace elements, of which the function of some, as yet, is still rather unclear. A sampling of the health benefits of calcium—an important element abundant in raw milk—includes: reduction in cancers, particularly of the colon; higher bone mineral density in people of every age; lower risk of osteoporosis and fractures in older adults; lowered risk of kidney stones; formation of strong teeth; and reduction of dental cavities, to name a few.[29,30]

ENZYMES

The sixty-plus (known) fully intact and functional enzymes in raw milk have an amazing array of tasks to perform, each one of them essential in facilitating one key reaction or another.[31] The most significant health benefit derived from food enzymes is the burden they take off our body. When we eat a food that contains enzymes devoted to its own digestion, it's that much less work for our pancreas.[32]

BENEFICIAL BACTERIA

Through the process of fermentation, several strains of bacteria naturally present or added later (lactobacillus, leuconostoc, and pediococcus, to name a few) can transform milk into an even more digestible food.[33]

Use Caution

There are countless reasons to look into this nutrient dense food, but there are also reasons to be cautious. In America there are approximately twenty states that allow farm-raised raw milk for sale. You will need to consult your state's dairy council to see if your state allows the sale of raw milk to individuals or through retail stores. The purpose of this information is to show you how intricately God designed foods given to us for health. The purpose is not to make you a criminal by purchasing raw milk in states where it is illegal.

I received raw milk from a friend of mine as a gift, since she owned a cow and I wanted to experience it. At first I was a little squeamish about the thought of drinking raw milk. When I brought it home the fat had risen to the top. I skimmed it off and put it in the blender with a little salt. In one minute, voila! I had butter! The milk tasted very creamy and had a delicious flavor.

Proverbs 30:33 says, "Surely the churning of milk bringeth forth butter, and the wringing of the nose bringeth forth blood" (KJV).

DIGGING DEEPER: Read more about milk in the *Treasures of Health Nutrition Manual.*

Fun foodie idea: Find raw milk and make your own butter. Then take milk you brought home from the store, pasteurized and homogenized, and try to make butter with it. Does it work? No. Why not? The milk we buy from the store is no longer in the form God designed for our health.

Nursing and God's Design

What about nursing? Take a look at some facts about breast feeding from Dr. Rex Russell.

Most scientists claim that life came from random chance process and by natural selection. In nature, however, a chorus of voices rings with the message that this theory fits neither simple nor complex observations. To maintain health, the following must be present simultaneously and in proper balance: organic vitamins, minerals, essential fatty acids, essential amino acids, and unrefined carbohydrates. These are all present in human breast milk, as are the hundreds of other lesser-understood food factors. The longer scientists study the human breast and its milk, the more obvious it is that neither random chance nor survival of the fittest could explain its complexity.

The design of the milk is perfect in caloric content, amino acid concentrations, and enzyme concentrations. Both lipase and lactase are ideally concentrated, meeting the developing infant's needs much better than could any formula or other mammals' milk. The caloric content and the nutrient balance of the mother's milk change dramatically according to the infant's needs. Our most brilliant neonatologists using the best computers could not design a better-balanced product than breast milk, regardless of the infant's needs at whatever age or stage of development.[34]

Pasteurization

Pasteurization is heating food, in this case milk, to 161 degrees Fahrenheit for fifteen seconds, which destroys the enzymes and changes its protein structure, making if difficult for our bodies to assimilate and digest. There's no debate about the effectiveness of pasteurization for killing unwanted bacteria. There's also no doubt that pasteurization gives dairy products a longer shelf life by lowering the presence of bacteria that cause spoilage. But pasteurization also kills desirable bacteria found in fresh milk, and it denatures milk enzymes that may be active in the human digestive tract when fresh milk is consumed.

Pasteurization does not guarantee that the milk will be clean.[35] The FDA only requires a bacteria count of less than 75,000 per cubic centimeter of Grade A milk.[36] By heating or pasteurizing, the count is dropped to about 25,000, but the count may be back up by the time it is sold—and it will still be considered Grade A milk. You may get sick when harmful bacteria are present. Certified raw milk has to contain bacteria counts of less than 10,000—and raw milk can earn this certification easily if it is clean.[37,38]

Homogenization

Homogenization breaks down and blends fat globules in milk, which suspends them evenly in the milk. If milk is not homogenized, the fat globules are large enough to separate from the milk and thereby are less absorbed in the bloodstream. An example of this is cream separating and rising to the top of a container. Homogenized milk does not need stirring and lasts longer on the shelf.[39]

Beginning in the 1960s and continuing through the 1980s, an M.D. named Kurt Oster published a series of articles linking a connection between homogenization and the development of heart disease. Dr. Oster discovered an enzyme capable of digesting the lining of the arteries and causing ulcers inside our arteries. Homogenization could trigger immune reactions and cause damage to blood vessel walls. The result was described as plaque formation—the very same plaque formation that gives rise to atherosclerosis in many American adults.

Milk and the Three Principles

Think back to one of the tools needed for this journey—the Three Principles. Let's review them again and see if you can determine how milk and milk products fit into these principles.

Principle I—Eat only substances God created for food. Avoid what is not designed for food.

Principle II—As much as possible, eat foods as they were created—before they are changed or converted into something humans think might be better.

Principle III—Avoid food addictions. Don't let any food or drink become your god.[40]

How would you apply the Three Principles to milk?

Principle I _____

Principle II _____

Principle III _____

What conclusions can you make from what you have learned?

_____

Milk Allergies

Over the course of several months I had many conversations with a friend whose little girl was suffering from a rash. The intermittent rash was painful and itched continuously, causing her trouble particularly at night. We tried deciphering if it was related to cleaners used in the home, foods she was eating, pollen in the air, and so forth. Finally I asked my friend if her daughter consumed any dairy. The mother quickly said she does not eat *much* dairy. But just to be safe she eliminated all dairy for a trial of three weeks. After only a few days, the rash disappeared. The mother was quite surprised, since the doctors only had offered her a steroid and never considered a food allergy. Several years later the child has had no more rashes unless she consumes a dairy product by mistake.

Almost every home in America is plagued by allergies of one sort or another. Milk is a very common allergy, especially among children.

We will look at allergies sporadically throughout the different food groups and in more detail in week nine. But it is important to understand that certain foods are a culprit for allergies. Dr. Doris Rapp has done extensive research in the area of children's behavior and allergic reactions. She states that food-related allergies can cause a wide variety of complaints. In the intestines it can be in the form of abdominal discomfort, pain or cramps, diarrhea, constipation, nausea, vomiting, and at times blood or mucus in the bowel movement. In some people, irritable bowel, Crohn's disease, ulcers, mucous colitis, and even ulcerative colitis can be due to undetected allergies. Allergies can also present themselves in areas unrelated to the intestines. For example, headaches, nose or chest complaints, fatigue, hyperactivity, depression, agitation, muscle aches, chronic ear infections, skin rashes, joint tightness, heart irregularities, and problems remembering or thinking are sometimes caused by food allergies. Milk has been proven to be a cause for concern. If you believe you or your children may have a milk or dairy allergy, the test is simple and cheap. Eliminate all dairy from the diet for a minimum of two weeks, but preferably for one entire month. Then document the reaction when the foods are reintroduced slowly.[41]

Taking this treasure to heart: It makes sense that God-designed milk would bring health. But how are you doing with the milk from God's Word? Are you ready to trust God in all areas of your life, including your health? Are you ready to trust Him in his choices for food? Write out your responses in a sentence prayer. Let God know your concerns, questions, and praises.

Applying this treasure at home: Few of us have access to raw milk, so if milk is on your grocery list, organic would be a better choice than regular milk. Rice milk and almond milk are also great substitutes in recipes and for drinking, especially if you have family members who are allergic to dairy.

Fun foodie idea: Visit a dairy farm with your family and encourage everyone to milk a cow. See if the farmer has raw milk that you can taste. You may be udderly amazed at the flavor!

DAY THREE—THE JOY OF JUICE

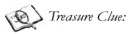 *Treasure Clue:*

Yes, the Lord answered and said to His people, Behold, I am sending you grain and juice [of the grape] and oil, and you shall be satisfied with them.

—Joel 2:19 AMP

Affirmation: My Father sends me all the provision I need to be satisfied in life and do what He has called me to do. I carry with me the anointing—an ability to function successfully in every area of my life.[42]

Write an affirmation of your own using Joel 2:19.

_____

_____

The Joy of Juice

Hardly anyone gets enough fruits and vegetables in his or her diet, so why not try juicing? The American Cancer Society recommends we eat five to nine servings of fruits and vegetables daily to prevent cancer. For most of us, this is hard to fit into our diet, and that is where juicing fits in. Fresh fruits and vegetables are full of phytochemicals, antioxidants, and enzymes. These enzymes actually increase the rate at which food is broken down and absorbed by the body. By getting enzymes from fruit and vegetables, you save your body's enzymes to digest other foods.

These enzymes are mostly destroyed during cooking and processing. Bottled and packaged juices are pasteurized, which destroys the enzymes.

Juicing fruits and vegetables gives you all the nutritional value of the original raw food, including the water content. Even those vegetables that are sometimes hard to get in each day can be added to your fresh juice. When you are eating a healthy diet full of fiber, juicing fits in quite nicely. Do not replace eating all fruits and vegetables with juicing, since fiber is vital for our colon health. Some unique and tasty juices can be made with carrots, cucumbers, and celery. For a refreshing change, throw in an apple or a banana. Just about anything that is grown in the garden can be juiced. Juicing fruits is always a treat, but be careful of the high sugar content. What are two factors to keep in mind for balance in your menu when it comes to juicing?

_____

_____

Fun foodie idea: Have a "Juice Night." Ask each person to bring three vegetables and three fruits to your home. Then with a blender, juicer, or a Vita-Mix machine, invent your own concoction and see which juice is your favorite. (If you're using a blender, you may need to add some organic juice for a liquid base.) You will be surprised how you can hide different vegetables in fresh juice!

Grape Juice or Red Wine?

"Thus says the Lord: 'As the new wine is found in the cluster, and one says, "Do not destroy it, for a blessing is in it"'" (Isa. 65:8 NKJV). For years, researchers have advocated the benefits of drinking wine as a preventive measure against heart attacks. More recently, though, studies have determined that the alcohol content in red wine is not the factor responsible for reducing cardiovascular disease (CVD).

Instead, researchers from all over the world are discovering that the antioxidants—called flavonoids—are the protective agents helping fight CVD and many other disease-related problems. And where can you find these helpful flavonoids? Purple grapes.

Patrick J. Bird, Ph.D., of the University of Florida says, "Plants manufacture some 1,000 different flavonoids. But one—resveratrol—most commonly from the skin of the red grapes, seems to be most effective in the battle against heart disease. Resveratrol acts by decreasing the stickiness of blood cells that aid in clotting. Grapes are the richest source of resveratrol. Besides offering some protection against heart disease, it has been shown to decrease the activity of free-radical reactions that are linked to several cancers."[43]

In November 1998, the American Heart Association released this good news: "Purple grape juice seems to have the same effect as red wine in reducing the risk of heart disease."[44] Research has gone on to discover that resveratrol is not the only ingredient for promoting health found in the grape. Recent research has discovered the Georgia-grown muscadine grape produces a unique phytochemical, ellagic acid. Dr. Joseph Maroon, in his book *The Longevity Factor*, explains this unique ellagic acid that is in muscadine grapes is virtually absent in other grapes. It has a powerful antioxidant and anti-cancer properties. The polyphenols in muscadine grape skins have been shown to have positive effects on heart disease, high cholesterol, diabetes, metabolic syndrome, and other inflammatory conditions. One of the more interesting effects of the muscadine is its ability to repair the aging of DNA in our cells.[45]

Another scientist, Dr. Steve Chaney, professor at the University of North Carolina, had this to say in a personal interview:

> Ellagic acid, found in the muscadine grape, blocks an enzyme that is involved in the formation of advanced glycation end products (AGE proteins), one of the central four mechanisms of cellular aging. (In layman's terms, it helps repair damaged cells at the DNA level—that is science at its best!) Resveratrol has no effect on this enzyme, but does block the other three key mechanisms of cellular aging.[46]

There are numerous supplement products promoting resveratrol in juices, pills, powders, and more. With the scientific research coming from scientist Dr. David Sinclair from Harvard Medical School, resveratrol has become the hottest supplement on the market. Pharmaceutical companies are very interested in these ingredients because of their hopes for controlling diabetes. The future will tell us the complete story but for now keep watching.

DIGGING DEEPER: Read more about resveratrol and its health benefits in the *Nutrition Manual.*

In further defense of grape juice over wine, one researcher John Folts, Ph.D., at the University of Wisconsin had this to say: "Wine only prevents blood from clotting at levels high enough to declare someone legally drunk. With grape juice, you can drink enough to get the benefit without worrying about becoming intoxicated. What's more, alcoholic drinks don't improve the function of cells in blood vessel linings the way grape juice does. And alcohol generates free radicals—unstable oxygen molecules that can actually cause damage to blood vessel tissues—dampening any of the benefits that red wine's antioxidant may offer."[47]

Fresh juice is a gift from God to be enjoyed. The only caution would be to monitor the volume consumed, particularly if someone has a tendency toward diabetes. The sugar content of one glass of juice is equal to three apples.

Cautions of Strong Drink

Read Ephesians 5:18. What command are we given here? Some versions use the word *dissipation*, which means overindulgence in the pursuit of physical pleasures or wasteful use.[48]

_____

Is the purpose of this statement for our spiritual or physical life, or both? Explain.

_____

_____

Let's look at the health concerns associated with strong drink.[49] From the moment alcohol enters the body, it acts like it has special privileges. Unlike foods that require time for digestion, alcohol needs no digestion and is quickly absorbed. About 20 percent is absorbed directly from an empty stomach and reaches the brain in one minute. When the stomach is full of food the process takes longer, but the alcohol will reach the brain eventually.

Take a look at some of the effects of alcohol. Circle the problems you were not previously aware of:

- Acts as a depressant
- Affects every organ of the body
- Can cause impotence
- Causes liver damage
- Causes brain cell death
- Causes dehydration
- Contributes to body fat
- Creates B vitamin deficiency
- Increases homocysteine
- Increases inflammation
- Increases the risk of menstrual disorders and spontaneous abortions
- Lowers production of red blood cells
- May increase risk of certain cancers
- Produces free radicals
- Slows or suppresses the immune system

The effects of abusing alcohol may be apparent immediately or they may not become evident for years to come. Among the immediate consequences, all of the following involve alcohol use:

- One-quarter of all emergency-room admissions
- One-third of all suicides
- One-half of all homicides
- One-half of all domestic violence incidents
- One-half of all traffic fatalities
- One-half of all fire victim fatalities

The facts are all around us, yet alcohol is still a subject of contention among some people. People bring up the fact that Jesus gave wine as a drink at the wedding feast. I was not there, and neither were the theologians that give this fact as an excuse to drink. For those who want an excuse, excuses are out there, but the goal of this study is to overcome health challenges and follow a biblical plan. God's plan is to build health; alcohol will never build health. To be more Christ-minded, our goal is to seek Him in everything we do. This includes what we drink and why we drink. For many people, alcohol fills a void. At the Last Supper Jesus spent with His disciples, He gave them a drink representing His blood that was poured out for them. Jesus was trying to show them that between the bread and the drink, He would be everything to them. Their lives would be full. When we don't allow or accept God to fill us completely, we are left with a void. Something will need to fill this void. Alcohol is used by some people to fill this void.

So how do you apply this lesson to your life? That is for you to pray about. This is one time I ask you not to share this concern with your foodie friend, if he or she is in favor of drinking. Find someone who is more neutral, or meet with God alone.

Here is how I view this subject. People usually drink for one of three reasons. First, they drink to fit in with their peers. If that is true, then I suggest finding new friends. Our only peer to determine what we eat or drink should be God and our goal should be to give Him the glory. Second, people drink for the supposed health benefits. We have already seen the health benefits are not solid enough to overcome the deficit. And third, people drink because they are addicted. We will address addiction more when we study fasting. Any food or drink can become an addiction. If you recognize it as an addiction, then you are able to overcome it.

I try to keep my relationship with Christ first in my life. I don't want anything to hinder it, and being under an influence of another nature other than God is detrimental to this relationship. I also don't want anything to hamper my ability to witness to others, and drinking alcohol, becoming drunk, and being out of control is definitely an obstacle. Third, I am seeking a body that is controlled by discipline, and I seek to gain health. Alcohol does not fit into this plan. It does not contribute to my health, and since I have an addictive appetite, the last thing I need is another food or drink that will add to this anomaly. The bottom line is there is nothing to gain by drinking wine or alcohol. But I will never let alcohol or wine interrupt a friendship; that would be worse than the effects of the wine.

From what you have learned, should we have alcohol in our treasure chest?

_____

There are many cautions when it comes to drinking. What conclusion can you draw from the effects of alcohol?

_____

_____

Jeremiah 33:3 says, "Call unto me, and I will answer thee, and show thee great and mighty things, which thou knowest not" (KJV). Many people suffer from an addiction to alcohol and other food or drink. As you review Jeremiah 33:3, write a prayer about what God is showing you in your personal life or the life of a family member.

_____

_____

_____

After each Principle, write how it should be applied to water, juice, and wine.
Principle I (eat only the foods God gave us):

_____

Principle II (eat foods closest to the way God designed them):

_____

Principle III (don't let any food or drink become an addiction):

_____

Taking this treasure to heart:[50] God chose the juice of the grape to symbolize the blood of Jesus Christ. When Jesus sat with His disciples at the Last Supper, He passed a cup filled with the "fruit of the vine," saying, "This cup is the new covenant in My blood; do this, as often as you drink it, in remembrance of Me" (1 Cor. 11:25 NASB).

The Greek word for "fruit of the vine" is *genematos*. It is the word from which we get "generation" and pertains to producing or bringing forth. Grapes are a life-giving form of fruit. Leviticus 17:14 tells us that blood is the life of all flesh. On the cross, Jesus willingly poured out His blood—His very life—for you and me.

Applying this treasure at home: Juice abuse is a common phrase among nutritionists. Juice bought from the store can be loaded with sugar. If this is a choice for your family, then you might want to consider diluting the juice with pure water. This will cut down on calories and sugar. Read the labels on all products containing juice. Make smart choices. Typically, when I buy juice my first choice is organic; my second choice is fresh pressed—not from concentrate—which is very difficult to find.

Day Four—Beverages Good and Not So Good

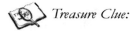 *Treasure Clue:*

But Jesus replied to them, You are wrong because you know neither the Scriptures nor God's power.
—Matt. 22:29 AMP

Affirmation: I have been given revelation knowledge of the Scriptures. I am ever mindful of the exceeding greatness of God's power that is at work in and through me.[51]

Other Beverages

We have learned the benefits of drinking pure water, raw milk, and fresh juice. But what about those pleasing and taste-enhancing beverages that are now the staples of our modern society? After all, they are made with water, so they should count in our treasure chest, right? When it comes to the chemistry in your body, water and fluids are two different things. As it happens, many of our favorite manufactured beverages contain some chemicals that alter the body's chemistry at its central nervous system's control centers. Even milk is not the same as water.

The body needs water—nothing substitutes for it. Coffee, tea, soda, alcohol, and even milk and juices are not the same as water.

Caffeine in Beverages

Caffeine is a natural product of the plants and seeds from which a drink is processed. If you apply the three principles to caffeine, you already know if it is healthy to consume. Principle III says to not become addicted to any food or drink. This is where caffeine can cause a problem. When too much caffeine is consumed, it can be toxic to the brain cells, can block the production of melatonin (sleep hormone), can eventually cause the loss of memory, may cause attention deficit disorder, and can exhaust the brain cells' reserves of energy. Studies also show that caffeine dehydrates the body.[52]

Caffeine-containing sodas with artificial sweeteners are more dangerous than those containing regular sugar. Artificial sweeteners are potent chemical agents that fool the brain cells by masking as sugar. Sweetness normally translates to the entry of energy into the body. The sweeteners, through the taste buds, program the brain to behave as if true sugar has been consumed and will enter the bloodstream, and the body reacts accordingly. Since there is strict control of the level of sugar in the blood, the brain calculates the outcome of the sweetness and instructs and programs the liver not to manufacture sugar from other raw materials. But since the body can't begin storing sugar that is nowhere to be found, the brain and the liver prompt a hunger sensation to find food and make good on the promise of energy. The result is a state of anxiety about food. Studies show that people who consume artificial sweeteners seek and eat more food than normal for up to ninety minutes after the intake of the sweetener.

The Miracle of Green Tea

Tea has been an important beverage for thousands of years and has been a huge part of culture in countries around the world, forming major parts of ceremonies, creating trade routes, and even starting revolutions. But tea isn't just appreciated for its good taste and worldwide appeal; it also offers numerous health benefits.

Is any other food or drink reported to have as many health benefits as green tea? The Chinese have known about the medicinal benefits of green tea since ancient times, using it to treat everything from headaches to depression. In her book *Green Tea: The Natural Secret for a Healthier Life*, Nadine Taylor states that green tea has been used as a medicine in China for at least four thousand years.

Today, scientific research is providing evidence for the health benefits long associated with drinking green tea. For example, the Purdue University researchers recently concluded that a compound in green tea inhibits the growth of cancer cells. There is also research indicating that drinking green tea lowers total cholesterol levels, as well as improves the ratio of good (HDL) cholesterol to bad (LDL) cholesterol.

To sum up this study, here are just a few medical conditions in which drinking green tea is reputed to be helpful:[53]

- cancer
- rheumatoid arthritis
- high cholesterol levels
- cardiovascular disease
- infection
- impaired immune function

What Makes Green Tea So Special?

The secret of green tea lies in the fact that it is rich in catechin polyphenols, particularly epigallocatechin gallate (EGCG). EGCG is a powerful antioxidant; besides inhibiting the growth of cancer cells, it kills cancer cells without harming healthy tissue. It has also been effective in lowering LDL cholesterol levels and inhibiting the abnormal formation of blood clots. The latter takes on added importance when you consider that blood clots are the leading cause of heart attacks and stroke. In a 1997 study, researchers from the University of Kansas determined that EGCG is twice as powerful as resveratrol.[54]

Why don't other teas have similar health-giving properties? Green, oolong, and black teas all come from the leaves of the Camellia sinensis plant. What sets green tea apart is the way it is processed. Green tea leaves are steamed, which prevents the EGCG compound from being oxidized. By contrast, black and oolong tea leaves are made from fermented leaves, which results in the EGCG being converted into other compounds that are not nearly as effective in preventing and fighting various diseases.

Harmful Effects?

To date, the only negative side effect reported from drinking green tea is insomnia due to caffeine. However, green tea contains less caffeine than coffee; there are approximately thirty to sixty milligrams of caffeine in six-eight ounces of tea, compared to over one hundred milligrams in eight ounces of coffee.

DIGGING DEEPER: Read about aspartame and tea in the *Treasures of Health Nutrition Handbook.*

Calculating Calories in Your Drink

We want to be healthy, so it is helpful to have an easy rule to calculate calories in a drink such as a homemade milkshake. Dr. Brian Wansink, author of *Mindless Eating,* came up with the 10-20 Rule.[55] Dr. Wansink conducted a beverage study to determine if people could estimate how many calories they drink. The result was they underestimated it by 30 percent. It doesn't matter whether it's a soft drink, milk, juice, or wine.

His lab developed a 10-20 rule of thumb for teaching people to estimate the number of calories in a drink. "Thin drinks" (like soft drinks, punch, juice, and milk) are about 10 calories per ounce and "thick drinks" (smoothies and meal replacement shakes) are about 20 calories per ounce. It's a ballpark, but it's better than mindless drinking. Just poured a 32-ounce Coke at McDonalds? Think 320 calories, including ice.

Taking this treasure to heart: The human body is entirely dependent on the many complicated functions of water for its survival. Water is free (basically). Salvation is free. Both are essential for life here on earth. You have heard it said the best gifts in life are free, and these are the two best gifts anyone could receive.

Take a moment now to pray, asking God to help you stay thirsty for His Word. Nothing will satisfy you more. Earlier this week we learned that people who are thirsty are dissatisfied. Is there dissatisfaction in your life? If so, write it out here. If not, write a prayer to God in thanksgiving for the hydration of His Word in your life.

_____

_____

_____

_____

_____

Just as the relief from chronic dehydration is to gradually add more water to your daily routine, the relief from dissatisfaction spiritually is to gradually get more time alone with God and His Word.

Write out one nugget of truth you learned from this week's study.

Applying this treasure at home: How are you going to apply what you have learned this week? What is one change you would like to make in regard to beverages: water, milk, juice, wine, tea, coffee, and soda? Making one simple change per week will take you farther longer than doing drastic changes right away. My prayer is that this is a life-changing process, not a diet that ends without results. Write your one simple change on your Action Plan sheet and share it with your foodie friend. If you feel daring, make more than one commitment.

FABULOUS FOODIE FRIDAY

A man went to visit his ninety-year-old grandfather, and while eating a breakfast of eggs and bacon, he noticed a film-like substance on his plate. The man said, "Grandfather, are these plates clean?"

His grandfather replied, "Those plates are as clean as cold water can get them, so go on and finish your meal."

That afternoon, while eating the hamburgers his grandfather made for lunch, the man noticed many little black specks around the edge of his plate. Again he asked, "Grandfather, are you sure these plates are clean?"

Without looking up from his burger, the grandfather said, "I told you those dishes are as clean as cold water can get them; now don't ask me about it anymore."

Later that day, they were on their way out to get dinner. As the man was leaving the house, his grandfather's dog started to growl and would not let him pass. "Grandfather, your dog won't let me out," he said.

Without diverting his attention from the football game he was watching, his grandfather shouted, "Coldwater, get out of the way!"

Water clearly is the best beverage of choice, pure and simple. Many people avoid drinking too much water for fear it will cause weight gain. They end up dehydrated, and it shows up in their dry, wrinkled skin.

Foodie Time

If water is boring, liven it up. Join your foodie friends this week and challenge each other to see how many flavors can be made from crisp clean water and the addition of vegetables, herbs, extracts, or teas. Add limes or lemons for a citrus flavor. Add a cucumber for a refreshing clear crisp taste; it is best if it sits for at least 10 minutes.

Iced tea is a healthy choice. Decaffeinated green tea or herbal teas are loaded with antioxidants, and if the tea does have caffeine, the amount is very low. When making green tea, do not boil the water at length, bring the water to just about boiling and then remove from the stove. Let the tea bags steep for 3-5 minutes. The shorter time will retain the highest amount of antioxidants.

Herbs such as lemon balm or mint added to ice and water make a delightful taste. Avoid buying into the marketing campaign of the flavored waters, sports drinks, and vitamin waters. Always drink the purest choice. As you begin to drink more water, you will recognize the signs of dehydration in your body. You will literally crave more water. Your taste for food will even be more pronounced. Drink to the God-filled life you were designed.

Check out the recipes on www.designedhealthyliving.com for beverages, including how to make your own almond milk, rice milk, and almond milk shake. These are very simple and tasty recipes.

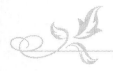

Grains

Day One—Bread of Life Adds Value to the Treasure

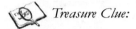 *Treasure Clue:*

I tell you the truth, he who believes has everlasting life. I am the bread of life. Your forefathers ate the manna in the desert, yet they died. But here is the bread that comes down from heaven, which a man may eat and not die. I am the living bread that came down from heaven. If anyone eats of this bread, he will live forever. This bread is my flesh, which I will give for the life of the world.
—John 6:47-51 NIV

Is It Any Wonder?

Who can forget the red, blue, and yellow balloons on the package of Wonder Bread or their slogan, "Don't forget the Wonder"? I remember envying kids who were given Wonder Bread sandwiches in grade school. Sometimes I would swap my fresh fruit for a piece of sandwich, especially if it was filled with peanut butter and grape jelly. The taste lingers in my memory. But the best amusement with Wonder Bread was when you could take the center, make a tight ball, wet it a little, and then toss it. This fleeting enjoyment was guaranteed to put you on lunch cleanup instead of going to recess.

Growing up, I used to wonder why my mom would purchase dark bread. Now I understand she was ahead of her time and tried to make better choices. Today we still try to make better choices, but it can be confusing to figure out what kinds of bread are healthy. Labels and knowledge will prove powerful as we discover the treasure of whole grains.

Building Our Pyramid and Filling Our Treasure Chest

Looking back at the Mediterranean Pyramid (see Week One, Day Four), you will see that grains, beans, nuts, legumes, and seeds fill the bottom portion and form the foundation. For many years, scientists and nutritionists have agreed that bread (whole grains) is the staff of life. Remember, this is not a new idea; God gave us this gift in the beginning of creation in

Genesis 1:29. Read this verse and compare it with John 6:32 where Jesus says that God gives us true bread—Jesus Christ.

Ecclesiastes 1:9 tells us there is nothing new under the sun. The oceans will continue to fill but never overflow, the rivers will continue to flow, generations will continue to come and go. The grains of truth and health that we seek have always been here, waiting for our discovery. Each day we hear of "new" ideas, "new" technology, and "new" medical advances, but are they really new? Now is the time to fill our treasure chest with foods that bring life. Seeds are the good example of life. Inside the tiny layers of the seed reside all the nourishment necessary to not only bring forth the life of a new plant but also provide the food to sustain that plant as it begins to grow. This remarkable nourishment for the seed is available to our cells as well.

Grains: a Symbol of Whole Life

Natural whole grains were abundant in the land God designed for Adam and his family. God also provided whole grains in the Promised Land. The many references to grains make it clear that it was vitally important and, quite literally, the staff of life. The ripe golden kernels contain carbohydrates, proteins, fats, minerals, and vitamins and can be considered the perfect food source. We typically think of wheat as the most popular grain, but there are many others, such as barley, rice, corn, buckwheat, amaranth, flaxseed, kamut, millet, oats, rye, triticale, and spelt.

Let's make a short journey through Scripture and glean truths about the use of grain and bread. As you review these scriptures, consider the application of bread in each situation. Many times bread is a symbolic reference. Below is a list of symbols referring to bread in Scripture. As you read the verses below, write down the matching symbol. You may need to read surrounding verses to comprehend the teaching.

- Forgiveness
- God the Provider
- Gladness
- Redemption
- Blessing
- Unity
- Fellowship

GENESIS

Genesis begins with God creating a land that is perfect. We have already talked about how God changed Adam and Eve's diet after they sinned, and how man's food source was changed again after the flood. But let's take a look later in Genesis to see what God has to say about grains in particular.

Read Genesis 26:12. How large was the harvest Isaac reaped? _____

Why did he enjoy such a bountiful harvest? "And the Lord _____" (N.ASB).

Which of the symbols listed come to mind when you read this story? _____

DEUTERONOMY

"Observe the commands of the Lord your God, walking in his ways and revering him" (Deut. 8:6 NIV). Moses taught the Israelites what Jehovah God commanded so that they would be blessed. Read Deuteronomy 8:1-11. Verse 3 states, "Man does not live on bread alone but on every word that comes from the mouth of the Lord" (NIV).

What is God teaching us in this passage?

_____

_____

What grains does God promise in this good land? _____

Which of the symbols listed come to mind when you read this story? _____

RUTH

A good romance novel is hard to pass up. Look at the Old Testament book of Ruth; if you have time, read the entire story. This Old Testament narrative takes place during the harvest time. This historical event was continuously shared at the Wheat Harvest Feast, which later became known as the Feast of Pentecost.

Ruth was a young Moabitess who gleaned in the wheat harvest of Boaz, a wealthy farmer. Her gentle and giving spirit and hard work came to his attention. He invited her to share a luncheon one day. Read about that meeting in Ruth 2:8-19.

What were Ruth and the other young women doing in the fields?

_____

What kind of grain were they harvesting?

_____

What was the first invitation Boaz extended to Ruth?

_____

What was the second invitation?

_____

What did they eat for their luncheon date in the field?

_____

Which of the symbols listed come to mind when you read this story?

_____

EZEKIEL

In Ezekiel 4, what are the ingredients that God instructed the prophet to make into bread (verses 9-11)? _____

How many days was he to eat this bread? _____

Today, variations of this multi-grain bread are made all around the world. It is called the bread of fasting. Later we will learn more about the complete proteins of the grains and beans in this recipe. When combined in a meal, they combine to equal a complete protein, and it has all the amino acids needed for the body to make healthy cells. This helps us understand why Ezekiel was in perfect physical shape when the time came to rise and walk away.

Which of the symbols listed come to mind when you read this story?_____

I SAMUEL

In 1 Samuel 17:17-18, what foods did Jesse ask David to take to his brothers, who were fighting the Philistines?

_____

Which of the symbols listed come to mind when you read this story? _____

In the *Healthy Treasures Cookbook* you will find a recipe for roasted grains. Some even call this a substitute for popcorn. In my opinion, the time it takes to prepare and experience these biblical foods is worth it.

In 1 Samuel 25, conflict arose between David and Nabal. In order to smooth things over after her husband, Nabal, had insulted David, Abigail chose a well-known and very effective element of conflict resolution: food. What did she take as a peace offering (verses 18-19)?

_____

Which of the symbols listed come to mind when you read this story?_____

How would your family life be different if you followed Abigail's example with conflict?

_____

There would be a lot more discipline to make sure insults never happen. I am sure that I would have been spending a lot of time in the kitchen before learning this lesson.

PSALMS

According to Psalm 4:7, what is one of the people's greatest joys?

_____

Which of the symbols listed comes to mind when you read this story? _____

MATTHEW

In Matthew 12:1, what "fast food" did Jesus and His disciples eat on the Sabbath?

_____

Many Bible students believe Jesus and His disciples were walking through the fields in the spring while the grain was still green. Green wheat is very soft to chew and is loaded with nutrition.

In Matthew 14:13-21, how many men were fed with five loaves of bread?_____

How much bread was left over?_____

Read Matthew 26:26. As Jesus broke the bread, what did it symbolize?

_____

Which of the symbols listed come to mind when you read this story?

_____

ACTS

Read Acts 2:42- 46. Who is eating the bread? _____

What is the purpose of this meeting? _____

Which of the symbols listed come to mind when you read this story? _____

Wheat and grain are used over and over again throughout Scripture as a sign of a gracious God supplying all our needs. The numerous biblical references to wheat and bread make it clear the importance they played in people's daily lives. The grain was used for nourishment, provided as an offering, and given as a gift. Grain and harvest time was used to determine the calendar and festivals. If the harvest was not ready, then a month would be added to the calendar.[56]

JOHN

Knowing grains were used in biblical days—and that God gave them to us to eat—reinforces them as a treasure. But the greater treasure is understanding the spiritual application.

Read John 6:26-40. What truths can you glean from the following verses?

Verse 29: _____

Verses 32-33: _____

Verse 35: _____

Give a practical application from the truths you learned.

_____

_____

Which of the symbols listed come to mind when you read this story? _____

Jesus Is Our Daily Bread

Read today's Treasure Clue again. Jesus is the "bread of life" and is sometimes referred to as our "staff of life." What do I mean by "staff"? In Bible times *staff* meant "bread." When we pray, "Give us this day our daily bread," we must remember that we are also asking Jesus to be our daily portion and our sustenance. We must come to Him and Him alone for everything we need to live the abundant life He has promised us.[57]

Sadly, many of us have become accustomed to spiritual junk food. Instead of being satisfied completely with His whole unrefined word—looking to Him to be our life—we look to the shallow, self-centered experiences of others.

Taking this treasure to heart: Read Matthew 6:11, and rewrite it here as a prayer to God.

_____

_____

_____

What is one nugget of truth you learned from today's lesson?

_____

_____

Applying this treasure at home: Are you giving your family not only whole grain bread, but also the whole truth of God's Word? Just as refining the wheat removes essential ingredients from the grain, so does refining Scripture. We need to read it for ourselves to get the "whole" truth and not let anyone remove the essential ingredients of our faith.

DAY TWO—WHOLESOME BENEFITS

Wholesome benefits of grain give proof of a designer. Further proof that grain was important to the health of those who lived thousands of years ago is shown in how it was grown in all inhabited lands. Consider Dr. Rex Russell's teachings that point to the fact that a benevolent Creator designed seeds and grains.

- A designer would make grains available to all people everywhere. Grains can be easily grown from the Arctic in the Northern Hemisphere to the Antarctic in the Southern Hemisphere.
- A benevolent designer would have designed grains to have good storage life. Farmers frequently store grains in elevators or on the ground until buyers can be found. In

the pyramids of Egypt, kernels of wheat found buried with the pharaohs can still be sprouted four thousand years later! What if this grain could only be sprouted one to five days? How would next year's crop be planted?

- In this complex world, we need different seeds and grains for different nutrients, climates, altitudes, and tastes. All the facts point to a creator whose diverse designs included barley and buckwheat, corn and millet, oats, rice, rye, sorghum (milo), wheat, sesame, and others. In addition, almost any seed can be used for grain.[58]

Summarize why grains prove there is a Creator.

_____

_____

_____

According to the Whole Grains Council, the medical evidence is clear that whole grains reduce risks of heart disease, stroke, digestive system cancer, hormone cancers, diabetes (Type 2), and obesity.[59] Other recent studies show benefits such as:

- Reduced risk of asthma
- Healthier carotid arteries
- Reduction of inflammatory disease risk
- Lower risk of colorectal cancer
- Healthier blood pressure levels
- Less gum disease and tooth loss

If a doctor offered you a pill that promised to do everything on this list without any side effects, would you take it? Few foods and no drugs that I am aware of can offer such diverse benefits as whole grain.

Whole grains are not all in the same botanical family but they all have a similar grain kernel. The kernel is comprised of three basic parts: bran, endosperm, and germ.

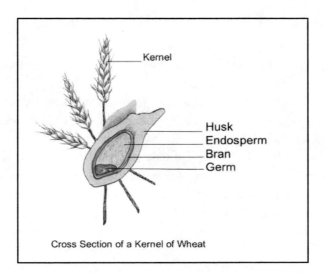

Cross Section of a Kernel of Wheat

- *Bran*—The bran enfolds and protects the kernel's inner layers. It is high in fiber and nutrients such as B vitamins, zinc, iron, and protein.
- *Endosperm*—The endosperm makes up about 83 percent of the kernel. The starchy carbohydrates and protein found there provide nourishment for the sprouted seed when it is planted. Only this part is used to make white flour.
- *Germ*—The germ is the part of the seed that brings new life to a plant. It is the richest source of natural vitamins niacin and riboflavin, potassium, magnesium, iron, zinc, copper, manganese, and vitamins E and K. In addition to all this, the germ is one of the best sources for vitamin B complex, enzymes, and high quality protein.

Special Added Benefits of Whole Grains

If you are not yet convinced that whole grains belong in our treasure chest, consider the following additional benefits.

FIBER

Fiber is the structural part of the seed and is located primarily in the bran. It is not a nutrient so it is not absorbed into the bloodstream. It is resistant to digestion and therefore passes through the digestive tract. In this passing, it has some remarkable effects on our health. Fiber will give you more energy, help you control your weight, and really make a difference in the prevention of disease.

Facts about fiber:

- Fiber decreases intestinal transit time. Fiber moves food more quickly through the GI tract; therefore, there is a lower chance for toxin buildup.
- Fiber creates a more favorable medium for intestinal microflora to live in.
- Increased sense of fullness after eating fiber helps one eat less and enjoy it more.
- Fiber acts like an ambulance driver, as it takes dead Candida out of the body.
- Fiber plays a key role in reducing the risk of Type 2 diabetes. It traps nutrients and delays their absorption; thereby glucose absorption is slowed. This helps prevent glucose surge and rebound associated with diabetes onset.
- When eaten with water, fiber helps prevent several GI disorders.
- Fiber prevents compaction, which could obstruct the appendix and permit bacteria to invade and infect it.
- Fiber stimulates the colon muscles so that they retain their strength and resist building out into pouches known as diverticulitis.

There are two types of fiber—insoluble and soluble—and both act as a toxin magnet. Insoluble fiber takes on the role of a broom for bowel regularity. Insoluble fiber acts as a sponge as it absorbs and holds moisture, thereby producing larger, softer stools and promoting regularity. Soluble fiber causes proper utilization of sugars and fats. Soluble fiber helps diabetics, hypoglycemics, and those with insulin resistance, cholesterol issues, and high blood pressure problems.

DIGGING DEEPER: To get a deeper understanding of fiber and its contribution to health read "Fiber and Field Guide to Fiber" in *The Treasures of Health Nutrition Handbook*. Look at ways to increase fiber in your diet. The best way to get the full range of dietary fiber is to make 45-60 percent of your calorie intake whole foods: fresh fruits, vegetables, and whole grains.

From what you learned by digging deeper, write out a sample dietary plan to get thirty-five grams of fiber in your diet.

Breakfast: _____

Lunch: _____

Dinner: _____

Snacks: _____

DIGGING DEEPER: Go to the Designed Healthy Living website (www. designedhealthyliving.com), click on "Nuts about Nutrition," and then click on "Dietary Wellness for Specific Body Parts." This very helpful chart will help you understand how different foods contribute to various parts of the body.

VITAMIN E

A rich supply of Vitamin E is found in the germ of a seed. This fat-soluble vitamin is extremely beneficial to the life of the new plant as well as to our bodies. Vitamin E contains a mix of tocopherols, which mix with selenium (also included in the germ) and contribute to the health of your heart, help prevent free radical damage as it slows the effects of aging, and help maintain healthy cell membranes.

B-COMPLEX

Refining whole grains into processed flour removes the vital nutrients, including B-complex. This was evidenced in the increase of Beriberi and pellagra that plagued the nation soon after this process began. Years later the manufacturers were encouraged to return the germ back into the milling process, but they choose to enrich the flour with synthetic vitamins that replaced some of the B vitamins. Adding a few B vitamins back into the flour reversed these health crises. Milling your own wheat will ensure that all nutrients, including the B vitamins, will be available for your body to assimilate. B vitamins help decrease PMS and stress symptoms, lower cholesterol, assist with poor coordination, help control your appetite, and much more. This is by far my favorite supplement since it is known as the "B-happy" vitamin, but I find that less supplementation is needed when I eat fresh milled bread.

CARBOHYDRATES

Carbohydrates are fattening…or so we've been told. Most Americans fail to appreciate carbohydrates because they are confused about what carbohydrates really are. Several years ago, the South Beach Diet came along with its new idea that bread is taboo, which only added to the confusion. Let's think about carbs like puzzles: they range from simple to complex, and they're either easy or hard to construct or take apart. Simple carbs are like those five-to-six-piece wooden puzzles for toddlers that have no tight, interlocking sides. The pieces will quickly come out when the puzzle is turned upside down. Simple carbs break down very quickly in our bloodstream and cause our body to react with insulin and energy. Too many simple carbs can lead to diabetes and a host of other problems. Sugars, canned fruits, honey, candy, soda, some processed foods, and quick, high-energy foods are examples of simple carbs.

Carrying on with the puzzle analogy, imagine those thousand-piece puzzles your family might put together over the holidays. The interlocking sides and intricate colors make putting this puzzle together a long, drawn-out affair. Similarly, when we eat complex carbohydrate food, it takes our bodies a long time to assimilate the nutrients. The high fiber and nutrition will delay the sugars from entering the bloodstream—thereby not raising our insulin. Whole grains, beans, legumes, nuts, seeds, and most vegetables and fruits are samples of complex carbs. These carbohydrates will also help fuel your body with energy in a time-release fashion to ensure steady blood sugar levels. Endurance athletes often "stoke up" on complex carbohydrates to fill up without filling out. Often people worry about getting fat from eating bread, but if you are eating whole grains with all the fiber and nutrients intact, those high carbohydrates are not fattening. Fewer than half of the calories in whole grain bread are contained in the fat. According to nutritionist Phyllis Balch in *Dietary Wellness*, research shows that women who eat whole grains and fiber with nutrients included recover more quickly from symptoms of premenstrual syndrome. The research goes on to say those with seasonal adaptive disorder (SAD) and depression benefit from eating complex carbohydrates as well.[60]

CHOLINE, INISOTOL & LECITHIN

Choline, inisotol, and lecithin are found in the wheat germ and keep blood vessels flexible and resilient. This serves to "burn out" the cholesterol, a fatty substance that collects in the walls of the veins and may help prevent hardening of the arteries. Today, however, these are removed since the wheat germ will spoil if not refrigerated or vacuum packed.[61] Only milling your own wheat guarantees the inclusion of all the nutrients and benefits designed for our health.

PHYTIC ACID

Phytic acid is found in the bran of grains and beans. It increases the body's ability to absorb the correct amount of minerals, especially calcium. If grains were balanced with much more bran than already present, we could develop calcium deficiency. The correct balance is evidently extremely important. A thorough understanding of phytic acid can be found in the article titled "Phytic Acid: Friend or Foe" by Sue Becker at the Designed Healthy Living website.

Whole Grain Bread Is Better Than Fruits and Vegetables

Many people are aware that fruits and vegetables contain disease-fighting phytochemicals and antioxidants, but they do not realize whole grains are often an even better source of these key ingredients. Whole grains have some valuable antioxidants not found in fruits and vegetables, as well as B vitamins, vitamin E, magnesium, iron, and fiber. God—our top nutritionist—designed the wheat kernel and other grains to perfectly store these nutrients. Other nutrients found in whole grains include phosphorus, potassium, sulphur, manganese, nitrogen, iodine, oxygen, hydrogen, fluorine, magnesium, chlorine, carbon, iron, sodium, and silicon. This is a list of the very core of life.

Once nutrients are broken, as in milling, the nutrients immediately begin to oxidize. Due to this, within about seventy-two hours, ninety percent of more than 30 nutrients are virtually gone. This helps us see again why God reminds us to "give us this day our daily bread." Whole grains are most nutritious at the time of milling.

To Sprout or Not to Sprout?

Do you remember planting a seed in a cup, placing it on the windowsill in your home, and then eagerly waiting for it to grow or sprout? How excited I used to get when I would see a plant emerge from the hard shell of the seed and become a soft, delicate plant. That experience isn't just for kids, though. People who want the rich nutrients in sprouts grow their own. Research continues to confirm that sprouting of grains can bring additional benefits. The *pulse* that is mentioned in Daniel's diet (Dan. 1:12 KJV) comes from the Hebrew word for "sown things," which would include grains and sprouts. Sprouts are a nutritional gold mine. Sue Becker, in her article "Phytic Acid: Friend or Foe," explains sprouting grains:

Of the many essential nutrients needed by your body to promote health and life, there are only four nutrients deficient in wheat: vitamin A, vitamin C, vitamin D, and the amino acid lysine. When grains and beans are sprouted, there is some loss in protein but vitamin A content increases by 300 percent and vitamin C by 500 percent. In fact, sprouted grains were used on long ocean voyages to prevent scurvy. Limes and lemons would eventually rot, but the storable grains would last the duration of the voyage and could be sprouted at any time. Sprouted grains can also be more easily tolerated by those who cannot digest gluten.[62]

DIGGING DEEPER: Read "Fiber Mystery Unfolded" and "Kernel of Truth" in the *Nutrition Manual*. Notice the loss of nutrition in flour that has had the bran and germ removed through milling.

Taking this treasure to heart: Our joy in the Lord can be found in the discovery of the smallest kernel of nutrition-packed wheat. Settling for anything less, such as processed white flour, leaves us deceived, tricked, and conned. Only the truth can set us free.

DAY THREE—TYPES OF WHOLE GRAINS

God's perfect plan means the highest quality foods are also the most affordable so everyone can enjoy abundant health. While wheat is the cheapest, sometimes adding other grains to the menu can bring a pleasing taste and equal nutrition. New grains can be added for low cost, and I suggest you start with a small amount to make sure it pleases your family's palate before investing in a large quantity. Later we will learn how to add these different grains into the meal plans, but first we will look at some of the varieties of whole grains.

Grains in Scripture

Let's take a look at the two most common types of grain found in Scripture—wheat and barley.

WHEAT

"Celebrate the Feast of Weeks with the first fruits of the wheat harvest, and the Feast of Ingathering at the turn of the year" (Ex. 34:22 NIV). Wheat is the most popular and economical grain. It is divided into six classes: hard red winter, hard red spring, soft red winter, durum, hard white, and soft white wheat. Each wheat class has particular qualities, and they each work differently in your recipes. In whole food recipes, similar to those found in the *Healthy Treasures Cookbook,* you will find ingredients referring to these different flours. When you alter recipes, it is helpful to understand what makes each type of wheat different and which ones work best for a particular end result.

DIGGING DEEPER: Read Grains of Value in *The Treasures of Health Nutrition Manual.*

BARLEY

References to barley are scattered throughout Scripture. It was the most plentiful grain of Palestine. In 1 Kings 4:28, barley was used as food for the horses.

The most famous story containing barley is found in John 6:1-15, when Jesus fed five thousand men with just five barley loaves. Jesus used the most common food to perform this miracle. How did the people respond after they witnessed this miraculous feeding? (See verse 14.)

_____

_____

_____

Jesus is the Bread of Life, but the people only saw the miraculous feeding of thousands. In this study, we are learning that God's provision is perfect—both physically and spiritually.

Other Grains of Value

There are a host of valuable grains just waiting for our consumption. Check out the following list of whole grains and their uses.

- Amaranth—This grain has a nutty and somewhat sweet flavor. It works best in spoon breads, casseroles, loaves, or hot cereals.
- Quinoa—Quinoa is a great replacement for rice in your regular dishes. The Healthy Treasures Cookbook contains some enjoyable recipes using quinoa.
- Spelt—Today spelt is promoted for use by people with wheat and gluten sensitivities. It has a nutty aroma and flavor. The gluten content is more fragile than wheat and should be kneaded less in yeast recipes.
- Kamut—This grain produces excellent breads, pastas, and other baked goods. It has a light, slightly buttery flavor and a golden color. This is the grain that I mill to make fresh pancakes since it gives a deceptive Aunt Jemima flavor.
- Barley—Barley flour makes excellent pie crusts and cookies. It also mixes well with rice flour. It is the whitest of the whole grain flours and has a mild taste. It has no gluten and cannot be used with yeast.

- Brown Rice—Flour made from brown rice can be gritty in texture and taste but is excellent for thickening gravies and sauces. Baked goods made only from rice flour tend to be crumbly.
- Millet—This grain is often used as a morning cereal or in soups, stews, casseroles, stuffing, and puddings. However, millet flour tends to be heavy and bland in flavor.
- Oats—Oats are an ideal cold-weather crop. Since they have a slightly higher fat content, they produce a sense of warmness and stamina. Oat flour works well with cookies and in pie crusts.
- Buckwheat—Buckwheat is not related to wheat; it is actually a member of the grass family. The flour has a stronger flavor than many other flours and is most often used in pancakes, waffles, and quick breads.
- Corn—Corn is referenced in scripture ninety-four times and may refer to grains in general. When purchasing fresh corn, popcorn, and cornmeal always look for organic options, since a large portion of corn comes from crops that are genetically modified organisms (GMO).

As you can see from this list, great things come in little packages. What grains have you sampled?

Which grains can you include in your diet this week?

Seeds and Nuts

Leave the silverware in the drawer—these foods are to be eaten raw. The popularity of these seeds and nuts is increasing due to their concentrated burst of flavor and added crunch in breads and recipes. It is not unusual to find a sprinkling of sunflower, coriander, poppy, fennel, sesame, mustard, pumpkin, or cumin seeds on hot soups or cold salads.

Nuts and seeds are more nutrient dense than most foods. They are rich sources of protein, fiber, B vitamins, folic acid, calcium, iron, zinc, vitamin E, and selenium. Do you think nuts have too much fat to be part of a healthy diet? Wrong! Nuts do contain a lot of fat, but 90 percent of this fat is the heart-healthy unsaturated kind. These mono-saturated and poly-unsaturated fats help move cholesterol through the bloodstream, thereby lowering LDL cholesterol while protecting against cancer. Nuts were designed to be good for you.

Read Genesis 43:11. Which grain, nuts, or seeds are listed in this verse? What was the purpose of the food? You may need to read the surrounding verses to get the full story.

_____

_____

_____

Principle II states that we are to eat foods closest to the way God designed them. Keeping that in mind, raw nuts are always the best choice. Roasted nuts have been found to carry carcinogens. In addition, while heating or roasting nuts does enhance the flavor and reduce spoilage, it also may alter some of the fatty acids. This is why processed nuts are less likely to go rancid, but the trade-off may be a loss of healthy nutrients. Seeds and nuts contain vitamin E, a natural antioxidant, which protects the oil from going rancid. Processing or altering the seeds removes some of the natural antioxidants in the nuts and seeds.

There are numerous kinds of seeds and nuts. As they have come from the Creator, they are a healthy addition to all menus. It only takes a small serving to meet the oil requirement necessary for a healthy diet. So be stingy when pouring them on your favorite salad or cookie recipe.

Highlighting Flax Seed

Flax saved the Israelite spies while they hid on Rahab's roof. You can read about this in Joshua 2:1-14. While we may not need to hide any spies in our home, flax is still beneficial to us. This seed is loaded with several essential nutrients, like calcium, iron, niacin, phosphorous, and vitamin E, and it is a rich source of Omega-3 fatty acids. Whole flax seeds do not digest well because of their hard shell. To get their nutritional benefits, the seeds must be cracked or ground in a blender or coffee grinder. Once ground, flax seeds go rancid quickly, so use daily or store in the refrigerator.

Legumes

Legumes are grown worldwide in thousands of varieties. Their shared characteristic is a pod filled with edible seeds. Beans, dried peas, and lentils are all considered legumes. Peanuts, clover, alfalfa, and fenugreek are legumes also. Both in Old Testament times and at the time of Jesus, legumes—the most famous of which were lentils—seem to have been the second most important component of diet after grain. One ancient authority numbers more than twenty kinds of legumes, the most important of which were lentils and chickpeas.[63]

Legumes are among the most versatile and nutritious foods available. They are typically low in fat, contain no cholesterol, and are high in folate, potassium, iron, and magnesium. They are also a good source of protein and can be a healthy substitute for meat, which has more fat and cholesterol.

Genesis 25:27-34 is a well-known Bible story that includes the consumption of lentils. As you read this story, you will see that lentil stew and bread were such an enticement that Esau was willing to sell his birthright.

What was the only concern on Esau's mind?

_____

Do we sometimes act the same as Esau? Why?

_____

Due to our hurried lifestyles, we are often only concerned with getting something to eat quickly instead of thinking about the consequences of our choices. We may not be selling our birthright, but instead we may be making unwise choices for the health of our body. It takes time to invest in your health and the health of your family, but it is time well spent.

Read 2 Samuel 17:27-29. What foods were brought to David?

_____

How are the people described in verse 29?

_____

Were the provisions brought by David enough to satisfy their biological needs?

_____

LENTILS

For many of us, lentil stew is not part of our weekly menu, but this little grain packs a powerful punch. The protein content in lentils makes it a dish both nourishing and satisfying, especially when combined with grain. Other key nutrients in lentils include fiber, potassium, B vitamins, phosphorus, magnesium, manganese, iron, copper, vitamin A, and calcium. The best thing about this little pea-like grain is that it does not need presoaking and it cooks quickly.

Some believe that the word *lent* may be derived from the word *lentil*, as it became customary to refrain from eating meat during this time, and lentils could replace the needed nourishment.

Lentils could easily be stored and transported, which made them great food for most farmers and shepherds.

BEANS

Beans are a great food full of nutrition and are only 2-3 percent fat. There is less protein in beans than in a steak, but the percentage of usable protein is still over 50 percent.[64] For those on a budget, beans will stretch your dollars and give your family a hearty, healthy meal. Learning to cook dry beans is easy to do with a little practice. Canned beans can also be used, but they are more expensive and should always be rinsed well to avoid the additives.

DIGGING DEEPER: Read more about barley, flax seed, nuts, whole grains, and flours in the *Treasure of Health Nutrition Handbook.*

Taking this treasure to heart: God has provided an abundance of marvelous food sources for us and has given us permission to enjoy and use them. It is time to take a second look at our options. Not only can we start looking for foods that build health, but we can begin seeing God as our all-provider.

What is one nugget of truth you learned today?

_____

_____

Applying this treasure at home: Two treasures to add to your menu are hummus and tahini. Hummus is made from ground chickpeas, and tahini is made from ground sesame seeds. Both of these foods can be found in typical grocery stores. Add a bag of whole grain chips, and you have a great snack or appetizer. Tabouli is also an excellent choice, loaded with all kinds of goodness. Make your own from the recipe in the *Healthy Treasures Cookbook,* or you can buy it pre-made in the refrigerated section of many grocery stores.

DAY FOUR—FILL YOUR BASKET WITH GRAINS, SEEDS, AND NUTS

Shopping and Preparing

Your health is worth the extra work and expense to utilize the treasure of grains. Read Isaiah 55:2, and write it here.

_____

_____

Now rewrite it as a prayer.

_____

_____

Actually finding the grains we know we should eat can sometimes cause a dilemma. How easy is it to find whole grain bread in the store? Let's find out.

First, we need to know how to interpret the labels. The definition of *whole grains* is: whole grains—or foods made from them—containing all the essential parts (bran, germ, and endosperm) and naturally occurring nutrients of the entire grain seed. If the grain has been processed (cracked, crushed, rolled, and/or cooked), the food product should deliver approximately the same rich balance of nutrients that are found in the original grain seed.

Notice that a grain doesn't have to be wholly intact to be a whole grain. It just has to have all three parts (bran, germ, endosperm) still present in their original proportions.

Grain Packaging

You will encounter many terms on grain packaging. Let's take a moment to look at which ones describe whole grain, and which do not.

- Whole Grains—The following terms describe grains that contain *all* parts of the grain, which means you are getting all of the nutrients: whole grain (name of grain), whole wheat, whole (other grain), stone ground, brown rice, and oats (oatmeal, old-fashioned, instant, and wheat berries).
- Maybe Whole Grains—These words are accurate descriptions of package contents, but because some parts of the grain *may* be missing, you are likely missing out on

the benefits of whole grains: wheat flour, semolina, durum wheat, organic flour, and multigrain (may describe whole grains, several refined grains, or a mix).
- Not Whole Grains—These terms *never* describe whole grains: enriched flour, degerminated, bran, and wheat germ.

Note that words like *wheat, durum,* and *multigrain* can (and do) appear on good whole grain foods, too. None of these words alone guarantees whether a product is whole grain or refined grain, so look for the word *whole* and follow the other advice here.[65]

Refined, enriched, and *whole grain* refer to the milling process and the making of grain products, and they have different nutrition implications.

- Refined—These foods have lost many nutrients during processing.
- Enriched—These products may have had some nutrients added back in, but not necessarily in their natural form. In the case of wheat, forty nutrients are removed and five or six are put back in. Some people refer to that as the Great Grain Robbery! The nutrients removed are then used as supplements that are in turn sold back to you so you get what was originally designed in the grain. In other situations the nutrients are used in animal feed.
- Fortified—Foods have nutrients added during processing, but in a fortified food, the added nutrients may not have been present in the original product. *Fortified* and *enriched* are used interchangeably.
- Whole grain—These products may be rich in fiber and have all the nutrients found in the original grain.

Enriching white flour helps prevent deficiencies of certain nutrients, but it fails to compensate for losses of many other nutrients and fiber. Only fresh-milled, whole-grain flour contains all of the nutritive portions of the grain.

Whole-grain products such as brown rice or old fashioned oatmeal not only provide more nutrients and fiber, but they often do not have the added salt and sugar of flavored, processed rice or sweetened cereals.[66]

Will the Real Bread Please Rise?

If you want the real stuff, there is only one way to get it. Mill the grain yourself and bake your own bread. When my friends first told me this, I thought they were off their rocker! I was picturing a horse and a stone mill in my backyard. I thought there was no way it was going to work, but I knew in my heart it was truth. Since it was truth, God would make a way to keep it from becoming an additional stress factor in my life. Working full-time and milling your own wheat is possible and, even more importantly, it is very rewarding. There are numerous testimonies from people who are doing this. Health problems are often erased. The best gift of all in milling is that God reveals Himself once again as the provider. The lesson to be learned, as we have explored this week, is that bread is the staff of life.

Who doesn't want to come home to the smell of baked bread, fresh-baked cinnamon rolls, or a hot bubbly pizza on a whole wheat crust? Does that make your mouth water?

Deciphering Ingredients

In case you are not ready to bake your own bread, here are some general tips for understanding bread labels.[67]

If the first ingredient listed contains the word "whole" (such as "whole wheat flour" or "whole oats"), it is likely—but not guaranteed—that the product is predominantly whole grain. If there are two grain ingredients and only the second ingredient listed is a whole grain, the product may contain as little as 1 percent or as much as 49 percent whole grain.

If there are several grain ingredients, the situation gets more complex. For instance, let's say a "multi-grain bread" is 30 percent refined flour and 70 percent whole grain. But the whole grains are split between several different grains, and each whole grain comprises less than 30 percent of the total.

The ingredients might read "Enriched white flour, whole wheat, whole oat flour, whole cornmeal and whole millet" and you would *not* be able to tell from the label whether the whole grains make up 70 percent of the product or 7 percent of the product.

Do you see why it is easier to make your own? Add it up: making your own bread gives you peace of mind and better health, saves you money, provides aromatherapy, and teaches your family biblical truths. No matter how you do the math, this is a bargain or a gold mine, depending on your terminology.

Health Challenges

Principle II states that we should eat foods in the form closest to the way God designed them or before man altered them beyond recognition. This has been hard for most people, since labels are so confusing and the facts about health are frequently nothing more than myths. Many of our foods have been altered so they can sit on the shelf for long periods. There is a synergistic effect of the nutrients God designed in the whole grain. When one or more of these are removed it becomes a problem, and the consequences can lead to allergies or autoimmune diseases.

What God designed for us was created perfect and we want our food to be as close to those foods as possible, but remember we are not looking back at what we can't change. Instead, we are looking forward to the rewards from this treasure hunt.

Avoiding Gluten on the Hunt

It's important to note that gluten-intolerant people *can* eat whole grains. In fact, there are many gluten-free grains available.

Grains with gluten include wheat, including varieties like spelt, kamut, faro and durum; and products like bulgur, semolina, barley, rye, triticale, and oats.

Gluten-free grains include amaranth, buckwheat, corn, millet, quinoa, rice, sorghum, and wild rice. Oats are inherently gluten-free, but are frequently contaminated with wheat during growing or processing. There are some companies who make gluten-free oats, and they are typically sold in the organic aisle.

Most people find whole grains to be a delicious way to improve their health, and they enjoy the pleasures of choosing among all the different whole grains.

Celiac Disease

The millions of people who can't eat gluten must choose their grains carefully. This includes the nearly three million Americans with celiac disease—an autoimmune form of gluten intolerance—who must eat a gluten-free diet for a better quality of life.

Other people may not have celiac disease but are allergic to wheat nonetheless, and must avoid all forms of wheat. A gluten-free diet sometimes is recommended as part of the treatment for children with autism.[68]

Substitutes for Gluten Grains

Many creative recipes have been developed for gluten-intolerant people using gluten-free grains along with foods like nuts, arrowroot, beans, chestnuts, mesquite, potato, soy, and tapioca. Some of these ingredients make appetizing healthy breakfast cereals and side dishes, while others are ground into flours for flavorful baked goods such as pizza, desserts, and breads.

DIGGING DEEPER: One of the main benefits of making your own bread is a lack of constipation problems. Read more about this topic in the *Treasures of Health Nutrition Manual.*

Applying the Three Principles to Grains

How do grain, seeds, lentils, and bread fit into the Three Principles?

Principle I (eat only the foods God gave us):

_____

Principle II (eat foods closest to the way God designed them):

_____

Principle III (don't let any food or drink become an addiction):

_____

Remember to guard your heart and mind; don't let Satan undo what you are learning.

Taking this treasure to heart: There are shelves filled with literature on the side effects of processed food and the detriment of bread. Our study this week has concentrated on the benefits of using whole grains. Our focus is to reveal the loving hand of our Father who offers this gift. Since there is a health revolution going on in our country, isn't this the time to introduce your friends and neighbors to the true Bread of Life that will satisfy both physical and spiritual needs? No more looking for answers. Our map—God's Word—gives us the answers.

Applying this treasure at home: What changes will you make regarding the grains and seeds your family consumes? Record this on your Action Plan.

Earlier this week you were asked to make a list of foods to eat daily in order to get an appropriate amount of fiber in the diet. If you have not completed this yet, now is a good time. It will help you to see how to get thirty-five grams of fiber in a diet. Once it is written down, you will see the simplicity of this diet change.

It is never too late to live happily ever after.

FABULOUS FOODIE FRIDAY

The Treasure of Whole Grains

A mother was preparing pancakes for her sons, five-year-old Kevin and three-year-old Ryan. The boys began to argue over who would get the first pancake. Their mother saw the opportunity for a moral lesson. She said, "If Jesus were sitting here, He would say, 'Let my brother have the first pancake. I can wait.'"

Kevin turned to his younger brother and said, "Ryan, you be Jesus."

To this day, in the Middle East, the "breaking of bread" with one's former enemy is an important symbol of the end of hostilities. This is one interpretation attached to the famous words of Psalm 23:5, "You prepare a table before me in the presence of my enemies" (NIV).

Is there someone in your life with whom you need to break bread?

Add More Legumes to Your Diet

Consider these ways to incorporate more legumes into your meals and snacks:

- Prepare soups, stews, and casseroles that feature legumes
- Use pureed beans as the basis for dips and spreads
- Add chickpeas or black beans to salads
- Snack on a handful of soy nuts, walnuts, almonds, or pecans rather than on chips or crackers
- Add garbanzos or other canned beans to your salad. If you typically buy a salad at work and no beans are available, bring beans from home in a small container.

If you can't find a particular type of legume in the store, you can easily substitute one type of legume for another. For example, pinto and black beans are good substitutes for red kidney beans. Cannellini, lima beans, and navy beans are easily interchangeable. Experiment to discover which types of legumes you like best in your recipes.

Foodie Time

Have a grain foodie feast. Try the following menu with your foodie friends. If your digestive system cannot tolerate beans, try using Beano™ or EZ-Gest®.[69] Recipes from the *Healthy Treasures* cookbook:

Appetizer—Bean Hummus with chips or raw vegetables
Main Dishes—Lentil-Barley Stew, Quinoa Pilaf, and Tortilla Bean Casserole
Salad—Zesty Rice and Bean Salad

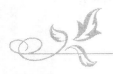

Vegetables and Fruits

DAY ONE—COLORFUL JEWELS IN THE TREASURE

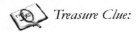 *Treasure Clue:*

Sow the fields, and plant vineyards, which may yield fruits of increase.

—Ps. 107:37 KJV

Strategies for Dodging Vegetables

Today's kids stick to the same classic vegetable-avoidance strategies their parents used. According to a study conducted by Green Giant, the three top strategies are:[70]

40 percent push vegetables around on plate so it looks like there's less
16 percent feed them to the dog
12 percent give them to a younger sibling or to a vegetable lover

It seems many families deal with the uncertainty of whether or not they can get enough fruits and veggies into their menus. For my household, my kids were not the biggest concern. It was my husband who would only touch corn on the cob, french fries, mashed potatoes, and popcorn. That was the full list of the vegetables in his diet. My kids were opposites; one loved vegetables and the other avoided them at all cost. This meant that I had to either sneak the veggies into the meal or show my family that God had a better plan. I am more in favor of the second idea, but I will never pass up an opportunity to make an addition to a favorite dish. If you come to dinner at my house, you may not realize that there is sweet potato in the chocolate cake!

Where Did the Good Come From?

Some food historians teach—along with many other fallacies—that food evolved from the miry clay. To avoid these false teachings, we will use our valued treasure map. The Holy Bible contains many scriptures about food, and the Fertile Crescent of the Holy Land is where all history started. While not mentioned by name, the Fertile Crescent is the area that arches over the deserts of what are now Jordan, Iraq, Iran, and Saudi Arabia. This land was very fertile, with the Tigris and Euphrates rivers and their tributaries running through it. Today, this land is known for growing various grains (like wheat and barley) and fruits (such as grapes, olives, figs, oranges, lemons, and pomegranates).

Egypt and its water source—the Nile—is at one end of the crescent. During Bible times, the vegetables and other food produced in Egypt were famous. "We remember the fish we ate in Egypt at no cost—also the cucumbers, melons, leeks, onions, and garlic" (Num. 11:5 NIV).

The Israelites were given a land that was abundant in food, specifically "a land of wheat and barley, vines and fig trees and pomegranates, a land of olive oil and honey" (Deut. 8:8 NKJV). Later in Scripture we read that Abigail took one hundred cakes of raisins and two hundred cakes of pressed figs to David (1 Sam. 25:18).

There are many references to food in Scripture, but it all started in Genesis. Here is a quick synopsis of what took place in the beginning of Genesis: God said, God created, God blessed, God gave, and God said it was good. God created us in His image, blessed us, and then told us what to eat. Then He said it was good. That same "good" is what we are going to see in our bounty.

Read Genesis 1:11. Describe the plants that God designed.

_____

_____

What does God declare about this part of the creation?

_____

_____

Look up Genesis 1:29, and write it down.

_____

_____

Look up Revelation 22:2, and write it down.

_____

_____

What conclusion might you draw from comparing these two verses and their locations in the Bible?

_____

_____

_____

Since there is no right or wrong answer to the previous question it would be interesting to share your notes with your small group or foodie friend.

From the beginning to the very end of Scripture, we see God's inclusion of fruits and vegetables and His desire to nourish and heal our bodies. Remember, Christ is the Alpha and Omega, the beginning and the end. In the beginning He created us, gave us food to eat, and declared it good. In the end He once again shows us that the same foods will bring healing.

Look up Psalm 85:11-12. What will God give us that is good?

_____

Look up Psalm 104:14. What does God supply for us?

_____

Can you can see in these verses that God has designed food for us and that "the Lord will indeed give what is good" (Ps. 85:12 NIV)? We also read that we are to cultivate the plants. In today's society that may mean finding the best stores to acquire the very best quality foods, visiting a local farm, or tilling up your yard to plant a flourishing garden.

Let's travel back in time and use our imaginations. You are in the Garden of Eden. As you walk you see every color of the rainbow brilliantly displayed in the bounty around you. Imagine picking up these treasures and feeling the textures: smooth, hard, fuzzy, horned, hairy, gnarled, dimpled, or prickly. If you were to pick one, which would it be? Or perhaps you are like me and want to just sample them all. Imagine taking a bite. Discover diversity in each one: tart, sweet, nutty, mild, tender, crisp, juicy, rich, fruity, and smokey.

Even today there are hundreds of varieties of fruits and vegetables, and we are going to barely scratch the surface of the soil with our study here. Let me encourage you to continue learning about new fruits or veggies after this study ends. Take a field trip to a local farm or farmer's market. Use your senses and enjoy the treasures. Each season brings new foods. The hunt can be as fun as the discovery.

According to History, "It Was Good!"

Now that we know food is good, let's see how much "good" you have been enjoying in the past few days. Write out your answers to this self-assessment test.

List the vegetables you ate in the last three days and what color they were.

_____

_____

List the fruits you ate in the last three days and what color they were.

_____

_____

How many servings of fruits and vegetables do you think the average person should eat daily? Circle the answer: 2-3, 4-10, 5-13, 8-10

Watch for the answer to this question as you read this week's study. Fruits and vegetables are some of the richest sources of nutrients you will find to build a healthy diet.

Fruits and vegetables provide a wide array of vitamins, minerals, complex carbohydrates, amino acids (from proteins), essential fatty acids, antioxidants, and phytonutrients. These phytochemicals and antioxidants work together with the vitamins and minerals to help protect against cancer, heart disease, and other disorders. Fruits and vegetables also contain soluble and insoluble fiber that allows our bodies to select what nutrients are needed. This fiber allows many unneeded calories to pass through the intestinal tract.

Unknown Food Factors

The natural foods we eat each day contain thousands of different natural chemicals—some known and well-studied, some known and unstudied, many completely unknown and immeasurable. So far, scientists understand the relevance of a small percentage of them. These unknown food factors are still being discovered, and they are continually found in the foods God approves. Once these nutrients are discovered, scientists are able to find ways to make a simulation (synthetic or chemical substitute) of them to add to our processed foods or supplements. It is said that imitation is a form of a compliment, and man is always imitating what God has given us. But aren't we blessed to have the real thing in the original design from our Creator?

Along with the known and unknown food factors are associated food factors, sometimes referred to as the synergistic effect of nutrients. These associated food factors have been shown to protect humans from vascular disease, bacterial infections, viral infections, cancer, and much more. As stated in the *Journal of the American Dietetics Association*: "Never before has the focus on the health benefits of commonly available foods been so strong. The philosophy that food can be health promoting beyond its nutritional value is gaining acceptance in the scientific community as mounting research links diet/food components to disease prevention and treatment."[71]

Synergistic means the total effect of the combined associated food factors and other nutrients has a greater effect when blended together than if the nutrients are isolated and used individually. Often these same isolated nutrients have little effect by themselves. It is like saying 1 + 1 = 3 when the food is eaten in the form God gave us. Here again, the total package of nutrients in any of the foods listed in Genesis 1:29 is greater than the sum of its parts.[72]

Cruciferous Plants

One of the fun discoveries I have made in this hunt was the meaning of the word *cruciferous*. Cruciferous refers to plants that have flowers with four petals that botanical historians describe as resembling the crucifix or cross; thus, they are called cruciferous. Many authors and health books refer to them as "The Magnificent Twelve" because of their ability to dramatically reduce and prevent disease. Only our God could design foods like that and then place a reminder on the plant that the ultimate healing was given to us on the cross!

The following are the Magnificent Twelve Cruciferous Vegetables:

Broccoli	Kale	Rutabaga	Brussels Spouts
Kohlrabi	Turnip	Cabbage	Mustard Greens
Cauliflower	Radishes	Watercress	Horseradish

These twelve vegetables are the power fighters against cancer and heart disease, the two top killers in our country. It is suggested that we consume three one cup servings from this list every day. Eat at least one cup raw and two cups slightly steamed, except for horseradish. Use horseradish grated fresh in sauces and spreads. Alternate the vegetables daily. You can find more detailed information on these twelve magnificent vegetables in the *Nutrition Manual*.

Beyond the Magnificent Twelve, the following are the most-agreed-upon top nutritious vegetables:

- All dark leafy vegetables
- Red bell peppers
- Carrots

- Peas
- Sweet potatoes
- Swiss chard
- Winter squash

More Health-Building Foods

Several other fruits and vegetables are great for building up your health. Check out these common foods.

FIGS

From the beginning in the Garden of Eden, the fig, with its astonishing health-giving and healing powers, is mentioned more than fifty times in the Bible. In fact, it is the first fruit specifically named (see Gen. 3:7).

Figs, either fresh or dried, have been prized since ancient times for their sweetness and nutritional value. Greek and Roman athletes ate figs to increase their stamina and improve their performance. Even today, in the Middle East, a compote of dried fruits is a popular dessert. Dried figs, apricots, and raisins are soaked overnight, boiled gently with a piece of cinnamon, and served cold with a sprinkling of orange or lemon juice.

GRAPES

"Then they came to the valley of Eshcol and from there cut down a branch with a single cluster of grapes; and they carried it on a pole between two men" (Num. 13:23 NASB). What a gigantic cluster of grapes! Such abundance was not unusual in the vineyards that were so important to the people of the Bible. Grapes were the first thing Noah planted after the flood. "And Noah began to be a farmer, and he planted a vineyard" (Gen. 9:20 NKJV).

Grapes were eaten fresh, or dried and eaten as raisins, just as they are today. Most of the crop of the vineyards was made into juice, wine, and vinegar, although grapes were also pressed into cakes.

GARLIC

Garlic is a food that will liven up any dish and yet its medicinal properties have been documented all the way back to Hippocrates. The Israelites missed the garlic in Egypt as they traveled around in the desert. It was used to treat plagues in Europe and as a cure for dysentery during World War I. Cancer, high blood pressure, cholesterol, and infections are just a few of the health issues believed to be relieved with garlic.

ONIONS

There was no onion breath in the wilderness. Onions were another food highly missed by the Israelites when they left Egypt. Egyptians used onions as currency to pay the workers who built the pyramids. They also placed them in the tombs of kings, such as Tutankhamen, so that they could carry these gifts with them to the afterlife. Onions have been revered throughout time not only for their culinary use, but also for their therapeutic properties. As early as the sixth century, onions were used as a medicine in India.

Foodie Fun Fact: All plant life has built-in protection against insects. These "protective pesticides" are usually found in micro amounts and are safe for human consumption. Isn't it amazing that the vegetable kingdom has a "defense system" designed into it, just like our bodies do?

DAY TWO—HEALTHY COLORS

"Eat your vegetables; they are good for you!" This wisdom is passed on from generation to generation. And yet today we continue to learn more and more about how a diet rich in the colors of fruits and vegetables can do wonders for our bodies, such as:

- Decrease the chances of having a heart attack or stroke
- Protect against a variety of cancers
- Lower blood pressure
- Help avoid diverticulitis
- Guard against cataracts and macular degeneration
- Add variety to your diet and enliven your palate[73]

Need proof? The story of Daniel is one that helps us see how the value of these foods can make a difference in physical and mental ability.

Read Daniel 1:1-16.

In Daniel 1:8, Daniel "made up his mind" that he would not go against the teachings from God's Word. This is the mindset that we need to consider adopting. Personally, I have found that if I intentionally decide to eat only certain foods on a given day, then I am less likely to overeat or eat the wrong foods. If I start a day without intentional plans, I sometimes lack the control to eat what is most healthful. Honestly, I deal with spiritual strongholds in the discipline of eating. However, we can all learn from Daniel that it is important to make up our minds before each day begins—or even before we go out to a restaurant—to eat foods that will bring life to our bodies. Such intentionality will make you will feel more energized and invigorated.

How did Daniel come into the king's care?

_____

Even though Daniel was taken from his normal life and placed into qualification training for service in the king's court, he still knew he was a child of the true King. He remained committed to the teachings he had received in his earlier years. Daniel made a conscious decision to follow God's commands.

How would you summarize verse 8 for your life today?

_____

_____

_____

How did God respond to Daniel's act of obedience regarding his diet and his relationship with the commander of the officials?

_____

_____

_____

What foods did Daniel eat for three years?

_____

_____

Continue to read through verse 21. Daniel made up his mind not to defile himself, and God granted Daniel His favor. Later in the book, we read that Daniel and his friends followed this diet for three years and were smarter and healthier than all the other youths who had followed the king's special diet. What conclusion for your own life can you draw from this verse?

_____

_____

_____

_____

_____

Daniel was a "youth." How might your kids benefit from following a plan like this for a week, month, or longer?

_____

_____

_____

In today's society it may seem extreme to "limit" our kids like this, but think back to Daniel and remember that he set his mind on following God's design. Possibly your kids are dealing with heath concerns. As the parent and guardian of those kids, how can you make a difference in their health by setting your mind on following God's laws? As they see us setting God's laws as a primary reason for choices we make, they will begin to imitate our actions.

As I look back at the health of my kids, I truly wish I had learned this truth earlier. Now I can apply this teaching to my grandkids. Some of you still have a chance to make a difference in your family. Frankly, the decision will continue to come back to us to decide what we will do with this information from God's Word.

Your Health Is Worth It

Many health problems are either brought on or made worse by a poor diet. Outside of cancer, the top three health problems are obesity, heart disease, and elevated cholesterol. Scripture alone is enough reason to concentrate on the foods God designed, but science has been able to help us understand the design of fruits and vegetables in relation to our health. We have an opportunity to take God at His word and start applying His truths.

CANCER

Vegetables contain many cancer-fighting substances. The statistics on cancer are frightening, yet vegetables and fruits may help lower this risk. According to the American Cancer Society (ACS), approximately 1,437,180 new cases of cancer were diagnosed in 2008.[74] All cancers involve the malfunction of genes that control cell growth and division. An interesting statistic from the ACS is that only about 5 percent of all cancers are hereditary. This means we have a way to avoid this disease. People die every day with cancer; it is second only to heart disease. The sad fact is that among children, almost 11,000 new cases of cancer were diagnosed in 2008, and cancer is the second leading cause of death, second only to accidents. These startling facts from the ACS were found in the same publication that states, "Inadequate intake of fruits and vegetables is listed as one of the primary risk factors that can lead to this diagnosis."[75]

DIABETES

Diabetes is no longer the "other person's problem." Diabetes (Type 2) has become an epidemic in America. Many people do not even know they have it or that they are close to having it (with pre-diabetes). The good news is that in most cases diabetes can be prevented. A healthy diet of at least three to five vegetables and two to three fruits a day, along with exercise and a healthy weight will help anyone avoid the pitfall of this disease.

HEART DISEASE

Adding food with plenty of colors protects against several forms of heart disease and stroke. Some exciting research shows that plant-rich diets can help prevent or control two of the main precursors of heart disease and stroke—high blood pressure and high cholesterol. A study completed by the *Journal of the American Medical Association* showed that those who ate the minimum of five fruits and vegetables a day were 15 percent less likely to have a heart attack and had a 30 percent lower incidence of the most common kind of stroke. The Ischemic stroke is caused by a blood clot blocking an artery in or to the brain. Even adding one extra fruit or vegetable a day can decrease your risk of developing a clot by 6 percent.[76]

Cholesterol levels also seem to respond to a diet with plenty of fruits and vegetables. These results may be because the participants replaced meat and dairy with vegetables or because of the high soluble fiber content that blocks the absorption of cholesterol from food. Either way you look at it, fruits and vegetables are a good investment for your heart.[77]

CATARACTS

We don't know about Popeye's muscles, but a new study suggests that he and other spinach eaters do have healthier eyes. Researchers at The Ohio State University have demonstrated in the laboratory that certain antioxidants found in dark leafy green vegetables—not only spinach but also kale and collard greens—can help prevent cataracts. This is another great reason to take a closer look at the foods God gave us.[78]

OBESITY

How many times do we reach for the apple pie while the lonely apple shivers in the crisper? Since obesity is a major contributor to almost all diseases, it might help to consider what foods add to this problem and how to choose better ones. Let's look at obesity in a new way—the energy density of foods. The apple pie is a high-energy-dense food, which means it has a high number of calories per serving. Therefore it contains more fat and calories and less satiety (feeling of fullness and satisfaction) when compared to a food that is a low-energy-dense food. Water and fiber in foods like an apple, increase volume and thereby reduce energy density. This simply means you would need to eat five apples (53 calories each) to equal the calories of a serving of apple pie (280 calories per serving). Yet the average person could not eat five apples because of the fiber, water, and bulk of the food. It would be too much. In their natural state, fruits and vegetables have high water and fiber content and are low in calories and energy density.

Studies that tested the influence of vegetables on feeling of satiety found that adding vegetables (such as carrots and spinach) to meals with equal calories enhanced the feelings of being full. These studies did not distinguish whether the effect was related to the vegetables' fiber and water content or to the reduction of energy density of the food. However, the ratings of fullness were correlated positively with the dietary fiber content, the water content, and the total weight of the meal.

Defining Energy Density

Energy density is the relationship of calories to the weight of food (calories per gram). There are several levels of energy density:

- High energy density foods have a large number of calories per serving. Examples include low-moisture foods like crackers and cookies or high-fat foods like butter and bacon.

- Medium energy density foods have a moderate number of calories per serving. Examples include hard-boiled eggs, dried fruits, bagels, broiled lean sirloin steak, hummus, grape jelly, whole wheat bread, and part-skim mozzarella.
- Low energy and very low energy density foods have the least amount of calories per serving. Examples include tomatoes, cantaloupe, broth-based soups, fat free cottage cheese, fat free yogurt, strawberries, broccoli, and skinless roasted turkey breast. Most fresh fruits and vegetables fall into one of these two categories, low energy and very low density. [79]

Decreasing Obesity

We can decrease obesity by eating more low and very low energy density foods. A great way to do this is by adding fruits and vegetables to your menu. Check out these steps for adding these colorful foods to your diet.

1. To lose weight, you must eat fewer calories than you spend. Adding fruits and vegetables to an existing eating plan that supplies sufficient calories or has more calories than needed can cause you to gain weight. Fruits and vegetables should be substituted for foods high in energy density.
2. To lower the energy density of foods, such as soups, sandwiches, and casseroles, substitute fruits and vegetables for foods such as high-fat meat, cheese, and pasta. For example, vegetables such as carrots, broccoli, mushrooms, and celery can be added to a chicken noodle casserole, thereby lowering the calories per serving of the original casserole. Lettuce, tomatoes, onions, and other sliced vegetables can be added to sandwiches while decreasing the amount of high-fat meat or cheese. Many different vegetables can be added to pasta sauce.
3. The way fruits and vegetables are prepared and consumed makes a big difference in their effect on weight. Techniques such as breading and frying, adding high-fat dressings and sauces, and as part of a high-calorie dessert greatly increase the calorie and fat content of the dish even if it includes fruits and vegetables.

Final Tips

Whole fruit is lower in energy density and more satiating than fruit juices. Pulp-free fruit juices lose their fiber content in the process of juicing. For weight control purposes, the whole fruit contains added fiber that helps us feel full.

Are canned and frozen fruits and vegetables just as good as fresh? Frozen fruits and vegetables are good options when fresh produce is not available. We need to be careful, however, when choosing canned. Choose those without added sugar, syrup, cream sauces, or other ingredients that will increase calories, thereby raising the energy density. Additionally, consumers should be aware that frozen and canned fruits and vegetables sometimes contain added salt, which is not found in fresh produce.

Vegetables tend to be lower in calories than fruit; thus, substituting more vegetables than fruit for foods of higher energy density can be helpful in a weight management plan. The Dietary Guidelines for Americans recommends that people eat more servings of vegetables than fruits in a healthy eating plan.[80]

Taking this treasure to heart: What nugget of truth did you pick from the garden today?

_____

_____

Applying this treasure at home: Think about different steps you can take this week to increase vegetables in your meal plan. Record the different colors of fruits and vegetables you are eating today. How colorful is your diet?

Red _____

Green _____

Yellow _____

Purple _____

Blue _____

Orange _____

Day Three—Confusion in the Garden

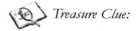 *Treasure Clue:*

Then God said, "I give you every seed-bearing plant on the face of the whole earth and every tree that has fruit with seed in it. They will be yours for food."

—Gen. 1:29 NIV

The Three Principles are easy to apply to eating fruits and vegetables. We can clearly see from Genesis 1:29 that we can eat the foods God gave us, according to Principle I. But Principle II will require a little more deciphering. Let's look at the difference between organic and conventional grown foods.

Choosing Organic or Conventional

Which to choose—organic or conventional—seems to be a popular question floating around in stores, magazines, and the marketplace. Some claim organic is the only right choice of food, but the cost may make it prohibitive. So what is the best buy?

Principle II says to eat foods as God has created them, before they are changed or converted. Once we know the difference between organic and conventional, following this rule will become a simple choice.

In the United States, organic farming began on small farms. In the mid-1970s these pioneering farmers came together to create regional grassroots networks in order to learn from one another and to educate the public about the benefits of growing and eating organically raised food. Original standards came from their dialogue and experience. While they shared some common principles, organic standards and requirements for certification varied among the different groups.

In 2002, the United States Department of Agriculture (USDA) implemented the National Organic Program (NOP), which established national standards defining *organic,* and laid out guidelines about how organic crops are grown and how livestock must be raised, processed, and handled. Today, organic produce farmers must follow strict guidelines that include such aspects as soil fertility, organic sourced seeds and plants, crop rotations, and weed, pest, and disease control. For the farmer there is a lot of paperwork, but for us there are many benefits. The conclusion of these standards is that "certified organic" fruits and vegetables must come from land that has not been exposed to the following materials for the immediately preceding three years: synthetic pesticides, herbicides, fertilizers, genetically modified seeds, irradiation, or fertilizer derived from sewage sludge. No, we definitely don't want the sewage sludge!

Principle II states to eat foods close to the way God designed them. That would mean eating organic, since the use of synthetic chemicals is prohibited in the production, transportation, and preservation of the fruits and vegetables.

How to Identify Organic Foods

It is not always easy to identify organic foods in the local grocery store. The following explanations will help you navigate through the different terms and types of foods.

- Single-Ingredient Foods—On foods like fruits and vegetables, look for a small sticker version of the USDA Organic label or check the signage in your produce section for this seal. The word *organic* and the seal may also appear on packages of meat, cartons of milk or eggs, cheese, and other single-ingredient foods.
- Multi-Ingredient Foods—Foods such as beverages, snacks, and other processed foods use the following classification system to indicate their use of organic ingredients.
  - 100% Organic—Foods bearing this label are made with 100 percent organic ingredients and may display the USDA Organic seal.
  - Organic—These products contain at least 95–99 percent organic ingredients (by weight). The remaining ingredients are not available organically but have been approved by the NOP. These products may display the USDA Organic seal.
  - Made With Organic Ingredients—Food packaging with this label must contain 70–94 percent organic ingredients. These products will not bear the USDA Organic seal; instead, they may list up to three organic ingredients on the front of the packaging.
  - Other—Products with less than 70 percent organic ingredients may only list organic ingredients on the information panel of the packaging. These products will not bear the USDA Organic seal.

Keep in mind that even if a producer is certified organic, the use of the USDA Organic label is voluntary, but the adherence to these standards is not. At the same time, not everyone goes through the rigorous process of becoming certified, especially smaller farming operations. When shopping at a farmer's market, for example, don't hesitate to ask the vendors how their food was grown.

DIGGING DEEPER: There is much to learn about the benefits of organic. Read Organic and Natural in the *Nutrition Manual.*

New Study Verifies Organic Is Better

On a 725-acre farm study in 2007, researchers at Newcastle University (UK) found that levels of antioxidants in milk from organic herds were as much as 90 percent higher than what was found in milk from conventional herds. They also found that up to 40 percent more antioxidants were present in organic vegetables than in conventional ones. In addition, they found that organic tomatoes from Greece had significantly higher levels of antioxidants, including flavonoids thought to reduce coronary heart disease.[81]

Review Proverbs 14:12. How can this verse be applied to what we are learning?

_____

_____

Pesticides

The growing consensus among scientists is that small doses of pesticides and other chemicals can cause lasting damage to human health, especially during fetal development and early childhood. Scientists now know enough about the long-term consequences of ingesting these powerful chemicals to advise that we minimize our consumption of pesticides.

What's the Difference?

The Environmental Working Group (EWG)[82] research has found that people who eat the twelve most contaminated fruits and vegetables consume an average of ten pesticides a day. Those who eat the fifteen least contaminated conventionally-grown fruits and vegetables ingest fewer than two pesticides daily. The EWG developed a guide to help us make informed choices to lower our dietary pesticide load. This information can be found in the *Nutrition Manual* or at the EWG web site.

Will Washing and Peeling Help?

Nearly all the studies used to create these lists assume that people rinse or peel fresh produce. Rinsing reduces but does not eliminate pesticides. Peeling helps, but valuable nutrients often go down the drain with the skin. The best approach: eat a varied diet, rinse all produce, and buy organic when possible.[83]

Foodie Fact: If you are serious about maintaining your health, organic, chemical-free, unaltered foods from God's garden will always be the best choice.

Would You Like Selective Breeding, GMO, and GE on the Menu?

Grapes became more enjoyable when the seedless variety became available. Seedless watermelons are now very popular also. The problem with this variety of watermelons is that we no longer get a good seed-spitting contest, which has livened up many a boring family picnic. The vast majority of our crops today have been bred for a particularly appealing characteristic. Even though these fruits have been changed, they can still be grown organically. There has been selective breeding in our food chain since the beginning of agriculture but this is different from what we are seeing today with Genetically Modified foods (GMO) or Genetically Engineered (GE) foods.

A strawberry that contains a flounder gene that makes it frost resistant, and a bacterial gene that confers antibiotic resistance, and a virus gene that "turns on" the other added genes, is different fundamentally from a conventional strawberry. Under normal circumstances, a strawberry can only acquire genetic material from other strawberries—that is, plants of the same species. With genetic engineering, scientists can give strawberries genetic material from trees, bacteria, fish, and pigs, even humans, if they chose to. Where the donor organism and recipient organism are from different species, the resulting genetically engineered organism is called "transgenic."[84]

This kind of strawberry—or any other genetically altered agricultural product—is called a GMO (Genetically Modified Food). This type of food production has been popular only since 1992. Far-reaching results may not be truly felt until we are two or more generations along. The most common GMO foods are soy, corn, and wheat. It is always safest to look for organic options when buying any of these three foods. I recently had a conversation with a local grocery store produce buyer. I was concerned about whether the labels on the corn were completely accurate. He said that unless the corn was labeled organic, there was a high probability that it was a GMO version. This includes all processed foods with corn in the ingredients, including high fructose corn syrup. Some of the common foods that may include GMO's in their ingredients include: tomatoes, beets, potatoes, alfalfa sprouts, dairy, canola oil, rice, meat, poultry, eggs, farm-raised fish, salad dressings, juice, soda, vitamins, and some condiments.

Sticky Labels on Your Fruit

Product Look-Up (PLU) codes are designed to benefit the grower and retailer in identifying the produce. The labels tell if the fruit was genetically modified, organically grown, or produced with chemical fertilizers, fungicides, or herbicides.

Here's how it works. For conventionally grown fruit, (grown with chemical inputs), the PLU code on the sticker consists of four numbers. Organically grown fruit has a five-numeral PLU prefaced by the number 9. Genetically engineered (GE) fruit has a five-numeral PLU prefaced by the number 8. For example:

- a conventionally grown banana would be: 4011
- an organic banana would be: 94011
- a genetically engineered (GE or GMO) banana would be: 84011

However, although these are the accepted labeling guidelines, I have never found a fruit or vegetable labeled with the 8. As I mentioned earlier, most corn is unlabeled GMO. The other numbers are used regularly and can be relied on for your purchases. Marion Nestle, author of *What to Eat,* has come to the same conclusion regarding the absence of GMO labeling.[85]

Fun Foodie Fact: The adhesive used to attach the stickers is considered food-grade, but the stickers themselves aren't edible.

Treasure Clue

Refer back to our Treasure Clue for today, Genesis 1:29. How does God describe the food we are to eat?

_____

_____

God gave us seeds and the plants they bear as our food. Do you think the changes man has made to the seeds will make an impact on our health?

_____

_____

Today's lesson included very little Bible study and a lot of research study. From what you have learned, how would you apply Principle II to fruits and vegetables?

_____

_____

Are there other verses you can recall that would apply to this lesson? If so, share those with your group or foodie friend.

Taking this treasure to heart: Our culture is all about changes and making things better. Changing our foods may not be the best choice. Thankfully, the winds of change are proving the intricacies of God's design and the health it brings. What kernel of truth did you learn today that may change how you view fruits and vegetables?

Applying this truth at home: Pick out a new organic fruit or vegetable to try this week. For a foodie test, compare the taste and texture to a non-organic food of the same variety.

DAY FOUR—FIND THE RIGHT FARMER

How Do You Like Your Fruits and Vegetables?

Many people wonder if frozen and canned vegetables are as nutritious as fresh vegetables. The answer depends on both the time between harvest and the canning and freezing process. Generally, vegetables are canned or frozen immediately upon harvest, when their nutrient content is at its peak.

Home preparation of vegetables can also affect the nutrient content. Vegetables of any type (fresh, frozen, or canned) that are boiled in large amounts of water for long periods of time lose much of their nutritional content compared with vegetables that are lightly steamed.

Vegetables fresh from the farm or just picked are more nutritious than their frozen or canned counterparts, but frozen vegetables are an acceptable nutritional alternative. But remember, don't overcook any vegetables; you want them to be slightly crisp, not mushy.[86]

Dried fruit is processed minimally by the sun or hot air. The water content is reduced from 80 percent to 20 percent. Dried fruit has a high concentration of minerals (iron, copper, and potassium), fiber, and beta-carotene. Be aware that dried fruit has a high percentage of fructose sugar, and that vitamin C is lost in the dehydrating process. There are some physicians who encourage their patients to eat organic food that's unprocessed, scavenger-free, and so on. It becomes obvious which patients follow their advice. They "lose" those patients to good heath, but gain their friendship.[87]

Read Philippians 1:11. How can you apply the spiritual analogy for fruit to what you have learned?

Doing things right (righteousness) and appropriating the righteousness of Christ yields fruits that are glorious and praiseworthy to God.[88]

In the Garden of Eden, the very best fruits and vegetables were abundant, and Adam and Eve could choose from a great assortment in this treasure chest. For now we don't have that privilege, but we have learned that in heaven, as referenced earlier in Revelation 22, we will again be blessed with the finest that God has to offer. Let's not let anything stop us or excuse us from looking for the best of the harvest. Our work and sweat may come from finding a local farmer, searching the farmer's market, or maybe even finding a farm to pick our own produce. These are foods that are proven to give us nutrients that will build life. If your schedule is too busy, then make time and decrease the obligations that are stealing your health by preventing you from taking time to find the best foods and prepare them.

Local Treasures

Produce tastes best when it's fresh. Nutritional value is higher when foods are picked fresh and delivered to a retailer within one hundred miles of your home. Fresh local produce is usually cheaper than non-local, and when you can't buy organic, local is a good choice. Retailers are now offering fresh produce that's grown by local farmers. Crops are harvested near peak ripeness and delivered to the store quickly—rich in flavor and freshness. Even stores like Wal-Mart are getting into the "local" scene: "We feel fortunate. There are so many local farms that supply a wide variety of produce to our stores. These farms form the backbone of our local economies. And these farmers are people that live in our local communities. People that take pride in hard work. People that share in our commitment to customer satisfaction. People that believe in the highest standards of quality."[89]

Buying local from a farmer at a produce stand, a farmer's market, or a CSA (Community Supported Agriculture) gives you a chance to ask how the food was produced and determine if it meets your standards.

What About CSA's?

CSA's (Community Supported Agriculture) are an increasingly popular alternative to other food purchasing choices. A CSA offers great benefits for the farmer and the consumer. Many farms offer produce subscriptions, where buyers receive a weekly or monthly basket of produce, flowers, fruits, eggs, milk, meats, or other farm products.

A CSA is a way for the food buying public to create a relationship with a farmer. By making a financial commitment to a farm, people become "members" (or "shareholders" or "subscribers") of the CSA. Most CSA farmers prefer that members pay for the season up-front, but some farmers will accept weekly or monthly payments. Some CSA's also require that members work a small number of hours on the farm during the growing season.

A CSA season typically runs from late spring through early fall. The number of CSA's in the United States was estimated at fifty in 1990, and has since grown to more than 2,200. To find a CSA in your area, go to www.localharvest.com.

In general, remember these tips when shopping for local produce:

- Use all your senses—sight, smell, taste, and feel. You'll also need to listen to the farmer.
- While you, as the buyer, have a right to inspect the produce, be careful not to damage it. It is the farmer's product until you buy it.
- Talk to the person behind the stand. Ask for a taste of the product. Ask when it was picked, where it was grown, and what types of fertilizers and pesticides were used. They also can tell you some ways to use the produce.
- If you find farmers whose produce you like, get to know them better. Tell them how you use their produce and what varieties you like. Growers use that feedback to better serve their customers.

How to Pick the Best Produce

Consider the following tips when choosing produce:

- Avoid buying produce with blemishes, wrinkled skin, mold, or a waxy look. Instead, look for food that is firm and has a continuous color that is appropriate for the food.
- Pick up all cartons and see if there is any visible mold on the bottom. All cartons should be dry and not have juice in the bottom.
- Citrus fruits should not be chosen based on color unless they are organic; otherwise they typically have the color sprayed on them.
- Buy watermelons by weight. They should be heavy for their size and the bottom should be yellow tinged.
- Remember to use your sight, smell, touch, and taste (if allowed) to find the very best treasures.

While at the store, look for food storage bags that will lengthen the life of your produce. These come in food-specific varieties. I have learned from personal experience that they really do extend the life of the food. I am notorious for having great menu ideas when I purchase a basket of fresh fruits and veggies, but then as the week goes by I don't always take the time to fix what I bought and the produce can go bad quickly. The bags are worth the investment, and they are reusable.

Grow Your Own Victory Garden

"Then the Lord God took the man and put him into the garden of Eden to cultivate it and keep it" (Gen. 2:15 NASB).

During World War I, the US government recruited people to grow "victory gardens" to help take the place of food sent to the war zone. Colorful rationing posters showed a big garden and Uncle Sam encouraging everyone to "garden to cut food costs." We are not far from a similar scenario today. Although we are not in a state of rationing, it is still a day to conserve food for our families. Our victory garden can be one that supplies the treasures God designed for our health. As we see in Genesis, gardens have existed from the beginning to provide food. It may not be possible for you to till up your yard, but it can be rewarding to pick your own tomato from a hanging basket on your deck or to clip fresh herbs from a container on your kitchen window.

A rewarding book to help you design your garden without letting it control you is *All New Square Foot Gardening* by Mel Bartholomew. The author will help you design a garden of your own in a four-by-four-foot section of your yard. This style of gardening is the revolutionary way to grow more in less space.

Gardening with a Friend

Foodie friends are not just for cooking anymore! If your yard is not suitable for a personal garden, then gardening with a friend might be an option. Sharing the space, time, and labor will allow you to share the bounty as well.

Seasonal Foods

Eating foods that are in season and have not traveled far are always going to be your best source for the highest amount of nutrition. God has a plan and a reason for each season. We may not always understand His reasoning, but it is comforting to know that He speaks about the seasons in Psalm 1:3, ". . . which yields its fruit in its season" (NASB).

Recipes

Great recipes for fruits and vegetables can be found in a myriad of places, including the following:

- *The Healthy Treasures Cookbook*—This cookbook includes many recipes that use fresh fruits and vegetables.
- *Simply in Season* by Mary Beth Link and Cathleen Hockman-Wert—This book gives you wonderful recipes that are categorized by season and availability. I have found many treasures in this book.
- Garage sales—Sometimes the best recipes are found in old cookbooks buried in an old box at garage sales or used book stores. My old Betty Crocker cookbook has a great assortment of recipes for using cruciferous vegetables.
- Internet—Every recipe imaginable can be found on the Internet. When you find one you like, print it off and keep it somewhere handy. I like to put mine in a scrapbook and organize my favorite menus all in one place.

God Saw That It Was Good

"The earth brought forth vegetation, plants yielding seed after their kind, and trees bearing fruit with seed in them, after their kind; and God saw that it was good" (Gen. 1:12 NASB).

How would you apply the Three Principles to fruits and vegetables?

Principle I: _____

Principle II: _____

Principle III: _____

Share your applications with your foodie friend or group this week.

Taking this treasure to heart: As you look at this treasure chest, what do you see that God has provided for you? Take a moment to write out a prayer of thanks to God for what He has provided.

_____

_____

_____

Applying this treasure at home: What commitment are you going to make to include more fruits and vegetables in your diet? Share your commitment with your foodie friend and record it on your Action Plan sheet.

FABULOUS FOODIE FRIDAY

The Treasure of Vegetables and Fruits

> My daughter, Anna, was almost three years old when, one night at dinner, she asked me if Jesus really did live in her heart. Not wanting to go into the theology of salvation, I simply answered, "Yes." She responded with, "I don't think He likes carrots."

International Love of Food

Researching foods for this book allowed me to collect insights on how other countries view the contentment of eating. Everyone agrees eating is one of life's greatest pleasures. Clearly, eating provides more than just food for the body. Foods bring pleasure through their flavors and they promote family time together. In Great Britain's food guideline, the first rule is to simply "enjoy your food." The Netherlands also presents a simple message: "food + joy = health." The Greeks' health guidelines advocate that you "eat slowly, and in a pleasant environment." The Germans want you to "make sure your dishes are prepared gently and taste well" and to "take your time and enjoy eating." Japan's guidelines capture the spirit of enjoying food and family together: "Have delicious and healthy meals that are good for your mind and body. Enjoy communication at the table with your family and participate in the preparations of meals." Vietnam's guideline delivers a similar message—serve "healthy family meals that are delicious, wholesome, economical, and served with affection."[90]

It appears we all agree. Eating should be a pleasure. Let me encourage you to take time out of your busy schedule and select fresh fruits and vegetables. Prepare them creatively. And always give thanks for the bounty.

Foodie Time

Gather your foodie friends and throw a rainbow dinner. Pick a color and have everyone bring a food made from that color. I used to do this for St. Patrick's Day and made all the food green. Of course, we no longer use food coloring, so if I were to do it again, the colors would need to come from the food itself.

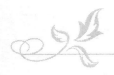

Herbs, Spices, Oil, and Vinegar

DAY ONE—CHERISH THE GEMS OF FLAVOR

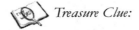 *Treasure Clue:*

To everything there is a season, and a time to every purpose under the heaven: A time to be born, and a time to die; a time to plant, and a time to pluck up that which is planted.
—Ecc. 3:1-2 KJV

At a health food store a man asked for an all-around herbal combination. The owner recommended one he said he'd sold for more than sixty years.

Dubious, the fellow took the bottle to the cashier, a really stunning young lady. As he was paying, he asked, "Has your boss really been selling this stuff for sixty years? He looks younger than I am."

"Can't really say, sir," replied the young woman. "I've only been working with him for forty years."

Fountain of youth? Who knows if herbs are the answer to youth, but with all the coverage they have received through throughout history it appears many believe it. Herbs themselves have been one of God's special blessings. They have provided people with flavors, fragrances, and medical benefits. As we go through this study, I hope a renewed understanding of the importance herbs played in our Savior's life will bring them to the forefront of your curiosity as they did mine. This may lead you to becoming an herbalist and starting your own biblical herb garden. Think of the lead-in to stories of Jesus' life as you share the stories of the importance of herbs. Imagine your treasure chest overflowing with new aromatic herbs that fill your home with pleasing scents while changing the most ordinary food into a memorable meal.

What herbs can you remember from stories in the Bible? Write them here and then see if we cover them in our study.

Enticing Aroma

Bees, butterflies, and hummingbirds travel hundreds of miles in search of the aromatic perfume of their favorite flower. Exotic spices from faraway lands can turn the heads of kings. Our Lord's head was anointed with the costliest of perfumes in preparation for burial. Spices, herbs, oils, and vinegars have been with us since the beginning of time. Yet today they are viewed as if they are a new discovery unearthed in a foreign land.

Herbs or Spices—Which Do You Prefer?

The words *herbs* and *spices* can be used interchangeably. Their medicinal and culinary value are equal. Herbs refer to all parts of the plant—roots, stems, leaves, flowers, seeds, essential oils, bark, and fruit. As you read the scriptures and references in this study you will understand how strong herbal knowledge was at the time.

Beginning in Genesis, herbs are mentioned four times in the King James Version. Other versions use the terms *sprouts, vegetables,* and *plants yielding seeds.* Read these verses in the King James Version and then another version to see the similarities: Genesis 1:11, 12, 29, and 30.

In the Garden of Eden, nothing needed to be planted because the Lord had already set everything in motion. Every plant was designed to produce after its kind. This means the plants we have today are similar to the way they were first created. The above verses in the King James Version show that there was a definite distinction made between the herbs and other plants of the fields. It appears, according to the Bible, that they were created to be distinctive.

Read Genesis 3:1-7 and 17-19. Adam and Eve sinned against the Lord. The Lord gave them a new plan for living because of their sin. Adam was reduced to eating bitter herbs from a cursed ground; and the Bible says he would eat of it in sorrow. Paradise would be filled with sorrow, sweat, and struggle. However, in the midst of the sorrow the Lord brought deliverance. Genesis 3:21 says, "Unto Adam also and to his wife did the LORD God make coats of skins, and clothed them" (KJV). Thank God that He provides a covering.

Popular Herbs in Biblical Days

What herbs were mentioned specifically in the Bible? Let's investigate some of them.

FRANKINCENSE AND MYRRH

Probably the most remembered herbs in the Bible are frankincense and myrrh, as they were two of the gifts the wise men brought to the baby Jesus (Matt. 2:11). Frankincense represents holiness, while myrrh is very aromatic and resinous and is obtained from thorn trees. Many believe the myrrh was to symbolize the suffering that would come to Jesus in the future, perhaps referring to the "crown of thorns" He would wear on the cross. Myrrh was used as a spice to make inexpensive wine more palatable. It was common to offer this mixture to criminals in Roman times and, indeed, was offered to Jesus when He was on the cross. Frankincense is used more as a fragrance rather than a spice for food.

ALOE

Read about aloe in Numbers 24:6. Experts say that the aloes of the Bible are derived from the sap of the eaglewood tree. Aloes retain their fragrance for many years, a characteristic that would make them useful for anointing the dead, because of the Jewish custom of often entering a tomb for ceremonies or the subsequent burials of additional family members. American aloe, or agave, is succulent, and is not to be confused with the biblical aloes.

Compare John 19:38-42 and Psalm 45:8 and reflect on them here.

_____

_____

GALL

Gall is an herb whose Hebrew name translates to "bitterness." It is mentioned several places in the Bible, but most famously at the crucifixion of Jesus. At that time it was mixed with wine and offered to those crucified to relieve pain, as it is actually the juice of an opium plant and therefore used as a narcotic.

Read Matthew 27:34. What ingredients were in the drink offered to Jesus?

_____

Did Jesus consume the drink? _____ The immediate reaction to that statement is that Jesus did not drink because of the taste, but further examination of the life of Christ shows that He refused in order to fully endure the cross.

MUSTARD

Mustard is another famous New Testament herb, mainly mentioned to note comparisons about size. "For truly I say to you, if you have faith the size of a mustard seed, you will say to this mountain, 'Move from here to there,' and it shall move; and nothing will be impossible to you" (Matt. 17:20 NASB).

Numerous books have been written on faith with the comparison to the mustard seed. We are just skimming over the various herbs, but this is definitely a topic to camp out on when you have time. There are some key words in this verse: *if* and *nothing*. If you have faith, *nothing* shall be impossible for you. Mustard—a small herb with a huge impact.

Foodie Idea: Visit your local grocery store and find mustard seeds in the spice aisle. Look at the size of the seed. As you observe it, think of the size of the seed versus the size of your problems in life. Then reread Matthew 17:20. How much faith is God asking us to have in our lives?

Herbs Out of the Kitchen

The value and usefulness of herbs led to them being an object of bartering as part of trade and taxes. "Woe unto you…hypocrites! For you tithe mint and dill and cumin, and have neglected the weightier provisions of the law: justice and mercy and faithfulness" (Matt. 23:23 NASB). The tithing of herbs dated back to Mosaic Law, for in Deuteronomy 14:22 it is commanded, "You shall surely tithe all the produce from what you sow, which comes out of the field every year" (NASB).

The version of this scene given in Luke 11:42 specifically mentions "mint and rue and every kind of garden herb" (NASB). Rue was used as medicine and in cooking. It is very aromatic and is also a stimulant. It is also known as the "herb of grace." Brushes made from rue were once used to sprinkle holy water at mass.

Read Luke 11:42. The emphasis placed on these herbs in Jesus' rebuke shows their importance to the people of that time. He wanted them to realize that it was more important to offer up justice, mercy, and faithfulness.

The Old Testament is seeded with verses referencing herbs, such as coriander, garlic, hyssop, saffron, and wormwood.

CORIANDER

Coriander has numerous Old Testament references. The manna sent from heaven in the wilderness was compared to it in Exodus 16:31. "The house of Israel named it manna, and it was like coriander seed, white, and its taste was like wafers with honey" (NASB). Coriander was used medicinally and as a spice.

GARLIC

Garlic is mentioned only once in the Bible, but it is done so in a way that makes the reader very much aware of how much the Israelites missed this culinary food. "We remember the fish which we used to eat free in Egypt, the cucumbers and the melons and the leeks and the onions and the garlic" (Num. 11:5 NASB).

HYSSOP

Hyssop is also referred to frequently in Scripture. Hyssop was known as a holy herb that was used to cleanse sacred places. "A clean person shall take hyssop and dip it in the water, and sprinkle it on the tent and on all the furnishings and on the persons who were there" (Num. 19:18 NASB). It is for its cleansing properties that in Psalm 51:7 David uses hyssop in a prayer of forgiveness, "Purify me with hyssop, and I shall be clean; wash me, and I shall be whiter than snow" (NASB).

SAFFRON

Along with other herbs and spices, saffron is mentioned in Song of Solomon 4:14-15, when he is expressing his affection to his lover. "Nard and saffron, calamus and cinnamon, with all the trees of frankincense, myrrh and aloes, along with the finest spices. You are a garden spring" (NASB). In those days, to be compared to herbs and spices was a prized compliment. How would you feel today if your spouse called you a cinnamon bun? Can you think of other fun food names you could use to speak well of your spouse?

WORMWOOD

Wormwood is often mentioned in instances where "intense bitterness" is the point being made. "But in the end she [an adulteress] is bitter as wormwood, sharp as a two-edged sword" (Prov. 5:4 NASB). Southernwood, which is often grown today for its fragrant properties, is a species of wormwood. This would not be a good term of endearment!

CINNAMON

"I have perfumed my bed with myrrh, aloes, and cinnamon" (Prov. 7:17 NKJV). Cinnamon was often used as a medicine, as well as a spice. It is a delicious spice long desired for its aromatic qualities. Cinnamon was used in the holy oil in the tabernacle to anoint priests and sacred vessels, as mentioned in Exodus 30:22-25.

Herbs During Passover

Read Exodus 12:1-51. This is the entire story of the Passover and God's instructions to the Israelites. As God instructs Moses and Aaron, we see specific mention of herbs. They are instructed to use bitter herbs with the unleavened bread and to remember the afflictions of slavery in Egypt. Today horseradish is used for this herb. As we learned in the chapter on vegetables, horseradish is a cruciferous vegetable. Do you remember what cruciferous means?

Many times after an affliction has healed we no longer remember the intensity of the pain. This is God's great design to help us forget certain situations or predicaments. In this instance, God did not want the Israelites to forget the deliverance from Egypt. Forgetting the pain of slavery leads to forgetting the great works He did to remove them from that situation and bring them to the Promised Land. God asked the Israelites to remember this act by telling each new generation and by celebrating with a Passover meal (sometimes referred to as the Feast of Unleavened Bread). It has become a memorial of redemption.

In Deuteronomy 11:10, the children of Israel are given a promise of great blessings that are in store for them, and herbs are prominently mentioned in it. In some versions the text will say *vegetable* instead of *herb*.

Read 1 Kings 21:2. Could this have been the beginning of today's kitchen herb gardens?

Besides the herbs mentioned specifically by name in scripture, botanists have traced many herbs we grow today to those found in the Holy Land. Many people are adding herbs to their gardens as "plant-scapes." In outdoor entertainment areas they add a fragrant aroma that no home gardener should be without.

Taking this treasure to heart: Read Ecclesiastes 3:2. What truths have you learned regarding herbs that you would like to plant in your mind, to treasure them always?

Applying this treasure at home: What is one practical step you can take with your new knowledge of herbs? Record this on your Action Plan. Think of ways you and your foodie friend can share herbs.

Day Two—Herbal Medicine

2000 BC Eat this root
1000 BC Roots are heathen. Say a prayer.
AD 1850 Prayer is superstition. Take this potion.
AD 1900 That potion is snake oil. Take this pill.
AD 1940 That pill is useless. Take this antibiotic.
AD 2000 That antibiotic is no longer effective. Eat this root.[91]

Herbs have come full circle. Centuries before our time, they were the immediate choice when a person became ill. Now we have a plethora of drugs that beg for our attention. How do we choose? We know God created everything necessary to bring life on this earth. We know He is the ultimate Healer. It is also clear that God designed for man to cultivate the earth.

Read Psalm 104:14. Who causes the grass and vegetables to grow? _____ If you have time, read all of Psalm 104 and see how the Lord cares for everything He has made.

"And their fruit will be for food and their leaves for healing" (Ezek. 47:12 N.ASB). Chemists have identified thousands of ingredients in herbs, many of them very powerful. Until 150 years ago, all medicine was derived from natural materials. Most of these fell under the heading "herbs." Generally, herbs were thought of as beneficial for health and healing, with little harm. There are numerous books written on the benefits to our health by incorporating herbs into our diet. This makes sense, since God created them and gave us several scriptures to tell us they are healing to our bodies.

The pharmaceutical industry has always isolated valuable ingredients from plants, making them available in purer forms. In 1975, 25 percent of all drugs still came from herbs, but today that amount is much less.

The transition from herbs to drugs was accelerated by the world wars that interrupted the international trade in herbs, which made synthetics attractive. Making synthetic drugs became more reliable and cost effective than depending on a natural resource.

As far as pharmaceuticals being better than herbs, that is sometimes hard to say. James A Duke, Ph.D. in botany and well-known herbalist, states, "In some studies, herbal products clearly perform better. Ginger, for example, has been shown to be superior to Dramamine as a preventive therapy for motion sickness. More research is needed that tests herbs against pharmaceutical drugs. Until that happens, we simply won't know which is better."[92]

In *Nutrition Today,* Dr. Linda Tapsell listed many reasons why herbs should be considered when trying to improve your health. Her article stated that herbs and spices are plant foods with a high concentration of phytochemicals (plant nutrients), which may increase the antioxidant power of the meal. The evidence also shows protection against inflammation.[93]

Buy Standardized Herbs

If you are going to use herbs before trying a drug, it is best to know what properties need to be met in your search for the right herb. "Standardized" means the herbal products have been processed to guarantee a known minimum level of one or more of the major active ingredients. In other words, they are the best quality. Herbs found in bins, jars, and gardens will vary in active ingredients, whereas standardized herbs come from reputable supplement companies. Standardized herbs also take the uncertainty out of herbal preparations. You know exactly how much of the active ingredients you are getting. Unfortunately, standardization makes herbs more expensive than the bulk herb. Even so, the expensive standardized herbal extracts are only about a tenth as costly, on average, as the pharmaceuticals that treat the same condition, so you are still way ahead, and there will be no toxic side effects.[94] Herbal products are not required to be labeled as "standardized," but researching the company manufacturing the product will give you the evidence you need. Only buy from a company that has "peer review double blind research" on their products. Anyone can sell herbs, but I would not suggest buying from just anyone.

Although herbs were used for medicinal values in years past, many uses were more folklore and legend than fact. Today, with modern advances in medicine, it is best to check with your doctor before considering any herbal remedies. Caution needs to be taken when combining herbs and drugs. Interactions may occur, so consult with your doctor if you are currently on a prescription and want to incorporate herbs into your diet or health plan.

FDA Consumer Magazine warns, "If you gather your own herbs to brew a cup of tea, be absolutely 100 percent certain that the herb you pick is the herb you seek....There are half a million known plant species, less than 1 percent are poisonous. But it takes only one error."[95]

Sweet or Bitter—Which Do You Prefer?

In ancient times, sweet spices were often treasured as gifts. In Genesis 43:11, Jacob used them to win the favor of the Egyptian Pharaoh. He wanted to obtain relief from the famine. They were also used as holy oil by the priests under the Old Covenant (Ex. 30:34-35). Typically, sweet herbs can be used with little or no risk and have considerable benefits. But what about those bitter herbs? For centuries, bitter herbs were thought to be poisonous and caused people to be cautious. Since there are some bitter herbs that are poisonous, this is the proper response.

Sour and bitter foods may protect against diseases, but are less appealing to the taste buds. A recent review by Dr. Adam Drewnowski at the University of Washington (UW) Nutritional Sciences Program reports that phytonutrients (found in foods such as Brussels sprouts, cabbage, mustard greens and arugula), although associated with cancer prevention and other health benefits, taste bitter, acrid, or astringent.[96] Humans and animals have always associated bitter or sour flavors with spoiled or poisonous food, which is why food manufacturers routinely remove these compounds from plant foods through selective breeding and a variety of debittering processes.

The solution, Drewnowski states, is in following the example of Mediterranean cuisine. For generations, cooks in Greece, Italy, and France have coped with bitter vegetables by seasoning them lightly with salt and dashes of olive oil. The oil in particular blunts the bitter flavors of phytonutrients.

The Medicinal Action of Bitter Herbs

Bitter herbs may taste bad, but they have some great medicinal qualities. They can:

- Stimulate the appetite
- Stimulate the digestive juices needed to digest food properly
- Strengthen poor digestion
- Help the liver filter harmful substances from the body
- Help to metabolize fat
- Help in managing hypoglycemia and diabetes
- Help reverse stomach ulcers[97]

Weeds: Pull 'em or Eat 'em?

Most of us consider dandelions a noxious weed to be ruthlessly eliminated wherever it shows its beautiful golden blooms. However, the dandelion is not only a probable biblical plant considered as one of the bitter herbs, but for centuries around the world this herb has been valued for food. In fact, in many civilized countries dandelion leaves are prized for salads. The roots are dug, dried, and used for food or pulverized and used to make beverages. Perhaps we have been influenced by the power of chemical herbicide advertising and the enormous lawn care industry. Now we know we can save the money on the lawn care and enjoy a tasty salad at the same time.

Respect Your Spices

Have you ever wondered how long the salt and pepper have been sitting in those salt and pepper shakers in the corner restaurant? Salt, pepper, and the wide variety of spices and seasonings found in recipes need careful handling, storage, and usage. Many recipes call for freshly cut herbs, and you will want to use the same principles for handling and storing these herbs as you would for any fresh vegetable. When you use dried spices and seasonings, however, the following tips may be helpful.

- Do not store your dried spices and seasonings above the stove or near a source of heat or moisture. Even though they have been dried, spices and seasonings are heat sensitive. When they are exposed to steam, there is an increased risk of bacterial or fungal contamination.
- Don't keep your spices and seasonings forever; replace them at intervals of six months to one year, depending on the particular spice or seasoning. Seeds (like mustard seeds or dill seeds) are better at retaining their nutrients than leaves (such as bay leaves).
- Buy spices and seasonings from the bulk section of your grocery in small amounts, purchasing only what you will need over the next month. Replenish your supplies more frequently to keep your supplies as fresh as possible. When trying a new spice for a recipe, share it with your foodie friend.
- Use your sense of smell to evaluate the condition of your spices and seasonings. Periodically compare the aroma of your spices and seasonings to their aroma at the time of purchase. If the fullness and richness has been lost, replace the spice or seasoning with a full-aroma equivalent.
- Don't treat your spices and seasonings like they are part of your kitchen woodwork! Have fun using them.[98]

Remember that the dried contents of your spice containers were living plants, rich in nutrients, and are just as important as your staple foods in providing you the plan God designed.

Be Fresh in the Kitchen

Don't let culinary herbs intimidate you. If an herb is new to you, nibble on it. Then let your imagination fly with all the possibilities it can bring to your meals. Start with small quantities until you feel sure of yourself. And remember, it's hard to fail with fresh herbs.

Spice It Up, Dried or Fresh

Add flair to your cooking by using herbs and spices. Vary the seasonings to give your food attitude and style. Don't be afraid to experiment with combinations you might not normally consider. For example, nutmeg is a natural for sweets like cookies and eggnog, but it also makes magic with spinach.

Three easy-to-find favorites for enhancing herbs are lemons (which enhance almost any food), garlic (which partners with most meats and vegetables), and pepper—white or black (which adds sass to practically anything, including such fruits as strawberries, apples, and melon). Most herbs are very interchangeable; just experiment until you find what fits your needs and your taste. Be adventurous and have fun!

Taking this treasure to heart: Seasoning our life with herbs is a great addition to our treasure chest for ultimate health. Just as a pinch of an herb enhances our favorite meal, a pinch of Scripture goes a long way in our everyday life. When you consider there are over 31,000 verses in the Bible, if we just take one a day to treasure in our heart, our day will be seasoned with God's wisdom. Here is an herb of truth for you to treasure today: "I have chosen the faithful way; I have placed Your ordinances before me" (Ps. 119:30 N.ASB).

This verse can be changed into a personal prayer. "Lord, right now I am choosing the faithful way according to Your laws. I want to stay focused on Your laws; help me to choose the way of truth the rest of my days."

Write a prayer of your own here.

_____

_____

_____

Applying this treasure at home: How would you apply the Three Principles to herbs?

Principle I: _____

Principle II: _____

Principle III: _____

There is no "one herb" that is the magic cure for everything in your health. An assortment of herbs will give you an assortment of nutrients.

Day Three—Do You Need More Flavor?

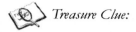 *Treasure Clue:*

You are the salt of the earth; but if the salt has become tasteless, how can it be made salty again?
—Matt. 5:13 NASB

The customer called the waiter over and said, while pointing to his steak, "Didn't I tell you, 'Well done'?"

The waiter replied, "Thank you, sir; I seldom get a compliment."

Compliments and complaints are often misunderstood. Let's read some verses to see what God is trying to teach us through the metaphor of salt and our speech.

Read Matthew 5:13. Who is the salt of the earth? _____

In Mark 9:50, salt is _____.

How can we be at peace with one another? _____

How would you summarize this verse?

_____

Colossians 4:6 What is the topic of this verse? _____

How would you summarize it? _____

_____

Read James 3:1-12. Could salt water produce fresh water in biblical days? _____

What is the topic in this chapter? _____

Do you see that all the references to salt in the New Testament refer to our speech? Christ is telling His disciples, and therefore us, that they are to go out and be the salt (voice) for Him. This is still our commandment today, but we need to choose our words wisely. Have you ever been able to eat just one potato chip when you are craving salt? Not usually. The hard part is not eating the whole bag. The same is true with our speech. We are to speak in such a way that when people hear us they will want to hear more. On the other hand, have you ever eaten something you thought was supposed to be salty and found out it was very flat and bland? You probably did not want to eat any more. When our speech and character are no longer adding flavor to those around us, it also becomes flat and flavorless to their ears.

On a scale of 1-10 how salty are you? _____

Ask your foodie friend or a family member their opinion of your saltiness. Record their answer. _____

We can add a better flavor to the life around us. We can bring healing to the hurting people in our family and community. Think back to the first day in this study. We learned that God would reveal His blessings through fellowship, food, fulfillment, family, and friends. These verses referring to salt can help in these areas. When our lives are seasoned with grace, our speech will bring peace to those to whom we are speaking. This, in turn, will benefit our family and friends. Our fellowship will be sweet, and we will have peace with one another.

The Quality of Salt

Salt has at least three unique qualities:

- A little salt sets the flavor in food. Likewise, we add a better flavor to the life around us. The fellows with whom I occasionally eat breakfast are always amazed when I take a salt shaker and sprinkle a smidgen in a cup of coffee. "I've never seen that before," they exclaim. "Why do you do that?" I answer, "It takes the bitterness and the bite out of the coffee."[99]
- Salt is a preservative. Our grandparents used salt to cure food to be used later. Ham, beef jerky, and salted fish were staples of their diets. Similarly, as Christians, we preserve the good of God's creation.
- Salt has healing properties. It kills most germs on contact. It burns when it hits a raw spot, but is very effective in cleansing a wound so it can heal. "Don't rub salt in my wounds," is a statement often heard when a person is hurt from good advice. We bring healing to those around us with words of comfort and encouragement.

A good Christian exhibits the qualities of salt.

DIGGING DEEPER: Read Salt and Fun Facts about Salt in the *Nutrition Manual.*

Hold the Salt Shaker

It's time to take inventory. Think back over the last three days and count how many of the following foods or ingredients you consumed: bouillon cubes, canned meats, canned vegetables, peanut butter, salad dressings (store bought), potato chips, corn chips, pretzels, processed cheeses, crackers, nuts, beans (canned), luncheon meats, deli meats, or butter. Write down the total: _____

If your number is below five, you are doing really well but it would be helpful to limit some more. If it is between five and ten, then you are getting more then you need in salt. If it is higher than ten, you need to consider a fast (assuming you are not a diabetic).

Salt is 40 percent sodium and 60 percent chloride, and both of these nutrients are essential in our diet. But salt is even more essential for the processed food industry. Adding salt to processed foods constitutes an "eat more" strategy all on its own; it makes food taste better because it heightens flavors, reduces bitterness, and enhances sweetness.

Salt is perfect for processed foods. It is cheap. It keeps foods from becoming discolored, and it extends shelf life. Even better, it binds water and makes food weigh more so you pay more for heavier packages.

Food made from scratch with real ingredients in their original form is relatively low in salt. Only about 10 percent of the salt in the American diet comes from salt added at the table; the other 90 percent is already added in processed foods, where it cannot be avoided unless you cook your meals using whole foods.[100]

Types of Salts

Most of today's salt is mined and comes from large deposits left by dried salt lakes believed to be left from a great worldwide flood. (Don't you love those facts?) The following are various kinds of salts you may encounter.

- Table salt is refined, fine grain salts with additives that make it free flowing.
- Iodized salt is table salt with iodine added to it. (See iodine section on the next page.)
- Kosher salt is an additive-free coarse-grained salt. It is used by some Jews and cooks to help remove blood from meat.
- Sea salt is the result of evaporation of sea water. It is also mined in the dried beds from the flood era, as mentioned above. Sea salt doesn't contain iodine or any other additives.
- Celtic salt is natural, solar-evaporated sea salt that has been hand harvested from the Atlantic marshes in France. It has a mellow, sweet-salty flavor.
- Rock salt has a grayish cast because it is not refined, which means it retains more of its minerals. It comes in chunky crystals and is predominantly used in making ice cream and for snow and ice removal.
- Seasoned salt is table salt combined with other flavoring ingredients, such as onion salt, garlic salt, and celery salt.

- Salt substitutes are products containing little or no sodium. They are typically chemical based.[101]

Iodine

Iodine comes to us in many foods, including dairy products, seafood, and many processed foods. This very important element helps keep the fluid regulated in our bodies. It is essential for the thyroid gland and the hormones it produces. Symptoms of iodine deficiency include dry skin, loss of hair, loss of memory, tiredness, and loss of muscle tone. Dr. Brownstein, in his book *Iodine—Why You Need It and Why You Can't Live Without It*, connects the increase in fibroid cysts and breast cancer to the lack of iodine in our diets.[102]

Iodine is one of the most crucial elements there is to preventing breast cancer. However, two decades ago a large amount of it was removed from our food supply when it was replaced with bromine—a known toxin—in baked goods. Incidentally, it was around that same time that breast cancer diagnoses skyrocketed! According to Dr. Brownstein, the breast is the largest storage area for iodine in the body, and it actually competes with the thyroid for iodine. If there is an iodine deficiency, it's the perfect setting for either thyroid or breast cancer to develop. Additionally, if someone is on thyroid medication for hypothyroidism and is iodine-deficient at the same time, it creates even more iodine deficiency, causing an even greater breast cancer risk.[103]

Soy Sauce

Add a spicy flavor to your stir-fry with soy sauce. Soybeans are a complete protein and are easily digested. I would not use just any soy sauce, however, since soybeans are a very debatable food source. On the good side, they are highly nutritious and assist with many health concerns such as hot flashes and cancer. When grown as a non-GMO (always stated on labels) and processed with a water wash, the health benefits are worth the additional enhancement to your meal. On the flip side, if the beans are GMO (not stated on labels) and processed with heat or alcohol, then you are consuming a possible health hazard. This is why the debate continues on this food product. In my kitchen you will only find Bragg's Liquid Aminos, since they follow the strictest guidelines in processing their soy sauce. Bragg's is a company that helped found the health movement in America. You will find this in many recipes in our cookbook.

Fake Flavorings

Herbs, spices, and salts have their own treasure of flavor, but due to the economics of our society, chemicals have replaced them with additives that simulate the flavors. Cooking with fresh herbs, dried herbs, and sea salt will eliminate the additives found in most mixes sold in the store.

MSG

"Avoid, abstain, and never go back" is the warning everyone needs to hear when it comes to additives such as MSG and Aspartame. Dr. Russell Blaylock, neurosurgeon and researcher, had this to say regarding these two ingredients:

> You need to abstain from all of these things. Aspartame is not a necessary nutrient, and neither is MSG. The weight of the evidence is overwhelming. If you want to avoid obesity, metabolic syndrome, and cancer, and if you don't want to make your cancer more aggressive, then you need to stay away from these products.
>
> The damage affects pregnant women, unborn babies, and newborns. It produces changes in the brain that are irreversible. What we've found is that it reprograms the wiring of the brain, particularly the hypothalamus, so it doesn't function normally. These children are abnormal for the rest of their lives in terms of their physiological function. [104]

What is MSG? Monosodium glutamate occurs naturally in many whole foods. Our concern is that it is a food additive developed in a lab—instead of the garden—that enhances flavors while having virtually no flavor of its own. How it adds flavor to other foods is not fully understood, but people do experience a more intense flavor from food containing MSG. It is a simple, inexpensive way for the food industry to enhance flavors, mask unwanted tastes, and hide undesirable flavors in foods.

DIGGING DEEPER: Read more about MSG and Aspartame in the *Nutrition Manual.*

Taking this treasure to heart: What herb of truth did you learn that makes a difference in your view of God's design?

_____

_____

_____

Applying this treasure at home: What Action Steps are you going to take today to apply what you have just learned? Are you going to look for MSG on labels?

Day Four—Dressing the Treasure: Oil and Vinegar

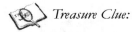 *Treasure Clue:*

A land of olive oil.

—Deut. 8:8 NASB

The Israelites were also on a treasure hunt. Their guide was a cloud by day and a pillar of fire by night. Can you just imagine an adventure like that? They took the journey without knowing their destination, but while remembering that God had delivered them from the bondage of slavery. Let's look deeper into Deuteronomy chapter 8.

Read Deuteronomy 8 and answer these questions:

Verse 1—Who was promised this land? _____

Verse 2—Why did God test them? _____

Verse 3—What does man live by? _____

Verse 4—How did God take care of them? _____

Verse 5—Does God discipline us? _____

Verse 6—In this verse are three conditions for experiencing God's blessings. Identify them and write them here.

_____

_____

_____

God had taught the Israelites how to live a fulfilling life.

As God led them toward the Promised Land He described it for them.

Verse 9—What will they lack? _____

Verse 10—How will they feel after they have eaten these foods? _____

How does God want us to respond to what He has given us?

_____

Verse 11—What warning does He give them?

_____

All throughout Scripture—specifically the Old Testament—God refers to the commandments He has given us. He continually asks us to always remember them, not because they are necessary for our salvation or our ticket to heaven, but because they are what is best. I love the fact that even in the middle of this chapter in Deuteronomy He gives treasures such as "a land of olive oil." We will be satisfied when we eat the foods God gave us, but we will continue to have problems when we try to refine Scripture or our food.

Fats and Oils in Scripture

In the Old Testament, there are references to both fats and oils. The references to oil all refer to the oil from olives. This oil was used for lighting, eating, anointing, and burning (see Ex. 25:6; 35:28; Num. 11:8). In the New Testament, oil is primarily used for lighting, eating, and anointing (see Matt. 25:3-4; Mark 6:13; Luke 7:46; Heb. 1:9; James 5:14).

Fats are another issue. References to fats in the Old Testament typically refer to their use in sacrifices and eating. Leviticus 3:17 says, "This shall be a perpetual statute throughout your generations in all your dwellings: you shall eat neither fat nor blood" (NKJV). Dr. Rex Russell writes, "When Leviticus 3:17 forbids eating fat, it is not referring to the internal, marbling fat in the meat of unclean animals, but to two other kinds of fat: the fat of unclean animals and the cover fat, including that of clean animals."[105] This verse raises other interesting questions regarding the issue of eating clean and unclean meat. You will not want to miss this intriguing teaching in Week Six.

_____

DIGGING DEEPER: Read Facts about Fats in the *Nutrition Manual.*

_____

Udo Erasmus, an expert on the science of fat, has this to say about it:

The fact is that some fats are absolutely required for health, while others are detrimental. Some fats heal, and others kill. Whether a fat heals or kills depends on several factors. What kind of fat it is? How has it been treated—is it fresh, has it been exposed to light, oxygen, heat, hydrogen, water, acid, base, or metals like copper and iron? How old is it? How has it been used in food preparation? How much was eaten? What balance of different fats do we get?

If we get the right amount of fats in the right amounts and balances, and prepare them using the right methods, they build our health and keep us healthy. The wrong kinds of fats, the wrong amounts or balances, or even the right kinds of fats wrongly prepared cause degeneration.[106]

In this previous statement by Udo Erasmus, his questions relate to the three principles. See if you can find the three principles and write them below.

Principle I _____

Principle II _____

Principle III _____

Clues to the answers: Principle I—*What kind of fat is it?* We want fats designed for our health. Principle II—*How has it been treated and how old is it?* We want fats before they have been altered into an unhealthy product. Principle III—*How much is eaten?* Did you find them all, or did you need these answers? Notice how we can apply these principles to all of our food choices.

Health Benefits of Oil

The oils mentioned in Scripture and found throughout our lands generate great healing properties. Check out the benefits of consuming virgin olive oil:

- Improves brain function
- Lowers high cholesterol levels
- Is anti-inflammatory
- Stimulates bile flow
- Improves liver and immune function
- Stimulates the production of fat-digesting enzymes
- Contributes to healthy cells
- Switching from refined corn oil to virgin olive oil can lower LDL and raise HDL
- Reduces the production of gallstones
- Improves digestion of fats
- Improves elimination of toxins
- Improves athletic performance

Keeping your body well-oiled is worth it. How many people do you know who have suffered from gallstones? Adding whole grain, fresh milled bread and olive oil to your diet may help eliminate those problems. Foods by God's design will always bring better health.

Oils in the Grocery Store

Today olive oil is the most prized of all oils, yet many people are unsure of how to find the highest quality in the store. Over the past 80 years the rules have changed so many times it's hard to know if you should eat butter or margarine; olive oil or vegetable oil. Let's refer back to the Three Principles and see if you can come up with the answers in reference to fats and oils.

Principle I _____

Olive oil made by simple traditional processes is known as virgin olive oil. It is made from whole, ripe, undamaged olives. Fresh olive oil should smell nutty, not rancid. It is made without heat. It is unrefined oil that still contains many natural factors unique to olives. Through industrial processes like degumming, refining, bleaching, and deodorizing, these natural factors are removed. Olive oil, which thereby loses its virgin quality, becomes non-virgin refined olive oil. But don't expect to find oils labeled "non-virgin" or "refined." If an olive oil is not labeled "virgin," it is non-virgin refined olive oil. The same is true for other oils—if they are not labeled "unrefined," they are refined, deodorized oils that lack the nutrients we need to build health.[107]

We should include the following oils in our diet: unrefined organic corn oil, olive oil, canola oil (see the *Nutrition Handbook* for canola controversies), and nut and seed oils. All choices should be organic and unrefined. In the US, the term "cold pressed" is not a legal term; you would need to verify its meaning with the manufacturer.[108]

Principle II _____

We have already learned to make good choices. Knowing the ill effects of an altered choice is helpful. Trans fats are now considered to be a health threat and are being removed from the shelves in stores. This is good news, but years of eating trans fats has not been good for our health. Trans fats are so named because they take a soft pliable fat molecule that is designed to fit into the cell and perform its pre-designed duty and make it a rigid molecule. Trans fats make your arteries spasm and cause dangerous inflammation.[109]

Why did we ever have trans fats in the first place? The answer is the same as most of our altered foods: convenience and shelf life. It is easier to ship and store solidified vegetable oils than liquid oils. Partially hydrogenated vegetable oils can be used in place of butter or lard. And a lesser degree of hydrogenation yields liquid oil that doesn't become rancid as quickly as unprocessed vegetables. Without this process, we wouldn't have had margarine or vegetable shortening, such as Crisco. We would have less heart disease.[110] Too much of the wrong kinds of fats is leading us to diabetes and heart disease. The American Heart Association and the American Diabetic Association both agree too much fat is contributing to health problems. Eating foods before they are altered is actually quite simple.

Principle III _____

Too much fat makes us fat. However, we are well-oiled machines when we get the right amount of fat in our diet. Milling your own wheat will give you fat, yogurt will give you fat, meat will give you fat. These are all healthful choices. Adding a little fat is good in the case of using olive oil in the dressing recipe or adding a little organic butter in a recipe. The problem, as we all know, is too much fat. Fat in processed foods comes with a lot of additives to enhance the flavor, which increases the desire to eat. If you feel you are addicted to fats, then a fast would be in order.

For people who eat whole-grain foods, the grain's germ can provide substantial fat quality and diversity. But the most undervalued foods—in terms of their ability to support health-promoting processes—are nuts, seeds, and their oils. These belong in the treasure chest as if you were in the Promised Land today.

DIGGING DEEPER: Read more about olives and olive oil in the *Nutrition Manual*. There are helpful shopping tips and fun uses for these treasures.

Vinegar

Vinegar is one of the oldest condiments in the world. It is believed to have been discovered quite by accident. Wine was exposed to air and, voila, "sour wine" or vinegar was invented. Too tart to drink, too precious to throw away, creative experimentation proved that soured wine had fascinating properties—one of them being the power to pickle!

Ancient Egyptians and Chinese used vinegar thousands of years before Christ, and its use is mentioned in both the Old and New Testaments. Traces of vinegar were discovered in an Egyptian vessel dating back ten thousand years. Babylonians used it for cleaning and preserving food, and in Rome legionnaires drank vinegar before battle, believing it gave them strength and courage. After the fighting was over, vinegar was applied as a disinfectant to cleanse wounds inflicted by swords.

Today vinegar—specifically apple cider vinegar—is touted as being a miracle cure. Whether that is true or false is your decision. One way to find out is to take the apple cider vinegar test: mix one to two teaspoons of organic apple cider vinegar with raw honey or agave nectar (to sweeten) in an eight-ounce glass of distilled water. Drink it first thing in the morning and one hour before lunch and dinner. Continue this for one month.

This tonic may cause the following results:

- Relieve chronic fatigue
- Relieve headaches

- Improve digestion
- Combat mucus
- Rid the body of toxins
- Strengthen the heart
- Fight kidney and bladder problems
- Help prevent constipation

Dr. Carol Johnston, professor at Arizona State University, just released a study proving that apple cider vinegar taken at bedtime favorably affects waking blood sugar in Type 2 diabetics and helps reduce glucose levels by up to 6 percent.[111] Johnston also discovered that her subjects were losing weight.

This is just a small list of the issues that can be alleviated with apple cider vinegar (ACV). Organic ACV comes as a brownish liquid with a cobweb substance known as the "mother" in the bottle. This is the highest quality of vinegar available. This treasure delivers enzymes, potassium, phosphorus, magnesium, iron, copper, trace minerals, essential amino acids, and many other powerful nutrients. Be aware that clear white vinegar has been refined and bleached. Some white vinegar is even processed from coal tar!

As far as the test goes, I did it and noticed a gradual weight loss of three pounds in one month. It might have been because my mouth was too puckered to enjoy my regular foods, but I am a believer in apple cider vinegar since it is made from organic apples and because the aging process enhances the nutrients.

> **DIGGING DEEPER:** Read about tips for using vinegars, making your own vinegar, and purchasing and storing your vinegars in the *Nutrition Manual*.

The key to cooking, and therefore living well, is using the best ingredients. Value quality over quantity.

Taking this treasure to heart: What is one drop of truth you pressed from today's lesson?

Applying this truth at home: What is one step can you take this week to add herbs, salt, olive oil, and vinegar to your pantry supplies? Record this on your Action Plan sheet.

Fabulous Foodie Friday

Foodie Time

Grab your foodie friend and go on an herb road trip. Herbs offer us a marvelous way to flavor and savor food. Begin your herb hunt at a local store, herb shop, or herb farm. After you have discovered which source has the greatest bounty, spend some time smelling the aroma of each one. Pinch the leaves. Which ones are the most enticing? Experience a new herb to liven up a recipe this week. It is a good idea to only buy a small amount until you are sure your family likes your choice. Herbs can be pricey, so the investment you make needs to be considered when testing new foods. Many herbs bear beautiful blooms and have marvelous fragrance for decorating and scenting your home. Throw away the plug-in, and add an herb garden to your centerpiece.

Try one of your favorite recipes and use fresh herbs instead of dried. You will notice a stronger aroma and possibly a more enticing flavor.

Adding Oil to Your Foodie Night

Another fun delight for your taste buds is to have an olive oil tasting event. Find your best quality grocery store and the highest quality olive oils. Many of these oils come with different delicate flavors. Even if they don't you are going to find a wide range of flavors among the wide assortment of olive oils on the market. If there is no strong olive flavor then quite possibly the olive oil you tasted is diluted with vegetable oil. Labels are not a good indication of this process of adding this filler. What brand is your favorite? Which one had a strong olive flavor or a light flavor? Use various varieties of bread for your tasting time. Add some cheese for a full delight.

Take this a step further and add your favorite herbs and garlic to your olive oil. Which herbs make the best dipping sauce for your bread?

Edible Flowers—Tips and Hints

Going natural takes on a whole new appearance when you serve a dish with these edible flowers. Try one or two for the fun of it. There are many flowers suitable for both gardening and consuming. In most cases both the leaves and the blossoms are edible.[112]

Edible flowers as a garnish make any dish look special on your table, but be sure the flavor of the flower complements the dish. Here are a few ideas to beautify your recipes and perk up your taste buds:

- Place a colorful gladiolus or hibiscus flower (remove the stamen and pistil) in a clear glass bowl and fill with your favorite dip.
- Sprinkle edible flowers in your green salads for a splash of color and taste.
- Freeze whole small flowers into ice rings or cubes for a pretty addition to punches and other beverages.
- Use edible flowers in flavored oils, vinaigrettes, jellies, and marinades.
- Asthmatics or others who suffer allergic reactions to composite-type flowers (calendula, chicory, chrysanthemum, daisy, English daisy, and marigold) should be on alert for possible allergic reaction.
- Never use non-edible flowers as a garnish. You must assume that if guests find a flower on a plate of food, they will think it edible.
- Use flowers sparingly in your recipes, particularly if you are not accustomed to eating them. Too much of a pretty thing can lead to digestive problems.

Some flowers to avoid (not a complete list): azalea, crocus, daffodil, foxglove, oleander, rhododendron, jack-in-the-pulpit, lily of the valley, and wisteria.

Fun Foodie Recipe

Are your family members foodies? If not, this may be a stretch, but have fun trying this recipe anyway. Dandelions are everywhere unless you are reading this in the winter, in which you may need to wait or order them online.

Dandelion Greens Delight

Ingredients:
1 pound dandelion greens
½ cup chopped onion
1 clove garlic, minced

1 whole small dried hot chili pepper, seeds removed, crushed
¼ cup cooking oil
Salt and pepper
Parmesan cheese

Preparation:
Discard dandelion green roots; wash greens well in salted water. Cut leaves into 2-inch pieces. Cook greens uncovered in a small amount of salted water until tender, about 10 minutes. Sauté onion, garlic, and chili pepper in oil. Drain greens; add to onion garlic mixture. Taste dandelion greens and season with salt and pepper. Serve dandelion greens with grated parmesan cheese. Serves four…and they will never forget it!

Be sure to send your comments about this recipe to the office of Designed Healthy Living. You can find our contact information on our website: www.designedhealthyliving.com.

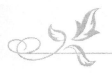

Protein and Meat

Day One—Where's the Beef in the Treasure Chest?

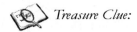 *Treasure Clue:*

Open my eyes, that I may behold wonderful things from Your law.

—Ps. 119:18 N.ASB

Focus and Desire

"Charlie Brown," Lucy begins in her philosophizing way, "life is a lot like a deck chair. Some place it so they can see where they're going. Others place it to see where they've been. And some so they can see where they are at the present."

Charlie sighs, "I can't even get mine unfolded!"[113]

Many of us can identify with Charles Schultz' character Charlie Brown. Life can get complicated, and this chapter may reflect that at first.

The more I listen to people and their justification of eating the more I realize we have taken detours in our hunt for health. Have you ever thought God could quite easily have made every single food on earth good for you? God could have made everything taste as good as chocolate and be as nutritious as spinach. But He didn't.

God may have designated certain foods as unclean as part of His bigger plan to simply build our faith. He wants our trust and obedience in Him to mature. He wants us to get to the point where we have complete confidence that His desire is beyond our understanding.

What does He ask of us? He wants us to experience joy that comes from following Him because we love Him and want to do all things to bring glory to Him—not for what He can do for us. God's desire is more than just offering us salvation or better health. John Piper, in his book *Desiring God*, shared a poem he wrote to his wife that explains his drive to desire God. Here is a small excerpt:

> His goodness shines with brightest rays
> When we delight in all his ways.
> His glory overflows its rim

When we are satisfied in Him.
His radiance will fill the earth
When people revel in his worth.
The beauty of God's holy fire
Burns brightest in the hearts' desire.[114]

What is your desire? How deep is your desire to glorify Him in everything you do?

_____

Have you ever considered desiring Him in your eating? _____

When our focus is on desiring Him, our choices become easier. In Leviticus, shellfish is considered unclean. Of all foods to change in my eating plan, I thought eliminating shellfish would be the hardest. What I had to do was change my focus. When my focus was on desiring to know God better, eliminating my once favorite fried catfish and shrimp scampi was no longer a regret but a heart desire. It was freedom. If I looked at laws as rules, then I would go right into rebellion, or I would think, "I will do it just this once since it's a holiday." My whole viewpoint changed. Eating became a way to desire Him more.

Since we are learning about health, why do I bring up desires when we're talking about meat? The answer is clear. If you are looking for good health, you can find opinions in any book at any store. We need to go back to why we are looking to Scripture for health. Dr. Rex Russell put it this way: "I am urging you to look at these laws for the purpose of glorifying God through acknowledging His desire and design for our health."[115]

Do you desire to truly understand why God has given us His laws?

_____

_____

Have you ever considered following the laws God gave us as a way to desire Him more?

_____

_____

Eating healthy by God's design is not a list of rules; instead it is a way of seeing how much God cares for us. Since He made us, He knows what keeps us ticking.

Many people wonder why God gave us the Old Testament law. Look up Deuteronomy 5:29 and write out your answer.

Dr. Adrian Rogers explains how these laws actually free us.

Have you ever thought that if you lived according to God's laws that you were going to miss out? Truth is, if you don't live according to God's law, you're going to miss out! God's laws are for your welfare. God is not a tyrant in heaven making a bunch of laws to make you squirm like a worm in hot ashes as you try to keep those laws. God loves you. Every time God says, "Thou shalt not," God is simply saying, "Don't hurt yourself." And every time God says, "Thou shalt," God is saying, "Help yourself to happiness."[116]

Happiness and joy are fruits that come from our focus on desiring God.

Dietary Laws—Fact or Fiction?

Read Jeremiah 26:4-6. Describe God's view of the law.

_____

_____

Read Psalm 19: 7-11. What is the benefit of keeping the law?

_____

_____

God gave us many laws. Jesus became the ultimate fulfillment of the law when He died on the cross. Before He died there was a curtain in the temple that separated the people from the most High Place. On that day when Jesus hung on the cross, the curtain was torn in two from the top to the bottom. The split curtain was a visual display to everyone that we are no longer separated from the true High Priest—Jesus. We no longer need an earthly priest, because we have the High Priest to hear our prayers. We no longer need to go through the ceremonial law to get to the Father.

The dietary laws will not bring us this salvation. His desire is for all of us to be in a personal relationship with Him—to desire Him.

But what does that mean about the Law? Jesus is the fulfillment of the Law. But how much of the Law did He fulfill?

Read Matthew 5:13-19. What do these verses teach you about the law?

_____

_____

Remember, following these dietary laws will not grant you a seat in heaven. We study these laws to better understand how God designed our bodies and to bring glory to Him.

Good Food/Bad Food List

Many diets today include a good foods list and a bad foods list. Today we will read the original good vs. bad—or clean vs. unclean—list.

> *"You must distinguish between the holy and the common, between the unclean and the clean"*
> —Lev. 10:10 NIV

Israel's history shows us a time when the laws were being established. God was building and solidifying Israel into its particular uniqueness. The distinction between "clean" and "unclean" became more sharply drawn. God wanted to preserve His people for his own purposes—to teach them to separate themselves from idolatry and to trust and believe in Him alone. His reputation depended on the validity of the Law.[117]

Read Leviticus 11:44-45. Write out verse 44a (the first sentence) and verse 45.

_____

_____

_____

_____

_____

What is God telling you in these verses?

_____

_____

Clean means separated *for* God, purity, holiness, acting in an ethically and righteous way, and being set apart.

Protein and Meat

Unclean means separated *from* God, death, putrefaction, unholy, lewdness, demons, pagans, idolatrous rituals and beliefs, and any meat with its lifeblood in it. (See Lev. 11-15, Zech. 13:2, Lev. 19:4; Ps. 106:37-39, Ezek. 22:3)

Why, in the middle of a list of foods, would God ask us to be holy?

_____

_____

Read the entire chapter of Leviticus 11.

What is the requirement for land animals to be considered clean?

_____

_____

What is the requirement for water animals to be clean?

_____

What is required of insects?

_____

List each animal under either the Clean or Unclean list.

Clean	Unclean

_____

_____

Which foods surprise you?

_____

_____

_____

Will road-kill be on your menu anytime soon?

Fabulous Foodie Fun Night: Rub your back legs together and join the "I Ate a Bug Club"! Chocolate-covered crickets and grasshoppers are available online and in some specialty stores. They also come in packages flavored with salt and vinegar, sour cream and onion, and various other flavors. See which flavor is your favorite. The good news is there's no waistline problem—without the chocolate, a serving of seven crickets only has nine calories!

Taking this treasure to heart: What is one truth or nugget God is teaching you today?

_____

_____

Rewrite today's Treasure Clue as a prayer.

_____

_____

_____

DAY TWO—WHAT'S FOR DINNER?

Principle I—Eating the Foods God Designed for Us to Eat

According to the grocery list found in Leviticus, clean meat is what's for dinner. The flesh of clean meat was given to us as food after the flood in Genesis 9. Meats contain proteins, iron, zinc, and vitamins. Another nutrient is omega-3 fatty acids, which are essential for life. Essential means that you must obtain it from your diet; your body cannot manufacture it. Many land animals God designed for food provides this additional benefit when they are raised in fields and allowed to graze.

The design of these animals' digestive tracts is especially significant. For example, a cow's stomach contains four rumination pouches in which various kinds of bacteria help to digest grasses and grains. These bacteria compete for nutrients, crowding out harmful bacteria, viruses, and parasites. They also destroy many toxins before they reach the cow's flesh.[118]

The purified nutrients, free of bacteria, are presented to the flesh of the cow. This healthy rumination process allows deposits of healthy omega-3 fatty acids into a grazing animal's flesh. These fatty acids protect whoever consumes them from the harmful effects of triglycerides or cholesterol.

How would you describe God's design in the cow's digestive tract?

_____

_____

Many loving parents who want to help their kids build strong bodies tell their kids they must eat meat in order to get protein. As we know, protein is essential to life.[119] But what does protein really do?

- Protein is the single most important food we eat.
- It provides the structure for all living things.
- It is a necessary part of every living cell in the body.
- After water, protein makes up the greatest portion of our body weight.
- Protein makes up muscles, ligaments, tendons, organs, glands, nails, hair, hormones, and many vital organs.
- It is needed for vitamins and minerals to be absorbed and assimilated.
- Protein provides energy directly to muscles.

The Protein Alphabet

Proteins are made from amino acids. Most studies believe that there are twenty amino acids that make protein in our bodies. Dr. Bruce Miller, in his book *Protein, A Consumers Concern*, describes protein in this simple way.

> Amino acids hook together to form proteins much like the pieces of a jigsaw puzzle. The twenty different amino acids combine in various ways to form our different proteins necessary for life. These twenty amino acids make up to 100,000 different proteins.
>
> These numbers are difficult to visualize, so let's compare it to the alphabet. There are twenty-six different letters in the alphabet, but those letters are used to make hundreds of thousands of words in the English language. Just as these twenty-six letters are the building blocks to the alphabet so the twenty amino acids are the building blocks for all our proteins.[120]

The body makes these different types of proteins as the need arises. It is necessary to have all twenty amino acids present at all times. If our daily diet does not contain all essential amino acids, we can show signs of deficiency ranging from depression to indigestion to stunted growth. Contributions to protein deficiencies include:[121]

- Impaired absorption
- Infection
- Trauma
- Stress
- Drug use
- Age
- Imbalances of other nutrients
- Lack of Vitamin C
- Lack of Vitamin B

I believe that the signs of protein deficiency are becoming more prevalent in America. As you read over this list below, you may even recognize some symptoms that you or a family member may be experiencing. Signs of protein deficiency include:[122]

- Fatigue
- Loss of vitality
- Poor wound healing
- Depressed immune system
- Unusual hair loss
- Poor nail growth

- Skin problems
- Water retention
- Poor muscle tone
- Slow or lack of growth in children

Sources of protein include: meat, dairy and vegetable products. Each has about seven to eight grams of protein per one-ounce serving. Vegetable sources of protein include legumes (such as soy), beans, and peas. Nuts (including peanuts, walnuts, pecans, and almonds) and seeds (such as pumpkin, sunflower, and flaxseed) are also excellent sources of protein.

With all these sources of protein, why should we eat meat? Meat—animal foods raised naturally—is the best source of a complete protein. This means that all nine amino acids, those essential in the diet and not formed in the body, are in the food and our body can make healthy cells. Soy is another complete protein. It requires less digestion than meat to get the nutrients available for the body to absorb. Other plants do not give the complete package.

DIGGING DEEPER: Read "Protein/Amino Acids," "Adding Protein to Your Health Program," and "Joy of Soy" in the *Nutrition Manual.*

Omega-3 Fatty Acids

Various studies have shown that essential fatty acids, such as omega-3, fight arterial plaque and detrimental clotting in blood vessels. They also slow the spread of breast cancers, lower blood pressure, and relieve inflammation.[123] These fatty acids are found in good supply in clean fish with scales and fins, as well as in the flesh of cows, chickens, and other clean animals.

Dr. Rex Russell, on his farm in Arkansas, raised longhorn cattle after reviewing this study by Dr. Floyd Byers of Texas A & M University.

Longhorn cattle have 30 percent less muscle fat and 15 percent less saturated animal fat than modern breeds of cattle; but they have a higher quantity of the omega-3 essential fatty acids.

Additionally, the cholesterol counts in longhorn beef are actually less than in the flounder fish—which is the ideal low standard for measuring cholesterol in animals. The longhorn may be unique, but other breeds that are kept lean probably could achieve the same numbers.[124]

Foodie Food Search: Will the real food please stand up? When science reveals that specific nutrients benefit our health, we then find those nutrients added to processed or altered food in various amounts. In other words, some egg suppliers have increased their omega content.

As you walk through the grocery store, count how many foods list omega-3 as a benefit from using their processed product. Was omega originally in the food, or was it added by giving feed to the animal, by adding flaxseed to the ingredients, or by fortifying it with supplements? There are other ways to add omegas to your food; see how many different ways you discover.

Fish

Read Matthew 13:48. What do you think the bad fish were?

_____

_____

A possible answer could be dead fish. Could it also be that Jesus was still acknowledging the dietary laws by stating the obvious: some fish are unacceptable? There are some who believe that Jesus came to do away with the whole law, but in this example Jesus was still following the law. What is good enough for Him is good enough for me.

Read Luke 24:41-43. After the resurrection, Jesus reveals Himself to His disciples. What request does He make? What do the disciples give him?

_____

_____

_____

Fish oil was once something of a joke among many nutritionists. No one is laughing today about the healing powers of fish. The reason, it seems, is that the natural oils found in fish appear to curtail the body's overproduction of a couple of hormone-like substances called prostaglandins and leukotrienes. Overactive prostaglandins and leukotrienes can cause blood clots, inflammation, and serious glitches in the immune system. Omega-3 oils halt these destructive reactions before they get out of control—something that is critical in preventing heart disease.[125]

There are three villains lurking deep inside our bodies that cause heart attacks and strokes. They are the plaque that clog arteries and dangerously restrict blood flow, the accumulation of platelets (sticky pieces of blood cells) that clump together and form clots, and the sudden, unexplained spasms of blood vessels that can throw the heart out of kilter or halt the flow of blood to the brain, causing strokes.

Studies on fish oil show it works wonders in reducing or eliminating all three risks. People who eat lots of fish seem to have thinner blood, which is less prone to clotting. Omega-3 oils also reduce triglycerides and dangerous LDL cholesterol, and that, say the experts, may be why fish is such a powerful ally in the battle against heart disease.

DIGGING DEEPER: In the *Nutrition Manual,* read "Fish," "My Fish Started Crawling," and "Parasites in Marine Fish." Learn more about essential fatty acids, EPA, and omega-3.

The Incredible Edible Egg

How long have we been told eggs have too much cholesterol? Think back to the Three Principles. Principle I teaches us to eat foods that God has given us for food. This means that eggs are a food God gave us.

Few verses reference eggs. Read Luke 11:10-13.

What foods are mentioned? _____

Jesus used two food comparisons. In each one there is a clean food and an unclean food. Jesus refers to these clean foods as good gifts.

Eggs are a balanced, rich source of nutrients. They are designed for making new birds; therefore they contain all the minerals, vitamins, proteins, and fats necessary to create a fully-formed, hatchable, living chick.

Chickens in the wild will eat grains, seeds, grasses, and living insects. Commercially grown chickens are fed a scientifically designed food that must withstand processing, transportation, and shelf life. This means the high quality of perishable living nutrients are no longer part of their diet. With the lack of plant sterols in this new feed, commercial eggs contain more cholesterol than homegrown barnyard eggs. As Udo Erasmus says, "Chickens in concentration camps don't perform their best, because they are lacking sunshine, whole fresh foods, fresh air, and room to move. They then lay unhealthy eggs."[126]

Studies indicate that the egg yolk has a considerable amount of cholesterol, but the yolk also contains lecithin, which breaks down and probably negates any ill effects. Michigan State University released a report in 2000 in the *Journal of the American College of Nutrition* that states, "Egg consumption made important nutritional contributions to the American diet and was not associated with high serum cholesterol concentrations."[127]

Keep in mind, we are looking for eggs from hens and other clean fowl. You will not need to snatch eggs from serpents, buzzards, and scavenger birds.

The conclusion: foods designed and given to us by God will always build health. Eventually the studies will prove it. A study done by the American Cancer Society showed that eggs protected against heart attack and strokes.[128] But even if studies did not prove God's Word, I will follow it anyway. Remember, God is omniscient—all knowing—and man is not.

Foodie Fact: Eggshell color is not an indicator of nutritional value. Like brown eyes, brown eggs are determined by a gene. The nutritional value of the egg depends on what the chicken ate and her living quarters.

Chicken

Which came first, the chicken or the egg? No matter what your answer is, they are both considered clean meats. Chickens, just as cows, are nutritious when raised properly. Free range chickens raised in a fresh pasture (and supplemented with organic grains when necessary) equals healthy meat. Typically chickens are not raised this way by high-volume farmers.

I recently visited some local farmers. The first farmer was a certified organic farmer of livestock and eggs. His chickens were kept safe in cages to prevent the foxes and hawks from having a feast, but the cages were large enough that the chickens could roam around all day and not even cross the same piece of ground twice. The farmer would move these pens to a new area of the field every couple days. His chickens were never given antibiotics, growth hormones, or steroids. The other farmer was not interested in "the organic thing." Although his chickens were definitely free range, since I had to walk around them to get to the door, he said chickens will eat seeds, feed, and another chicken's poop. He wanted to know how you can certify an organic chicken when their diet consists of these things. That was an interesting question.

Chickens have a digestive system known as the craw, which is similar to the rumination pouches of the cow. When raised in natural surroundings, chicken flesh should be great. When antibiotics, hormones, crowded living conditions, and steroids are included in the equation, the result is a detriment to our health. This was proven by Dr. Byers at Texas A & M University. He proved the omega-3 fatty acids are changed to omega-6 fatty acids when animals are fed excessive grain, antibiotics, or hormones. When the ratio of fatty acids changes, we lose the benefits.[129]

Foodie Experiment: Find local farmers in your area or ones that deliver to your local stores. See if you can visit a chicken farm. How are the chickens raised? Does the farmer supplement the chickens' diet? Purchase some meat and eggs for an experiment. When you get home, crack open a fresh egg from the farm in one bowl and then crack open another egg from the store (preferably the cheapest brand, since that is what most people purchase). Do you notice any color differences? Did the shell have the same hardness? Is the smell any different? Now cook some of each type of egg either by scrambling or hard boiling them. Then do a taste test. Which one has more flavor? In my experiments, the farm-fresh eggs have a richer yellow color and a more flavorful taste. The farm-fresh eggs make a more colorful platter of deviled eggs.

Taking this treasure to heart: What is one nugget of truth you learned today about protein and meat?

_____

_____

DAY THREE—MESSING WITH THE ANIMALS

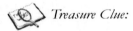 *Treasure Clue:*

*Discipline yourself for the purpose of godliness; for bodily discipline
is only of little profit, but godliness is profitable for all things, since it
holds promise for the present life and also for the life to come.*

—1 Tim. 4:7b-8 NASB

Principle II—Altering Our Meat

Eating meat was once reserved for the rich. In the post-depression era, everyone was eating meat—and lots of it. When we look at Principle II, it is helpful to understand what alterations have been made when it comes to meat and protein. The alterations and confusion come from our interpretation of Scripture. Typically there are three misunderstandings when it comes to eating meat considered unclean: we have better cooking techniques today, the law is no longer valid, Peter's vision means we can eat anything, and we give thanks before our meals. Let's review each one of those areas.

COOKING-BETTER TODAY THAN YESTERDAY?

If meat is cooked properly, then we are OK, right? That is a comment I hear all the time concerning eating meat. However, take a look at Job 14:4, "Who can bring a clean thing out of an unclean? Not one" (KJV).

Some people believe cooking methods were not as advanced in biblical days as they are now. Thereby, the caution God gave in Leviticus 11 was because of the means by which people cooked. Since we have advanced technology in our cooking, we should be healthier, right?

Consider that thought for a moment. The cooks in the Bible were excellent at making bread. The temperature for making bread can be very tricky—ask anyone who has mastered this art. We find the disciples eating fish cooked over an open fire. We do the same today when we roast the catch of the day over a campfire. Both of these examples show that the cooking temperatures we cook with today are very similar to earlier times.

Pork, rabbits, and shellfish are known carriers of parasites and disease. Cooking does not remove all of these problems. For instance, microwave ovens heat unevenly, which may allow some of the parasites to survive until consumed. Many outbreaks of vicious infections have developed in so-called cooked food. If the food is unclean, don't count on cooking to protect you. Some of the most toxic poisons are not destroyed by heat.[130]

VALIDITY OF THE LAW

Read Matthew 5:17. Did Jesus come to abolish the Law? What does that tell us about the Law?

_____

_____

_____

We have covered the Law in other areas of our study. Some say that because Jesus "fulfilled" the Law, we do not have to keep it. If this were true, why would He encourage His disciples to keep the commands and teach others to observe them in the very next verse? Besides, if He fulfilled the law that says we shouldn't murder, does it mean that we are now free to murder? This may seem like an extreme example, but I think you get my point. Even though Jesus fulfilled the Law, I do not feel free to ignore it.

Instead, since heaven and earth are still around, I believe Jesus came to expound on the Law and fit it fully with its complete meaning. Rather than giving me a reason for letting go of the Hebrew Scriptures, Jesus has made it more interesting and inviting to me.[131]

PETER'S VISION

There are members of my own family who discredit my eating style, since Peter's vision says we can eat anything we want.

Read the full account of Peter's vision in Acts 10 and 11.

Cornelius was a Gentile. What else do you learn about him?

_____

_____

What was Cornelius doing when he saw a vision? _____

Peter was Jewish. In verse 9, why did he go to the housetop? _____

In verse 10, what was Peter's physical desire? _____

Peter claimed he had never eaten anything unclean. True or false? _____

Does this mean he never had any ham or bacon? _____

In verse 20, the Spirit gives Peter assurance regarding the men who have come for him. Do you think this relates to the "unclean" vision? _____

Peter's dream is nestled into a pivotal section of Acts that clarifies God's intentions about Jews and Gentiles in fellowship together. Up to this point, some of the Old Testament laws had constructed a very real barrier between the Jews and their neighbors. Peter's dream was indeed a revelation from God—but it was not about food.[132] Peter didn't literally eat these unclean animals. Elmer Josephson, pastor and author of *God's Key to Health and Happiness*, gives this insight:

> Now did the words "Rise, Peter, kill and eat" mean that God was repealing the dietary laws? Is God reversing Himself on physical hygiene and sanitation in His requirement that a clean people have clean food? Did Christ's work on the cross perform a biological miracle in these filthy animals that made their flesh harmless to eat and fit for human consumption? Did the dispensation of grace and the coming of the Gospel so alter the gastric processes and digestive apparatus of man that all unclean meats will now build healthy bodies instead of producing disease and results in death as they did before?[133]

How would you answer these questions? _____

The answer is no. The animals did not change, the digestive system of man did not change, and neither did the laws. Peter's vision had nothing to do with clean and unclean foods! It was clear to Peter the Lord was now welcoming the so-called unclean Gentiles into the family of God. That's what this lesson is all about. No longer was there to be a spiritual separation. Read Acts 11:18 for the response by Peter's fellow Jewish believers after Peter confirmed the purpose of the vision. They praised God.

GIVING THANKS ERASES THE UNCLEAN

"But the Spirit explicitly says that in later times some will fall away from the faith, paying attention to deceitful spirits and doctrines of demons, by means of the hypocrisy of liars seared in their own conscience as with a branding iron, men who forbid marriage and advocate abstaining from foods, which God has created to be gratefully shared in by those who believe and know the truth. For everything created by God is good, and nothing is to be rejected if it is received with gratitude; for it is sanctified by means of the word of God and prayer" (1 Tim. 4:1-5 NASB).

Recently, outside of a convention for a large Christian organization, a group of animal rights advocates were trying to get the people at the convention to see that Jesus was a vegetarian. The Bible is clear about this issue in Matthew 14:19 and John 21:12-13. The picketers also believed that if Christians were pro-life, then they should not kill any animal either. These groups have grown in force in the last decade, but is there truth to what they are saying? Once again, we must always look to our treasure map as our guide. I agree that animals should be treated humanely, which is why I only purchase meats from natural free range farms that I have personally investigated. Kosher guidelines require the same butchering that was practiced in biblical times, which eliminates needless suffering. However, Scripture is clear on the issue of whether or not we can eat meat.

Every text needs to be seen in context. In 1 Timothy 4, God is speaking of meats He has created. There are those who were saying it was wrong to eat even clean food that God has created. This is simply not true. Verse 4 says that every creature of God is good, but that doesn't necessarily mean they are to be eaten. The pig and vulture were created for a good purpose, but not for our dinners. Are you ready to eat poisonous reptiles, wild beasts, rats, cockroaches, spiders, bats, dogs, or cats? And God is certainly not approving cannibalism! We must discover the truth in the light of all of God's Word.

Understanding Why Some Animals Are Unclean

Why did God make the unclean animals? Many were created as scavengers; as a rule they are meat-eating animals that clean up anything that is left dead in the fields. Scavengers were not created for human consumption. Modern science has discovered that even the scale-less fish and all shellfish (including lobster, oysters, clams, and shrimp) are disease-producing because of inadequate excretion. These are the scavengers—the garbage containers—of the waters and the seas, just as pigs are the collectors of the field.

A clean or unclean animal is defined by:

a) What it eats—The clean animals are herbivores (plant eaters). In general, they do not eat the flesh of other animals, thereby avoiding many parasites and diseases that are present in the flesh and blood of the animals. The unclean animals are omnivores, eating both vegetation and animal flesh. Omnivores will, by their biological nature, eat anything.

b) The cleanliness of its digestive tract—Clean animals have long digestive tracts that are usually six to twelve times the length of their bodies. This ensures that they will completely process and eliminate toxins and poisons. Unclean animals' digestive tracts are much shorter than herbivores because the decaying flesh and its byproducts are toxic and need to be removed quickly from the body.

The pig's digestive tract is similar to ours and the stomach is very acidic. Pigs never know when to stop eating; therefore they are gluttonous. Their stomach acids become diluted because of the volume of food, allowing all kinds of toxins to pass through this protective barrier. Parasites, bacteria, viruses, and toxins can pass into the pig's flesh due to overeating. These toxins and infections can be passed on to humans when they eat pork.[134]

Jayne Hurley and Bonnie Liebman offer a warning to pregnant women about pork, "To play it safe, women who are pregnant shouldn't eat a steady diet of hot dogs, bacon, or sausage that's cured with sodium nitrite (check the label). Several studies have found a higher risk of brain tumors in children whose mothers ate cured meats frequently."[135]

Frustrated Foodie: If leaving bacon behind is not for you, then follow this cooking tip: Always cook pork (including pork sausage) to at least 160°F to kill any *Trichinella*, a parasite that can cause abdominal pain, diarrhea, and (two or three weeks later) muscle pain, fever, and swelling.

Processed Meat & Stomach Cancer Risk

Swedish researchers evaluated nine studies involving 4,704 people over forty years old and found that regular indulgence in deli products (such as ham, bacon, franks, and sausage) posed an "unequivocal" cancer risk.

As little as one small hot dog or four pieces of bacon a day translates to up to a 38% increased likelihood in developing stomach cancer, which is responsible for one in ten cancer deaths. The study, published in the *Journal of the National Cancer Institute*, echoes earlier research that linked regular consumption of cured meat products to a 67 percent increase of pancreatic cancer. Some experts point to the fact that processed meats are loaded in salt—excess amounts of which have been linked to stomach cancer. Others point to carcinogenic compounds used in processed meat preparation [136]

Nitrates

This past year I have visited several cancer specialists with a family member. At each appointment I asked if diet had anything to do with cancer. Each one said that diet did not play a role or the role was very minute. But my next question to them was, "Do you eat the typical American diet?" Each one said they did not! One was a foreigner and he said he would not touch American meat; it was loaded with chemicals and nitrates. Another physician said he avoids nitrates but eats pork and shellfish. So what is it with the nitrates that physicians are avoiding but not telling us to avoid? This preservative appears in most luncheon meat, bacon, and processed meats. Sodium nitrate reacts with the powerful acids in your stomach to form nitrosamines—one of the most cancer-causing agents known to man.

In 1982, the National Academy of Sciences issued a report warning the medical community and the American public that these processed meats contain two chemicals shown to cause cancer in laboratory animals: nitrosamines (sodium nitrate) and polycyclic hydrocarbons. The association between these chemicals and cancer is so strong that it would be foolish to dismiss this warning.[137]

Shellfish Pose Dangers

Shellfish are the scavengers and janitors of the sea. When a tragic accident happens at sea, as gross as it sounds, these scavengers are the ones who clean up the accident—bodies and all. Pathogenic bacteria from human and animal wastes do not persist within shellfish tissues beyond a few days, but viruses such as hepatitis A can persist within their tissues for several weeks or more. This is because shellfish filter large amounts of water and tend to leave large quantities of bacteria and viruses behind, including the one responsible for hepatitis. These contaminated shellfish have caused significant outbreaks of human disease. And because of our international trading, contaminated fish viruses are showing up in various geographic areas.[138]

Oysters, clams, and other shellfish carry bacteria that can cause an infection called vibriosis. This bacterium is common in shellfish in the Gulf of Mexico. If the level of *vibrio vulnificus* in the blood becomes very high and causes serious infection, you can become very ill. At certain levels, it can even cause death. In fact, half of these vibriosis cases result in death.[139]

Red tide is caused by naturally occurring algae that produce a toxin that shellfish absorb as they feed. The toxin doesn't affect the shellfish, but consuming mussels or clams affected by red tide can cause sickness and even death in humans.[140]

Taking this treasure to heart: God has a plan, and whether or not we understand His reasoning behind what is clean and unclean, science has proven that clean food is the best choice. What is one nugget of truth you can treasure in your heart?

_____

_____

DAY FOUR—HOW MUCH PROTEIN IS ENOUGH?

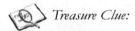 *Treasure Clue:*

Do not be with heavy drinkers of wine, or with gluttonous eaters of meat; For the heavy drinker and the glutton will come to poverty, and drowsiness will clothe one with rags.
—Prov. 23:20-21 NASB

Principle III—A Meat Addiction?

Steak, ribs, hamburgers, all-you-can-eat catfish—we are addicted to meat, both clean and unclean. When a wife comes to our classes and goes home to tell her husband that bacon is off the grocery list, there is typically a rebellion. Without the desire to follow God's laws for our betterment, there is no reason to look at the unclean meats from a biblical perspective. Those who are looking for God's laws to improve their life physically, spiritually, and mentally, and who will apply the teaching, will benefit greatly from it.

Obesity and heart disease are evidence we have an addiction to meat and fats. Consider meat a celebration or luxury food.

Calculating Your Protein Needs

Protein contains four calories per gram, and one pound is equal to 453.59 grams. Each one of us needs a different amount of protein in our diet. Here is the formula to calculate your needs:

Your weight _____ divided in half = _____ - 10 = _____.

This is the number of grams of protein you need daily. Refer back to Day Two's study for the list of reasons we need protein in our diet. A healthy diet would include 30 percent protein, 30 percent fat, and 40 percent carbohydrates.

Meat Quality

The quality of our meat is not what it once was. Fat is fattening. Fifty years ago beef was 5 percent to 10 percent fat, because cattle were allowed to graze on grass and mature for over three years. Today high-energy feeds and eighteen months of fast growth marbleize the beef with over 30 percent saturated fat. Meat production has become a huge economic enterprise, requiring more than 2,700 drugs including antibiotics, hormones, tranquilizers, and pesticides. More drugs are used by cattlemen than by medical doctors.[141]

By eating lean meats grown on open ranges and eating less meat per day or week, your health will greatly improve and the addictive cycle will end. God has carefully developed a perfect plan to protect us from many opponents. But if we allow the opponents to invade—if we don't block them out or avoid them—they will destroy His plan for our health. Protect yourself by studying God's plan for your health. Then put that plan into action by using discipline and enthusiasm. You may not succeed each step of the way, but keep striving forward.

Celebrate

In our family, birthdays mean the special person gets to choose his or her favorite meal—without any judgmental facial expressions from me. They look forward to this event. My husband will almost always choose his favorite barbecue beef ribs, my daughter will choose Honey Chicken and my son, lasagna. Remember, a celebration is more than food; we can celebrate the blessings God has given us—family, friends, fellowship, and fulfillment.

Taking this treasure to heart: Are you into the meat of the Word? Ask yourself these simple questions about your eating habits:

- Do I feel lethargic or full of energy—ready to face the challenges of the day?
- Am I eating a balanced diet?
- Should I cut down on the amount of meat that I am eating?
- When I cook chicken, do I leave the skin on? (The skin contains the fat and toxins.)
- What change can I make in my diet today that will make a difference in how I feel and look—today, tomorrow, and the rest of my life?

Yes, there are many difficult things in the Word of God. Will you give up because they are challenging, or will you go on to maturity through diligence and obedience? Ask yourself:

- Am I still sipping on the milk, or have I moved on to learn and understand the meat of God's Word?
- Am I challenging myself, or am I coasting through my Christian life?
- Am I sitting and soaking in church, or am I allowing myself to be squeezed and poured out as God's sacrificial love offering to the lost in my neighborhood, workplace, and family?[142]

FABULOUS FOODIE FRIDAY

Foodie Time

What was your favorite type of pizza before this week's study?

_____

Are you ready to try some new pizzas? Grab your foodie friends and family and have an "Anything Goes on Pizza Night"!

It's time to be creative with an old favorite. I have listed various types of pizza sauces, pizza toppings, and pizza dough for you. Mix and match until you find your favorites. Have fun!

PIZZA DOUGH

Add variety to your pizza dough by including fresh herbs, onions, garlic, honey, and various oils and flours into the dough. Recipes for dough, including a zucchini dough, are located on our website: www.designedhealthyliving.com. You can also find a whole wheat pizza dough recipe in the *Healthy Treasures Cookbook*.

PIZZA TOPPINGS

The most popular pizza toppings are pork sausage and pepperoni. How about branching out for a little bit of variety? There is no limit to what you may discover. Here is a list of toppings you may have not considered to place on your favorite pie:

Artichoke hearts
Avocado
Basil leaves
Bean sprouts
Celery
Chocolate
Chopped broccoli
Chopped fresh cilantro
Crushed fennel seeds
Peanut butter
Pie fillings

Pineapple
Roasted red peppers
Spinach leaves
Sun dried tomatoes
Meat Options:
Chicken
Roast beef
Salmon
Sardines
Tuna

PIZZA SAUCE

Are you ready to leave the tomato sauce behind and extend your taste buds? Try one of these sauces instead:

Barbecue sauce
Garlic/olive oil sauce
Italian dressing
Ranch dressing
Salsa (all varieties, including mango)
White garlic sauce
Worcestershire sauce

CHEESE

Don't forget the most favorite topping! Try one or more of the following:

Cream cheese
Farmers cheese
Feta

Gouda
Mizithra
Monterey jack
Parmesan
Provolone
Ricotta

Have fun enjoying the fellowship of making your own pizza. Outdoor pizza ovens are becoming more and more popular. You can even grill your pizza on your outdoor grill. Check out www.designedhealthyliving.com for special pizza recipes and tips for grilling.

Part I Conclusion—Just the Beginning

Did you ever imagine all these sumptuous foods filling our treasure chest? There is just an overflow of God's blessings and gifts in this treasure chest. Our life is not about what we cannot have; instead it is filled with the largest bounty ever imagined. Who could want more than the very best?

Yes, there will be days when the processed foods will be calling your name or your car will make a turn into a fast food parking lot, but remember what we learned in our teaching session about your health bank account. Is there enough in your account to cover the choices you are making?

Stand guard. We have just completed filling our chest, but you don't want to lose your treasure. There are many pirates and counterfeits awaiting you. They may invade from the inside like a Trojan horse or they might attack from the outside. What are these villains? Continue on to Part II of our study and you will learn not only how to protect this treasure but how to enhance it to a polished jewel.

PART II

GUARDING THE TREASURE

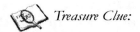 *Treasure Clue:*

"For I know the plans that I have for you," declares the LORD, "plans for
welfare and not for calamity to give you a future and a hope."
— Jer. 29:11 NASB

In Week One of this Bible study, we looked at 1Thessalonians 5:23-24 and saw how each one of us has three different components: body, soul, and spirit. So far we have learned how to feed our body the choicest of foods while building a healthy bank account. These foods and lessons have dealt with the body—the physical side of our life. We have filled the treasure chest with the finest there is to offer. Our next step is to protect it—to guard it from pirates. Pirates come in many disguises. Our most vulnerable areas for their entry are the soul (mind) and spirit. During the next six weeks we will put a hedge around all areas of our life so that we can let the villains out and the holiness in. Without this guard or hedge, we may fall prey to the very counterfeits that sidetracked us before we began. This will be the most important part of the treasure hunt.

Read the Treasure Clue above. Some people end with this first verse and claim that God has great plans for them without reading on to see how this is going to come to pass. Let's read on.

"Then you will call upon Me and come and pray to me, and I will listen to you" (Jer. 29:12 NASB). In this verse, underline the three action words God requires of us. Circle the phrase that tells us what God will do.

That sounds easy enough, right? We just need to pray, God will listen, and then we will have these great plans play out in our life. Have you tried this: prayed and then expected God to do what you want? This *is* a truth that God has given us, but maybe we should continue to read on.

"You will seek Me and find Me when you search for Me with *all* your heart" (Jer. 29:13 NASB, emphasis added). Underline the three action words that God requires of us. Circle the words that tell us to what degree we are to seek.

This verse is asking us to search for Him with *all* our heart. That means there is no part of our heart, life, or mind not included in the search. When we pattern our whole heart, mind, and soul after seeking His will, we will be focused on truly seeking what He wants instead of our own desires.

After telling us to seek Him with our whole heart, God gives us a promise: "And I will be found by you" (Jer. 29:14 NASB). Underline or highlight the promise God gives us when we search for Him with *all* our heart.

This is a pivotal clue to the treasure hunt: *our Lord wants us to find Him*. He wants us to seek Him. He wants to bless us in many ways. Through these blessings we can discover that physical healing is only a small part of the huge treasure chest we are discovering.

Take time now to pray, asking God to help you daily seek Him with your whole heart.

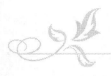

Fasting and Self-Discipline

Day One—God's Design for Fasting

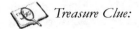 *Treasure Clue:*

But this kind does not go out except by prayer and fasting.
—Matt. 17:21 NASB

Several years ago my family was looking for answers to many health problems. Specifically, my husband Steve was dealing with a cholesterol count of 300, a triglyceride count of 940, high blood pressure, pre-diabetes, weight problems, early signs of glaucoma, irritable bowel syndrome, and continuous heartburn/indigestion. He was not a happy camper, to say the least.

So Steve began a partial fast, which included eliminating *all* animal products for one month. You have previously learned that clean animal products are not bad, but during a fast the digestive tract can heal better without these foods. So at the beginning of July Steve began his partial fast of omitting all animal products. He also started taking a fiber supplement specifically designed to bring down cholesterol.

Everyone knows July 4th is the biggest barbecue day of the year! So the question was, "Will Steve maintain his fast through this big holiday?" Not only did he make it through the holiday, he made it the entire month without breaking his fast.

The interesting part of this partial fast was that after three days he started feeling remarkably better and stopped taking his Prevacid™ for heartburn and indigestion. That was a wonderful relief after six years of taking a medicine his doctors had said he would have to take for the rest of his life.

At the end of the month, Steve went back to the doctor and had his lab tests run again. We were pleasantly surprised to find his triglycerides at 140, his blood pressure normal, and his cholesterol at 160. He had also lost fifteen pounds! Praise be to God!

Have you ever considered fasting to obtain total health?

Before we search deeply into the subject of fasting, what concerns do you have?

_____

_____

_____

_____

Take a moment now to pray about your concerns and ask God to open your heart to His response in regard to fasting. You may want to write your prayer here as a record of your feelings.

_____

_____

_____

_____

It is becoming more and more frequent that bodies and minds are breaking down under the stresses to which we subject them. We must begin to look at illness not as a failure, but as a sign that something is out of balance. God is a God of balance. His ways are life balancing. He has provided fasting as a way to total rejuvenation of the mind, body, and spirit.[143]

What Is Fasting?

Fasting can be found in both the Hebrew and Greek translations of the Bible, and both definitions refer to self-denial. In Stormie Omartian's book *Greater Health God's Way*, she states, "Fasting is a spiritual exercise and discipline. It is a denial of self. When you deny yourself, you position the Lord as everything in your life, and then there is no end to the wonderful possibilities for you. Deliberately denying you food for a set period of time in order to give yourself more completely to prayer and closer communication with God has great rewards."[1] Prayer is supposed to accompany fasting. In this respect, fasting should be distinguished from abstinence from food or activity.

Fasting has been used by many different religions, by great leaders both religious and political, and for special occasions. In fact, most nationalities have a tradition of fasting handed down from their ancestors. Hippocrates, the father of medicine, used fasting to combat disease more than two thousand years ago.

Many theologians believe fasting began as an expression of grief and may have come from the lack of appetite during times of great distress. Hannah, who would later become the mother of Samuel, was so distressed about her inability to have children that "she wept and did not eat" (1 Sam. 1:7 NASB). Later we read about David, who fasted to demonstrate grief at Abner's death (2 Sam. 3:35). Many references in Scripture describe fasting as "afflicting" one's soul or body (Isa. 58:3,5). Fasting came to be practiced as an outward expression of an inward feeling of remorse for sin.

People began to fast to turn away the wrath of God. Eventually fasting became a basis for petitioning God. David defended his fasting before the death of his son (by Bathsheba), indicating his hope that while the child lived David's prayer might be answered. When the child died David no longer needed to fast since God had sent His answer.

Fasting was practiced in the New Testament by various people, including Pharisees, disciples, Jesus, John the Baptist, Paul, and the New Testament church leaders.

Read Isaiah 58. In verses 1-5, what was wrong with the fasting of Israel?

_____

_____

_____

As you read these verses, it is as important to understand the kinds of fasts that do not please God as it is to understand the kinds of fasts He desires. God's people in Isaiah's day had been fasting, but without results. The reason, God says, is that they ignored the way fasting should change their lives; instead they treated it as an empty ritual.

Write out Isaiah 58:6 here:

_____

_____

_____

Verse 6 points out that fasting will help us "loose the bonds of wickedness, to undo the heavy burdens, to let the oppressed go free, and...break every yoke" (Isa. 58:6 NKJV). That should be enough reason for us to learn about fasting and how we can apply it to the treasure of healthy living.

What a Fast Is Not

Fasting is not an end in itself; it is a means by which we can worship the Lord and submit ourselves in humility to Him. We don't make God love us any more than He already does if we fast or if we fast longer. A fast is not a secret weapon that can be drawn on any situation we don't like. God retains His sovereignty and can still answer as He sees fit. We fast and pray for results, but the results are in God's hands. What we can know, assuming we are living in the center of His will, is that if we don't receive, it won't be because we didn't ask.

"Stand fast therefore in the liberty by which Christ has made us free, and do not be entangled again with a yoke of bondage" (Gal. 5:1 NKJV). Our goal for fasting, as with any discipline in our Christian walk, is freedom. If the result is not greater freedom, then something is wrong. There will be times in your life when fasting is necessary to break the bonds of strongholds such as gossiping, alcohol, food addictions, lack of trust, sinful behaviors, and so on. Turning your problems over to God and letting Him take control over these areas will bring this freedom and a great yoke will be lifted from your shoulders. Discipline always has its rewards.

Why Fast?

If fasting is so important to our spiritual and physical lives, why do many people avoid it? It seems we are currently living in a "feel-good religion" society and we don't want to be bothered with any thought of hunger or self-denial. Fasting is an act of discipline that means we will actually be denying ourselves and experiencing hunger.

I have been in church all my life and was rarely encouraged to fast. This left the impression that it must be for the deacons or ministers. I thought maybe the pastor fasted before he preached, but should I fast? Stories of great preachers like Jonathan Edwards, Billy Graham, and Bill Bright convinced me fasting was important for our leaders. Even the Pilgrims fasted the day before disembarking from the Mayflower. As I began to study the lives of these great men of God and how God used them, I realized I, too, wanted to be used of God. I wanted to be used in my family, my neighborhood, and my church. Fasting began to make an impact on my life, and I pray it will become natural in your life as it leads to healing and helps you to seek God with all your heart.

Scriptural Examples of Fasting

Scripture gives us many varied examples of fasting. Read the following scriptures and fill in the blanks below.

Matthew 6:16-18—_____ gave us instructions for how to fast.

Acts 9:8-9— _____ did not eat or drink after meeting Jesus on the road to Damascus.

Esther 4:15-16—Esther asked the _____ to do a three-day fast for her protection and their deliverance.

Deuteronomy 9:9, 17-18— _____ had two forty-day absolute fasts before getting the final _____ . His fast was to receive word from God.

1 Kings 19:5-8—Elijah ate _____ before a forty-day fast for protection.

Acts 13:2-3— _____ and _____ fasted and prayed before going on their first missionary journey.

Jonah 3:5, 10—The people of _____ fasted to change God's mind.

Daniel 10:2-3—Daniel did a _____ partial fast and sang praises to God during the fast.

Joel 2:12—God told the prophet Joel to turn to Him through _____ and _____ .

Luke 4:1-13—The Devil tried to tempt Jesus after His _____ . Jesus was fasting before carrying out God's plan.

Taking this treasure to heart: Fasting is found throughout the whole Scripture, and each time it is mentioned, the people involved already knew what it was and how to implement it. What is one truth you have learned today about fasting?

_____

_____

_____

_____

Applying this treasure at home: The first step in applying this treasure is to understand its importance. Begin praying about how God would have you implement the discipline of fasting.

DAY TWO—SPIRITUAL BENEFITS OF FASTING

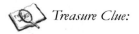 *Treasure Clue:*

Is not this the fast that I have chosen: to loose the bonds of wickedness.

—Isa. 58:6 NKJV

The spirit and body are so interrelated in God's creative design that fasting has both spiritual and physical benefits. By enabling us to surrender our lives to God in greater measure, we find fasting gives us more control over our tongues, our minds, our attitudes, our emotions, our bodies, and all our fleshly desires. Fasting also helps us to submit our spirits to God completely so that He can use them for His purposes.

Look back at Isaiah 58:5, 6, 8. It is recommended that each time you fast, you begin by reading Isaiah 58:6 so that you will be reminded of the promise God is giving you.

Listed below are the spiritual benefits from Stormie Omartian's book *Greater Health God's Way*. As you look at this list, read each item slowly and then lift each benefit up to God in prayer. Do not rush this assignment. God wants to do mighty things in your life, and He is waiting for you to spend time with Him so that He can accomplish His plan.

The following is an example of how to pray through the first benefit: "Dear Lord, You are the all-knowing, omniscient God. You know I need guidance in _____. Lord, I come to You and seek Your guidance in my life regarding fasting and how it may help me seek You more." Stormie Omartian's spiritual benefits of fasting are:[144]

1. To receive divine guidance, revelation, or an answer to a specific problem. We seek Him and His will when we fast. We acknowledge to God that He is God. Fasting releases us from the enemy's powers and strongholds.
2. To hear God better and to understand more fully His will for your life.
3. To weaken the power of the adversary. Some refer to fasting as getting a "holy oiling," and that because of it, the world, the flesh, and the Devil can't hold on to you. However, there is no scriptural reference for this viewpoint.
4. To cope with present monumental difficulties.
5. To have freedom from bondage.
6. To establish a position of spiritual strength and dominion.
7. To be released from heavy burdens (yours or others'). God may be calling you into consistent prayer for another person. Sometimes we need to hold up others' hands in prayer.
8. To break through a depression.
9. To invite the Lord to give you a clean heart and renew a right spirit in you.
10. To seek God's face and have a closer walk with Him

11. To seek the Lord when He is directing you to do something that you don't think you have the ability to do.
12. To be free of evil or debilitating thoughts.
13. To resist temptation—even from pornography.
14. To be set free from everyday sins—pride, jealousy, resentment, gluttony, gossiping, etc.
15. To help you when you are feeling confused.
16. To help you when life seems out of control.
17. To humble yourself.
18. To break the lusting of the flesh after anything.
19. To gain strength.
20. To invite God's power to flow through you more mightily.

Author and professor Elmer Towns, in his book *Fasting for Spiritual Breakthrough: A Guide to Nine Biblical Fasts*, goes into great detail about fasting for release of bondage.

Some people are unable to quit smoking or break their homosexual relationships. Although they weep, pray sincerely, and seek deliverance, they remain in bondage....By controlling what you eat, you determine that you will control your life for God's purposes. When you make a vow and reinforce it with a fast, you move in the strength of decision-making. You give up necessary or enjoyable food as a demonstration of the commitment of your will. When you make a choice to fast, you strengthen yourself to stand against a force that has enslaved your spiritual appetite.[145]

What is one area in your life in which you feel you are in bondage and would like to consider fasting for a breakthrough?

_____

_____

_____

God has put us in a circle of friends and other relationships. Fasting is not only for our benefit but can be done by us for the benefit of others. We can fast when we are seeking God's intervention in someone else's life. Is there someone you know who desperately needs God to work in his or her life and He may be calling you to intercede for him or her?

_____

Are you willing to fast for this person without he or she knowing? _____

This is where our spiritual discipline gets more difficult—to sacrifice our favorite foods for someone else and not even let him or her know. Don't be afraid to open up to what God is calling you to do.

> *Liberty is the right to discipline ourselves*
> *in order not to be disciplined by others.*

—Clemenceau[146]

Physical Benefits of Fasting

It is clear that Scripture speaks continually about fasting, but is it dangerous to our health? Why should we fast? What does denying ourselves our favorite foods actually do for us?

Over time, our body becomes overloaded with toxins. The system God designed for us will naturally detoxify itself, but with high levels of contaminants entering our body it is physically helpful to fast. Fasting is a safe and effective method that allows our body to "take a break" from the normal digestion process and use its energy to release toxins and rid them from our body. In fact, fasting is recommended for any illness, as it gives the body the rest it needs to recover. Acute illnesses, colon problems, allergies, and respiratory diseases are most responsive to fasting, while chronic degenerative diseases are the least responsive. If you have health concerns, a good starting point is a fast in which you omit a certain food or food group from your diet. This will be explained later in our study.

Fasting is also helpful during normal health. By fasting regularly, you give all of your organs a rest and thus help reverse the aging process and contribute to a longer and healthier life. During a fast, the following happens:

- The natural process of toxin elimination continues, while the influx of new toxins is reduced.
- The energy usually used for digestion is redirected to immune function and cell growth, as well as "cleaning up" our systems.
- The immune system's workload is greatly reduced, and the digestive tract is spared any inflammation due to allergic reactions to food.
- Physical awareness, clearer thinking, emotional stability, and sensitivity to diet and surroundings are increased.
- The body has an improved overall appearance.
- The body has more strength.
- There is more control over an out-of-control life.
- Fasting contributes to weight loss. It helps to retrain your desire for God's food and helps you to be more disciplined in how you eat.

- Fasting eliminates cravings. Dr. Rex Russell emphasizes that we should not let any food or drink become our god. It doesn't make sense to ask God to heal your body in a certain area, while at the same time continuing to consume foods that destroy your health. For example, it isn't logical for a mom to ask God to take away her child's hyperactivity when she won't eliminate refined sugar or processed foods from his diet.

Which one of these reasons listed above would give you reason to consider a fast?

_____

_____

_____

When you take control of your physical appetite you develop
strength to take control of your emotional appetite.

—Elmer L. Towns[147]

Types of Fasting

There are three main types of fasting: the normal fast, the absolute fast, and the partial fast.

1. Normal Fast—The normal fast is going without food for a definite period of time. The duration can be one day, three days, one week, one month or as long as forty days (as in the cases of Moses and Jesus). I do not suggest doing a fast for more then twenty-four hours until you have experienced it. Fasts that last longer than three days are extreme and might require the supervision of a qualified health care professional.
2. Absolute Fast—The absolute fast is going without food or water. This should be a short fast.
3. Partial Fast—The partial fast includes omitting one meal a day, or omitting certain foods for a certain period of time. Elijah partially fasted twice. John the Baptist and Daniel and his three friends also participated in partial fasts. People with hypoglycemia or other diseases could use this type of fast.

Depending on the length of the fast, different things can be accomplished. For example, three-day fasts help the body rid itself of toxins and cleanses the blood. A five-day fast begins the process of healing and rebuilding the immune system.

There are precautions to follow when considering a fast. For your first fast, do not fast on water alone. An all-water fast releases toxins too quickly, causing headaches and worse. Instead, follow an organic juice diet detailed below, as this removes toxins and promotes healing by supplying the body with vitamins, minerals, and enzymes. This type of fast is also more likely to lead to a continued healthy diet once the fast is over, as it will accustom you to the taste of raw vegetables and promote vitality.

How to Get Started

God wants us to demonstrate our commitment to Him. Take the following steps to show Him your intent.

- Determine in your heart and mind that you are going to fast.
- Set a date—in advance.
- Determine the spiritual reason you are fasting. (Refer to the list above.) Write this out on the fasting track sheet found in the *Nutrition Manual*.

To prepare for the fast, for three days prior eat only foods that God created in their purest, most natural form possible. This would mean avoiding processed food.

During the fast, consume the required amount of water for your body size. That would be one ounce for every two pounds of weight. A person who weighs 150 pounds will drink seventy-five ounces of water. Make sure the water is purified. Herbal teas and diluted organic juice can also be added. Do not drink orange or tomato juice, and avoid all juices made with sweeteners.

When you have completed the fast, follow with a one- to two-day diet of raw fruits and vegetables. The desired physical effects of the fast can be ruined by eating cooked foods immediately afterwards. The first meals after a fast should be small and frequent.

Taking this treasure to heart: What truth did you learn today that made an impact on your opinion of fasting?

_____

_____

_____

Day Three—Going Deeper into the Study of Fasting

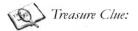 *Treasure Clue:*

Go and assemble all the Jews who are found in Susa, and fast for me;
do not eat or drink for three days, night or day.

—Est. 4:16 NASB

How Fasting Was Used in Scripture

Fasting is setting a time aside to devote more time to God in prayer. As we read about individuals in the Bible, we see how their faith and devotion to prayer made an impact on their lives and the lives of those around them. From studying biblical leaders who fasted, the one point that amazes me is fasts are mentioned as if the knowledge of them had been passed down for generations, but nowhere in Scripture is it explicitly spelled out with directions. Esther called for a fast, already knowing how to fast and what to expect. This attitude continues all throughout Scripture. We have lost the translation of *fast* in our current culture. Our children and grandchildren need to understand fasting as if it were as common as giving thanks at mealtime. Today let's go deeper into our study and see how these leaders understood and applied fasting.

ESTHER-FASTING FOR PROTECTION AND DELIVERANCE

If you are not familiar with her story, please read the short book of Esther now. The lesson from Esther is that if we fast for protection and deliverance from Satan, God will deliver us from evil. It reveals the power of a group of people fasting together to move the hand of God and to change the hearts of men.

Esther had everything to lose—including her life—but she put her faith in God. Through this time of fasting and prayer, hearts that had been bitterly turned against God were opened. This fast also shows how it can help hurting individuals turn back to God.

EZRA-FASTING TO SOLVE PROBLEMS

Read Ezra 8:21-36. Ezra needed protection while leading the Israelites to Jerusalem. He had previously bragged about his God to the king, so he did not want to ask for an escort. Instead he asked the Israelites to join him in a fast so that they might humble themselves before God and ask Him for a safe journey for them and their children, with all their possessions. Once again, the Bible reports how God answered the prayers of His people, who obtained spiritual results through fasting.

ELIJAH-FASTING TO BREAK CRIPPLING FEARS AND OTHER MENTAL PROBLEMS

Read 1 Kings 19:1-8. In this scripture Elijah is running for his life from the evil forces that were against Him. Read Ephesians 6:12. Confronted with the rage of evil forces, Elijah responded with fasting.

In the same way that God helped Elijah overcome evil forces, he has provided fasting as a powerful weapon to combat the spiritual forces that attack our minds and emotions as well. Through fasting, God will show us how to overcome negative emotional and personal habits.

We have many types of spiritual bondage from which fasting can help to deliver us. They include: negative attitudes, depression, despondency, fear, and anxiety. It is not suggested that you go on a forty-day water fast, but instead be willing to go to the Lord and see how you can add fasting to your walk with the Lord. He has promised us that if we call upon Him, He will hear us and heal our land. (2 Chron. 7:14)

DANEIL-FASTING FOR HEALTH AND PHYSICAL HEALING

Read Daniel 1:1-20. There are several occasions of fasting in the book of Daniel, but one of my favorite stories is the one about Daniel and his friends Shadrach, Meshach, and Abednego.

Daniel and his friends were given all the king's delicacies, yet they chose to eat a diet that was healthy. Daniel had proposed in his heart ahead of time that he would not defile himself. He avoided rich foods such meats, pastries, cakes, pies, cookies, alcohol, and any other food that is tempting to the flesh. As you read about Daniel and his friends, the Scripture explains how they were much healthier than the other Hebrew teenagers. This is a form of fasting in which Daniel just followed the scriptural healthy way of eating instead of eating the foods that are altered by man. His health was a testimony to the provision God has given us. When we fast for physical well-being, God will touch our bodies and enrich our souls.

Read Daniel 6. In this story about Daniel only bowing down to the one true God, he is thrown into a den of lions. The king was distressed over this situation because he loved Daniel. Therefore, the king spent the night fasting so Daniel's God would deliver him. In the morning, the king expectantly went to the den and found Daniel unharmed. This is a great example of how our witness to others enhances their ability to see God at work.

Personal Application

We have looked at examples, benefits, and instructions for fasting. Now it is time for you to write out a prayer asking God how He would have you apply this information to your spiritual and nutritional life. Are you ready to start a fast now? If not, pray about it.

_____

_____

_____

_____

_____

_____

As God directs, write out a plan for your first fast. Be specific on a date that will work best in your schedule and that is easy to remember, such as the first day of the next month. Also determine how long you will fast.

I will fast on _____ for _____ hours.

After you have a plan for the date and frequency of your fast, make a plan for how you will follow it. Write out what you will eat for the three days leading up to the fast. (For your first fast, it may be easier if you simply eliminate processed food in the days preceding the fast. This helps prepare your body for the different types of fasts that you learned about earlier.)

_____

_____

_____

The notes above will guide your first fast. As God leads you, it will become easier to follow and journal the prayers He will answer during this intimate time in your walk with Him.

In the _Treasures of Health Nutrition Manual_ or the website, you will find pages for journaling your fast. You may make copies of this and save them in a notebook to use with each fast. Some people find journaling unnecessary, but you are about to see God do amazing things in your life and you will want to share this experience with your kids and grandkids someday. Having it written down will be a reminder during those times when following a healthy living eating plan is not easy. You can look back and see all that God did for you during your fast.

"Jesus said to them, 'My father is always at his work to this very day, and I, too, am working'" (John 5:17 NIV). Your journal will document how God is working in your life and will give you great insight into His character. As your love relationship with the Father grows, your desire to eat unhealthy foods will go away. As we learned in the beginning of this chapter, we are to seek Him with *all* our heart.

There will be days when fasting is not what you want to do. I truly understand this, because it has been a challenge for me also. Let me encourage you to not punish yourself or feel bad if you don't follow through. Make a commitment to start again. There is no deadline—only rewards as God brings you through.

Write out how you feel physically before you fast. Then record your feelings during and after the fast. What Scriptures did God show you during the fast?

DIGGING DEEPER: Check out the Fasting Track Sheet in the *Treasures of Health Nutrition Manual*. This track sheet outlines the ideas mentioned above. You can make copies of this form and use it for each fast. This will track your success with the fast and the spiritual insights gained from the experience, as well as other notes for you to refer back to the next time you fast.

Taking the Daniel Challenge

Are you ready for a challenge? Let me encourage you to be the ultimate foodie friend to your study group and join a Daniel Challenge. This challenge involves doing the Daniel Fast for twenty-one days, beginning this coming Sunday. Your group can agree on another day to begin, but the important point is to set a date. Those who are up to the challenge should form a prayer group and meet for ten minutes each week for encouragement and support.

Those in the group who are not ready or physically not able should pray for those who are completing the fast. Let me encourage those who are not ready either physically, mentally, or spiritually to use these next twenty-one days to spend more time reading God's Word—our cherished treasure map—and pray about what God is teaching you. You could even fast from one food or food group. Whatever your choice, make it a matter of prayer and let God lead you.

The Daniel Fast is what I like to call "a whole body experience." You are setting aside this time for spiritual focus. You are putting your spirit in control of your soul as you discipline it and its cravings. You are eating healthy and wholesome foods for your body, and you will likely improve in health.

Read Daniel, chapter 10. Compare this chapter with chapters 1 and 6, which we read earlier. What foods did Daniel eat? _____

What did he drink? _____ What did he not drink? _____

Read Daniel 1:8. Who decided to follow God's plan? How do we know this?

_____

If we want to follow Daniel's plan, we must make up our minds to do it. If you are going to follow Daniel's plan, write out verse 8 as if it were you making up your mind. Write it as if you are writing to God.

_____

_____

In chapter 10, Daniel followed the fast for three weeks. We are going to follow his plan. The foods are simple and already in our treasure chest. Follow this simple plan:

- Eat fruits, vegetables, whole grains (not processed), nuts, seeds, and herbs.
- Drink water. Avoid beverages other than water.
- Avoid all meat, seafood, dairy, sugar, and processed foods.

Taking this treasure to heart: What is God saying to you regarding the fasts you read about or the Daniel Fast?

_____

_____

_____

Applying this treasure at home: In the Appendix of this book you will find the Daniel Fast Journal. This journal is a tool for you to use to record your challenges and praises. You may make copies for other members of your family to document their experience as they join you.

Day Four—Gaining Self-Control

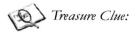 *Treasure Clue:*

Like a city whose walls are broken down is a man who lacks self-control.

—Prov. 25:28 NIV

Try going shopping and not see a child controlling his parents. Watch the news and see the drama of a killing in a metropolitan area. Listen to the morning news shows and hear about the epidemic of obesity—along with the newest cure. All around us we see evidence that we have a city whose walls are broken down by lack of self-control and discipline. The city may be our family, our neighborhood, or our own personal life. Self-control is the believer's wall of defense against the sinful desires that wage war against our mind and body.

The person you become is directly related to whether or not you choose to exercise self control over your life.

—Dr. Richard Couey

Michel Quoist, author of *Christian Response*, says, "If your body makes all the decisions and gives all the orders, and if you obey, the physical can effectively destroy every other dimension of your personality. Your emotional life will be blunted and your spiritual life will be stifled and ultimately you will become anemic."[148] Have you ever thought about how your actions involving self-control can determine who is master of your life? Quoist makes this distinction in his explanation, "If your body is in control your mental and spiritual life will greatly suffer." Anemic can mean "wishy-washy." How many times have you been wishy-washy in one area of your life, which led to being wishy-washy or weak in other areas?

The study of fasting revealed a need for self-control or discipline. Is this going to be easy? Probably not. God created our physical bodies and natural appetites, so they are not wrong or sinful in themselves.[149] But if left uncontrolled, we will find our bodies becoming self-indulgent—eating beyond our need, spending time in activities that are not beneficial, splurging on material possessions outside of our budget, and missing the true design God intended. Without learning and applying self-control, our treasure chest may be robbed and the hand-cuffs will be on us.

Whatever increases the strength and authority of your body over your mind—that thing is sin to you.

—Susannah Wesley[150]

Searching the Map for Truth

What does each of the following passages teach about self-control?

1 Corinthians 9:24-27

_____

_____

_____

1 Timothy 4:7-8

_____

_____

_____

2 Timothy 3:16

_____

_____

_____

Romans 12:1-2

_____

_____

_____

Self-control could be defined as avoiding excess or regulating our desires and keeping them in balance. Some of us, including me, have a tendency to overindulge our wants and consequently need to control them. How many times do we eat or drink just because it is tempting and not because we have hunger? But self-control involves a much wider range of attention than control of our bodily appetites and desires. We also must exercise control of thoughts, emotions, and speech. There is a form of self-control that says yes to what we should do as well as that which says no to what we shouldn't do. For example, I seldom want to begin a fast. Each time I plan a fast, I can think of all the food I would love to eat. Even foods that I don't normally eat become a temptation to me when I plan a fast. I usually have to draw a line in the sand—or in my case, the kitchen—and say, "For this amount of time I will not cross this line." Even Paul had issues, "I beat my body and make it my slave" (1 Cor. 9:27 NIV). There are times when I am drawn to gossip. I have to excuse myself from conversations so I will not be pulled in.

You will never discover the real you, never grow to be your unique self, until you are willing to exercise self-control.

—Dr. Richard Couey

Self-control is a vital character trait of the godly person. I am far from the godly person God wants me to be and I have continual struggles, but He helps me along the way just as He will do for you. Jesus told us, "If anyone would come after me, he must deny himself and take up his cross and follow me" (Matt. 16:24 NIV). Denying yourself is a form of self-control. There is no avoiding this commandment.

In his book, *The Faithful Life*, author and speaker Jerry Bridges defines self-control using two terms. The first is *inner strength*, which refers to moderation or temperance in the gratification of our desires or appetites. The second term is *soundness of mind* or *sound judgment*. It takes sound judgment to control our desires, appetites, thoughts, emotions, and actions. Working together, sound judgment helps us determine what we should do and how we should respond, and inner strength provides the will to do it. Sound judgment helps us regulate our thoughts and keep our emotions under control.[151]

Many times we know what to do, but we lack the strength to do it. Combining the two terms gives us the best definition: "Self-control is the exercise of inner strength under the direction of sound judgment that enables us to do, think, and say the things that are pleasing to God."[152]

Your Body Is a Temple

"Whether, then, you eat or drink or whatever you do, do all to the glory of God" (1 Cor. 10:31 NASB). We recently looked at one of the most powerful yet smallest words in the Bible—*all*. All means there is no part left out. Every single thing we do—if we have a desire to please God—should be done for His glory. Yet we are dealing with areas that need to be addressed, such as self-control. Our body is affected by what we eat and drink, laziness, our clothing, and sexual purity. All of these areas affect the health of our body and our ability to give glory to God.

We spent six weeks learning about the highest quality of biblical foods designed for our health. But even having this knowledge, we can still have a self-control problem of eating too much or desiring foods that bring harm to our body. How are we going to overcome this?

1 Timothy 6:17 helps us remember where the good comes from. ". . . God, who richly supplies us with all things to enjoy" (N.ASB). So why do we continue to look elsewhere for substitutes?

The apostle Paul emphasized the need to keep our natural desires under control. He spoke of his body as his opponent, as the instrument through which appetites and lusts, if left unchecked, would war against him. He was determined that his body would be his slave, not his master.

Write out 1 Corinthians 6:12.

_____

_____

_____

Paul further urged us to present our bodies as a living and holy sacrifice, acceptable to God, and to not be conformed to this world (Rom. 12:1-2). Jerry Bridges, in his book *Pursuit of Holiness*, explains this.

> Quite possibly there is no greater conformity to the world among evangelical Christians today than the way in which we, instead of presenting our bodies as holy sacrifices, pamper and indulge them in defiance of our better judgment and our Christian purpose in life.
>
> Overeating and overindulging in the wrong foods is common among many people today in our churches. Some show evidence in the shape of their body but there are others whose bodies don't reveal their secret of overeating. Either way—whether your body shows it or not—it is still wrong. Each of us should examine ourselves as to whether or not we eat or drink to the glory of God.
>
> For us to obey the scriptures on discipline usually requires change in our lifestyle. Our sinful nature has developed sinful habits.[153]

Consider this story about the difficulty of breaking bad habits:

> An overweight business associate decided it was time to shed some excess pounds. He took his new diet seriously, even changing his driving route to avoid his favorite bakery. One morning, however, he arrived at work carrying a gigantic coffee cake. We all scolded him, but his smile remained cherubic.

"This is a very special coffeecake," he explained. "I accidentally drove by the bakery this morning and there in the window was a host of goodies. I felt this was no accident so I prayed, 'Lord, if You want me to have one of those delicious coffeecakes, let me have a parking place directly in front of the bakery.' And sure enough," he continued, "the eighth time around the block, there it was!"[154]

This business associate definitely developed habits, and the coffeecake is evidence. How do we break these habits? Discipline is required to break any habit. If a golfer has developed the wrong style of swinging his club, he cannot just decide to change instantly. He has developed a certain habit, and much discipline—much correction and instruction—is required to break that bad habit and develop a new one.

In the same way, our patterns of disobedience to God have been developed over a number of years and are not broken easily without discipline. Discipline does not mean gritting your teeth and saying, "I'll not do that anymore." Rather, discipline means structured, planned training. Just as you need a plan for regular Bible reading or study, so you need a plan for applying the Word to your life.

We need to continue our goal in this hunt to be intentional—intentional in following God's design for our body. Intentional in self-control means having a plan and following it. If we say, "I am going to do this," without a plan we are setting ourselves up to fail.

Make a Plan

Follow these specific action steps to gain self-discipline:

1. Continue following the map—God's Word. As you read the Bible, ask yourself what each passage is teaching you concerning God's will for a holy, self-controlled life.
2. How does your life measure up to that scripture? Where and how do you fall short? Write out specific answers.
3. Record the intentional steps you need to take to obey these scriptures.

List areas in your life where God is giving you success. Rejoice over these successes.

_____

_____

_____

_____

Putting It into Action

Suppose you were meditating on 1 Corinthians 13, the great love chapter. As you think about the chapter you realize the importance of love, and you also see the practical outworking of love: love is patient and kind and does not envy. You ask yourself, "Am I impatient or unkind or envious toward anyone?" As you think about this, you realize you are envious toward Suzie from work who seems to be getting all the attention. You confess your sin to God, being very specific to name Suzie and your sinful reaction to her good attention. You ask God to bless her even more and to give you a spirit of contentment so that you will not continue to envy Suzie, but will instead love her. You might memorize 1 Corinthians 13:4 and think about it as you see Suzie at work. You even look for ways to help her. Each day you continue in this pattern until you finally see God working a spirit of love in your heart toward Suzie. The feelings toward her will never change unless you put forth a plan and follow through. Be specific—intentional—about your plan.[155]

Perseverance—A Necessary Ingredient of Discipline

Look at the definition of perseverance—steady and continued action or belief, usually over a long period and especially despite difficulties or setbacks.[156] Any training—physical, mental, or spiritual—often begins with failure. We fail more often than we succeed. But if we persevere, we will see progress until we are succeeding more often than failing. When we try to change our ways, at first it seems we are making no progress, so we become discouraged and think, "What's the use? I can never overcome that sin." That is exactly what Satan wants us to think.

It is at this point when we must exercise perseverance. We want instant success, but holiness doesn't come that way. Our sinful habits did not happen overnight, and it will take time to remove them. Determination is required to make any change in our lives.[157,158]

> *For though a righteous man falls seven times, he rises again,*
> *but the wicked are brought down by calamity.*
>
> —Prov. 24:16 NIV

Don't give up and don't give in. Keep going, keep persevering, and be intentional about your goals to a healthier life—a holy life. There is no limit to the rewards!

Taking this treasure to heart: Write out some areas in your life that need discipline.

_____

_____

_____

_____

_____

Applying this treasure at home: This week we have covered fasting and self-discipline. What is one step you are willing to do in at least one of these areas? Record this on your Action Plan.

FABULOUS FOODIE FRIDAY

Plant Your Gardens

It's time to plant our gardens. As you plant, may I suggest the following rules for your garden planting?

Plant three rows of squash:

1. Squash gossip
2. Squash criticism
3. Squash indifference

Plant three rows of peas:

1. Purity
2. Patience
3. Perseverance

Plant five rows of lettuce:

1. Let us be unselfish and loyal.
2. Let us be faithful to duty.
3. Let us search the Scriptures.
4. Let us not be weary in well-doing.
5. Let us be obedient in all things.

Foodie Time

Join your foodie friend and let's see how many recipes can be included in the Daniel Fast. The Designed Healthy Living website (www.designedhealthyliving.com) has a full twenty-one-day menu and shopping list if you need suggestions. Remember, raw foods are highly nutritious. They should constitute a minimum of 50 percent of this fast. What a great time for experiments in the kitchen! Also note that salad dressings should not include any milk products. Be adventurous and make your own.

Plan out three weeks of menus for your Daniel Fast.

Day	Breakfast	Lunch	Dinner	Snacks
Day 1				
Day 2				
Day 3				
Day 4				
Day 5				
Day 6				
Day 7				

Day 8				
Day 9				
Day 10				
Day 11				
Day 12				
Day 13				
Day 14				
Day 15				
Day 16				
Day 17				
Day 18				
Day 19				
Day 20				
Day 21				

You finished all three weeks! Congratulations, and praise be to God!

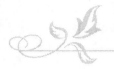

Sweets

Day One—Sweet Antiquities

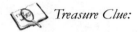 *Treasure Clue:*

Pleasant words are as a honeycomb, sweet to the soul, and health to the bones.
—Prov. 16:24 KJV

This week our treasure chest will fill with a popular favorite—the goodness of sweets. Before we cut into your favorite pie, let's review the middle part of this verse, "sweet to the soul." Do our words penetrate the soul as deeply as honey builds healthy bones?

This Treasure Clue is a sweet reminder of the savory taste of honey and how it compares to the words we speak to others. What words do we speak to those around us? Are they words that will sweeten the other person's day and possibly lighten their load?

List the people you talked with or could have spoken to in the last twenty-four hours.

_____

_____

_____

_____

How many chances did you have to speak sweet words? _____

How many of those times did you use words of encouragement? _____

Was there an opportunity you missed that you wish you could redo? _____

List the people in your life that are an encouragement to you:

_____

_____

_____

_____

Take a moment now to offer a prayer of thanks for those people and let them know how they encourage you. If your list was blank, then hold on and we will try to uncover why in the next few weeks.

Now list the people in your life who need encouragement from you:

_____

_____

People all around us need sweet words of encouragement. Think about the mail carrier, the cashier, a neighbor, your child's teacher, your aerobics instructor, your dentist, and so on. What about your family? Does your child, no matter what age, need encouragement? How about your parents? Many people are longing for encouragement, even when we don't recognize it.

Proverbs tells us that sweet words are healing to our bones. Physically, our bones benefit from the collagen found in honey, but emotionally, when words of encouragement and love are spoken there is a healing in our bodies much stronger than any food or supplement. What are some words that have been spoken to you that have made an impact on your life and made you feel good about yourself?

_____

_____

How did those words make you feel?

_____

Take a look at this list of short phrases that may change a person's day:

"I admit I made a mistake."
"You did a great job."
"What is your opinion?"
". . . if you please."
"Thank you."
"We can do this."
"You are not alone."

"I love you."
"I appreciate you."
"How can I pray for you?"

Let no unwholesome word proceed from your mouth, but only such a word as is good for edification according to the need of the moment, that it may give grace to those who hear.
—Eph. 4:29 NASB

Honey, I Love You

Yes, I love honey, and hopefully you will too when we get finished today. Honey should be treasured. For many reasons—mostly because it tasted so good—honey was one of the most popular foods among the people of the Bible. It became a symbol for abundance and God's blessings, which is why the phrase "a land of milk and honey" is found in Scripture more than forty times.

Let's glance at some of the messages on our map to gather knowledge regarding honey.

Honey was sent as a present:
Genesis 43:11—"And their father Israel said unto them, If it must be so now, do this; take of the best fruits in the land in your vessels, and carry down the man a present, a little balm, and a little honey, spices, and myrrh, nuts, and almonds" (KJV).

1 Kings 14:3—"And take with thee ten loaves, and cracknels, and a cruse of honey, and go to him: he shall tell thee what shall become of the child" (KJV).

Honey illustrates the Word of God:
Psalm 19:10—"More to be desired are they than gold, yea, than much fine gold: sweeter also than honey and the honeycomb" (KJV).

Psalm 119:103—"How sweet are thy words unto my taste! yea, sweeter than honey to my mouth!" (KJV)

Honey illustrates wisdom:
Proverbs 24:13-14—"My son, eat thou honey, because it is good; and the honeycomb, which is sweet to thy taste: So shall the knowledge of wisdom be unto thy soul: when thou hast found it, then there shall be a reward, and thy expectation shall not be cut off" (KJV).

Isaiah 7:15—"Butter and honey shall he eat, that he may know to refuse the evil, and choose the good" (KJV).

Honey is good for food:

Proverbs 24:13—"My son, eat thou honey, because it is good; and the honeycomb, which is sweet to thy taste" (KJV).

1 Samuel 14:29—"Then said Jonathan, My father hath troubled the land: see, I pray you, how mine eyes have been enlightened, because I tasted a little of this honey" (KJV).

Song of Solomon 5:1—"I am come into my garden, my sister, my spouse: I have gathered my myrrh with my spice; I have eaten my honeycomb with my honey" (KJV).

Luke 24:42—"And they gave him a piece of a broiled fish, and of an honeycomb" (KJV).

Matthew 3:4—"And the same John had his raiment of camel's hair, and a leathern girdle about his loins; and his meat was locusts and wild honey" (KJV).

It is not good to eat too much honey:

Proverbs 25:16—"Hast thou found honey? eat so much as is sufficient for thee, lest thou be filled therewith, and vomit it" (KJV).

Honey is food for the Promised Land:

Ezekiel 20:6—"On that day I swore to them that I would bring them out of the land of Egypt into a land that I had searched out for them, a land flowing with milk and honey, the most glorious of all lands" (ESV).

Scripture reaffirms honey as a gift and a blessing. God confirmed this with a special spot on our tongue to enjoy the sweet taste.

Foodie Fact: From the Promised Land to America…honeybees came with the Pilgrims to America in 1620. Can you imagine traveling with those bees on that voyage? Indians called them "white man's flies."

Honey in Your Medicine Cabinet

Move over, cough medicine, honey is coming on the shelf. In the past few years various children's over-the-counter medicine have been discontinued due to their adverse effects on kids. But this left parents in a dilemma if they did not know how to treat their kids naturally. In 2007, Penn State College of Medicine released a new study to give parents a safe and effective alternative. The study found that a small dose of buckwheat honey given before bedtime provided better relief of nighttime cough and sleep difficulty in children than no treatment or dextromethorphan (DM), a cough suppressant found in many over-the-counter cold medications.[159]

> The results are published by Penn State College of Medicine researchers, led by Ian Paul, M.D., M.S....In a previous study published in 2004, Paul and colleagues showed that neither DM nor diphenhydramine, another common component of cold medications, performed better than a placebo at reducing nighttime cough or improving sleep quality. However, honey has been used for centuries in some cultures to treat upper respiratory infection symptoms like cough, and is considered to be safe for children over twelve months old. Honey has well-established antioxidant and antimicrobial effects, which could explain its contributions to wound healing. Honey also soothes on contact.[160]

The medicinal benefits of honey date back to an Egyptian papyrus that contained a list of over five hundred remedies that used honey for various illnesses. It was particularly useful in the treatment of eye diseases, burns, and other wounds.[161] But what about today?

Honey is such a complex substance that, when eaten in moderate amounts, it contributes to our body's ability to metabolize foods rather than detract from it. Because raw honey is not cooked or processed, it contains all of its vitamins and minerals in their natural proportions. These vitamins, minerals, enzymes, and amino acids add up to more than 165 ingredients! This far exceeds sugar in nutrients alone. But it does more.

Honey contains eighteen amino acids, one of which is called proline. Proline is a major ingredient of collagen. Collagen holds the body together and is part of the matrix of which bone is formed. Many people with arthritis have found relief using honey in their diet.[162]

Home remedies for honey include using it as an anti-diarrhea mixture and also for sore throats. Once when we took a group of homeschoolers to hike the Grand Canyon, two of the girls came down with a sore throat. Our only resources were hot water with lemon and honey. The good news is that it really worked, the bad news for them was they did not get out of the ten-mile hike. From a mother's viewpoint, honey coats and lubricates the irritated linings of the throat, which makes swallowing easier. From the scientific view, the ingredient that makes it taste sweet also goes straight to the brain and signals the pituitary gland to start pumping out soothing endorphins.[163]

Foodie Tip: Honey has the power to make us feel better by improving our mood, and the power to think better by stimulating the part of the brain responsible for learning.

Other benefits of honey in our health are: calming frayed nerves, possibly helping to get a good night's sleep, helping with traveler's diarrhea, and sometimes helping with asthma.[164]

We continually see that the foods God gave us are filled with nutrition and help build health. It is sweet words to my ears to hear all the marvelous things honey can do when it comes to infections and other health issues. Each time I add more of God's foods to the treasure chest I feel privileged to know the One who gave us these foods.

Not everyone in the medical community agrees on the benefits of honey. When honey is heated and the comb removed, the nutrition level drops and the difference in nutrition between honey and white sugar vary only slightly.[165]

Honey to Avoid

Honey labeled "raw" is your best choice. If a label does not state "raw," then the honey is typically heated and pasteurized for a longer shelf life. Honey may also be altered with corn syrup and cheap sugars.[166] Some honey sources contain sulfa drugs and antibiotics used to control bee diseases. It will be worth your time to find a local beekeeper for fresh raw honey. It's definitely a sweet treasure to cherish!

What Is Honey?

Unlike table sugar, which is 99.5 percent sucrose, raw honey is a natural sweetener made of at least 165 identifiable components.[167] It contains amino acids, enzymes, vitamins, minerals, and at least twenty-five different kinds of sugar. Honey is a natural sweetener that requires no processing or refinement, unlike white table sugar. Sugar has no semblance to the raw cane sugar by the time the processing and refining are completed.

Honey has a complex nature. The exact composition of honey varies, depending on the nectars from which it is made. For example, bees collecting nectar from buckwheat blossoms produce a dark, strong-flavored honey that is richer in minerals than the white honey collected from clover blossoms.

The conclusion continues to amaze me. Foods created in God's design build health and meet our daily needs. So enjoy honey in small amounts. One tablespoon of honey is equal in sweetness to five tablespoons of sugar.

Digging Deeper: Read about honey in the *Treasures of Health Nutrition Manual.* You will find information about types of honey, how honey helps during pregnancy, and the crystallization of honey.

Taking this treasure to heart: God designed bees to work together as a team of more than 40,000 to make this delectable syrup. The birds and bees are in His care but the greatest truth is He cares for you even more.

Affirmation: I will let my sweet words to others be a reminder to me of how perfectly I am made in His image.

Applying this treasure at home: How can you apply honey to your treasure chest? Look for recipes that already have honey as the sweetener. Share these recipes with your foodie friend. Be bold; try to swap honey in a recipe for sugar. The *Healthy Treasures Cookbook* has suggestions for cooking with honey.

Day Two—Sweet Design

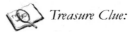 *Treasure Clue:*

Love the LORD your God with all your heart and with all your soul and with all your strength.
—Deut. 6:5 NIV

Circle the imperative verb in this treasure verse.
Underline or highlight the word *all* every time it is used.
What part of our life is not included in this command? _____

Since there is nothing left out for us to keep to ourselves, take a moment now and personalize this verse; rewrite it as a prayer to God. Here is an example: "Lord, I want to daily show You I love You with all my heart, all my soul, and with all my strength. I know my strength to accomplish this comes from You and You alone.

_____

_____

_____

This verse may seem a little out of place when it comes to sugars, but the purpose of reviewing it this week is to keep everything in perspective. We must love the Lord first, with everything we have. Then understanding how sweets fit into our plan will be simple. When we love the Lord with everything, our desire will be for foods that benefit our health. This will help us gain the strength for living. We have already discovered how honey fits into the Master's plan, so now we will add sugar cane to the chest.

Sugar Cane

An excursion from a cruise ship in the Caribbean allowed us the chance to visit an island with hundreds of acres flourishing with sugar cane. A local produce stand gave us the opportunity to purchase and experiment with fresh cut sugar cane. The sweetness had a lighter flavor than what is typically found in table sugar. It was also very fibrous to chew. If I had to work hard at getting sugar from a cane to put into my recipes, we would be eating fewer sweetened foods in our home.

Sweet Treats or Sweet Nothings

Three pieces make up the puzzle of our diet: protein, carbohydrates, and fats. Sugars are carbs—good or bad. Most textbooks say that since all carbohydrates are eventually digested and absorbed as glucose, the original food source—whether it's a bean or a candy bar—matters little. Sugar is sugar; sucrose is sucrose. This is not the whole truth. Sugars behave very differently in your body. An orange has sucrose that is chemically the same as the sucrose in your sugar bowl, but the orange comes packed with other nutrients, making it biochemically more friendly in the body. When you eat sucrose as part of a fruit or a vegetable, you not only get vitamins and minerals in the package but also fiber and complex carbohydrates that steady the absorption of sugar. Mothers always say, "Be careful of the company you keep; they will affect your life." That's also true with sugar. The other nutrients in food affect the way sugar is absorbed from the intestines and its consequent behaviors in the body. This explains why some sugars are bad and some are good.

Carbohydrates in the form of simple sugars are commonly known as glucose, fructose, and galactose. They are each absorbed differently in the digestive tract. Glucose and galactose are absorbed very quickly, while fructose (fruits sugars and honey) are digested slower. Blood carries glucose to our cells, where it is used for energy. Glucose is necessary for the amino acids that build enzymes, hormones, and many other necessary cells.

Metabolism requires glucose. If glucose is not available, the body uses fat or protein to supply energy for the cells. On the other hand, if the blood glucose levels are high, the glucose forms fat in our bodies.

Many diets lead people to lose weight, but at the cost of their muscles—not fat. Since there is less glucose in the diet, the body will metabolize protein. This contributes to muscle loss instead of fat loss. A healthy diet, agreed upon by many nutritionists, would have calories consisting of 40 percent carbohydrates (whole grains, vegetables, and fruits), 30 percent protein (lean organic meat or legumes), and 30 percent healthy fats (flax seed or olive oil). This contributes to protecting muscle mass and maintaining balance while making it easy to lose or maintain weight. We need healthy forms of carbohydrates in our diet in order to be balanced.

DIGGING DEEPER: To learn more about sweeteners, read "How Sweet It Is" in the *Nutrition Manual.* As we have learned, the Bible mentions honey numerous times, but it also refers to other sweeteners, such as freshly squeezed juice, dates, and sugar cane. If these sugars are dehydrated at relatively low temperatures, many of their ingredients are preserved.[168]

Natural Forms of Sugar

Sugar comes in many different forms and various colors. Remember, we are looking for foods that are the least altered. As you read through these various natural forms of sugar, write out a grocery list and try one new sweetener this month.

BROWN RICE SYRUP

Brown rice syrup is a balanced sweetener or complex carbohydrate. It has a mild taste and comes in different levels of sweetness. Because of its mild flavor, it blends well with stronger flavored sweeteners.

PURE MAPLE SYRUP

Maple syrup comes from the sap of maple trees and is a simple carbohydrate. Purchase maple syrup that is pure and produced without formaldehyde. The packaging should say if this chemical was used. Avoid maple-flavored syrups that are mostly colored sugar water. Store pure maple syrup in the refrigerator. This is a good choice to replace brown sugar.

STEVIA (sweet leaf, candy leaf)

Stevia is a natural alternative sweetener from the herb *stevia rebaudiana.* Though it hasn't gone through the FDA approval process for use as a sweetener, it is sold as a dietary supplement. It is available in powdered extract or liquid form. Be careful when purchasing the newer forms such as Truvia, as it may contain other ingredients not desirable. Read the label.

EVAPORATED CANE JUICE-SUCANAT, SAVANAH GOLD, HONEY CRYSTALS

You can find evaporated cane juice in some health food stores or grocery stores, or you can order it online through several sources. This product is formed by the evaporation of cane juice, which leaves all the nutrition intact for consumption. This allows our bodies to utilize the vitamins and minerals along with a slower release of the sugar in the bloodstream. By far this is the very best choice. Be careful in this selection, since sucanat has become a term grabbed by companies trying to make a sale. The sugar should not be crystallized but should have a slight tan color.

TURBINADO

Turbinado is only slightly better than white sugar. There is very little nutritional value to this product, since it is processed.

Enjoy the things created for food that contain natural sugars. Enjoy complex carbohydrates. If you must eat sugar, make sure you eat plenty of fiber and nutrients along with it.

Taking this treasure to heart: Just as hummingbirds are attracted to sweet nectar, so humans are pleased with sweet things. The Latin word *frutus*, which gives us our word "fruit," means "enjoy." If we eat fruits and vegetables in their natural state, the sweet flavors are beneficial because they contain fiber and other essential nutrients.[169]

Applying this treasure at home: Which sweeteners are you curious about trying?

Be on the lookout for these products in your grocery store or health food store.

Day Three—The Problems of Sugar

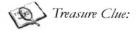 *Treasure Clue:*

Whether you turn to the right or to the left, your ears will hear a voice behind you, saying, "This is the way; walk in it."

—Isa. 30:21 NIV

If you are like me, you may have experienced the "Satan on your shoulder" trauma. I'm talking about those times when you are looking in the refrigerator or the pantry and your mind says, "I want another cookie," and you hear a voice from one side of your shoulder saying, "Go ahead. You deserve it. You've been working hard; you can lose weight tomorrow." Then the other voice says, "You know, that one is going to lead to two and then more and more until you have to throw away the box so no one knows how many you ate!" Then it says, "You will feel better if you don't eat…or maybe just eat some carrots." Which voice do you listen to?

We need to know where to turn and follow Isaiah's guidance: "This is the way, walk in it." Are we looking for quick comfort or a lifetime of feeling great? Turning to the right or left leads to quick comfort.

> *The first step towards getting somewhere is to decide that*
> *you are not going to stay where you are.*
> —John Pierpont Morgan

Today we are going to uncover what is on the right or the left. My prayer is that once you understand what happens when you make this turn, the choice will become easier.

First, let's take inventory so you'll know your starting point. Over the past three days, how many servings of sugar did you consume? Write down the number of servings of:

Pastries, cakes, cookies, and candy _____

Non-organic meat—especially hamburger and luncheon/deli meat _____

Fast food _____

Fruit and fruit juice _____

Beverages—sweetened, including flavored water and lattes _____

Salad dressing and condiments _____

Bread _____

Canned vegetables and fruits _____

Cereal _____

Processed foods _____

Total servings _____

Are you surprised by the amount of sweets you consume?

If there ever were a pirate stealing from our chest of good health, sugar would be the eye-patch-wearing scoundrel. Sugar tastes delectable and rewarding, but it is not always profitable for our health and longevity. In fact, all the calories from processed sugar are empty calories, containing virtually none of the nutrients your cells need so desperately. This makes sugar an anti-nutrient—eating sugar actually drains nutrients from your body. Certain nutrients are needed for you to metabolize sugar. B-vitamins are one of the nutrients necessary for simple carbohydrates to be digested and metabolized. All carbohydrate-rich foods have an abundance of B-vitamins so the body can assimilate them well. This is yet another proof of a divine design.

So what happens when we process sugar, thus removing the B-vitamins? The body has to supply them from other sources.

Since sugar is an anti-nutrient, it contributes to health problems such as diabetes, tooth decay, heart disease, osteoporosis, and immune dysfunction. If you want to avoid colds, or if someone in your family is "coming down with a cold," eliminate sugar from your diet to keep yourself healthy.[170]

Refined sugar causes calcium to be lost through the urine, forcing the body to remove calcium from the bones in order to replace the calcium lost. By removing the calcium from your bones, eating sugar contributes to osteoporosis. If you are concerned about or already suffering from osteoporosis, eliminating sugar from your diet would be a healthful decision.

Sugar can cause insomnia, according to Dr. Don Colbert, in his book, *The Seven Pillars of Health.*

> Many people eat too much sugar and highly processed foods before bed, keeping their nightly date with a bowl of ice cream, piece of cake, or bag of popcorn. These carbohydrates stimulate excessive insulin release from the pancreas. The result is a "sugar high" of energy. But later, usually in the middle of the night, your blood sugar hits a "low," which triggers the adrenal glands to produce more adrenaline and cortisol. Suddenly you are awake and feel hungry again.[171]

Sugar and simple carbohydrates put stress on the adrenal glands due to rapidly shifting blood sugar levels. By switching to vegetables, fruits, proteins, and high fiber carbohydrates, blood sugar remains more stable, providing less strain on the adrenal glands.[172]

Sugar Can Harm Us

The complex carbohydrates found in vegetables, grains, and fruits are good for you; the simple sugars found in sodas, candies, frosting, and packaged treats can do harm. Sugar can contribute to a host of problems, but on its own it is not the sole reason for each of these problems. Typically there are other factors involved such as lifestyle, exercise, and other foods consumed. The following details what can happen when we consume too much—or the wrong kind—of sugar.[173]

Excess sugar depresses immunity. Studies show that drinking two twelve-ounce sodas can suppress the body's immune responses by 50 percent. This was most noticeable two hours after ingestion, but the effect was still evident five hours later. As a result, you are more prone to bacterial and viral infections. In addition, sugar can actually feed cancer cells.

Sugar sours behavior, attention, and learning. Studies on children's behavior vary significantly, but the general consensus is that some children and adults are sugar sensitive, meaning behavior, attention span, and a learning ability deteriorate in proportion to the amount of junk sugar they consume.

Sugar promotes obesity. This doesn't need much explanation, but it helps to understand that fruits, vegetables, and even my homemade bread contain sugar, but they all come in a package with lots of fiber. This fiber helps the body to utilize the sugar so the pancreas and adrenals are not exerted. When you eat sugar, your body goes into fat-storage mode. That's why most diabetics gain weight when they begin taking insulin. Sugar creates a cycle of demand for more sugar, which raises insulin levels. Insulin is a powerful hormone that signals the body to store fat.

Sugar promotes sugar highs. This is proven daily in schools and day cares where kids are given sugar treats and then become unmanageable.

Sugar promotes diabetes. Sugar causes an elevation in insulin levels, which can lead to the cells becoming resistant to insulin. This leads to diabetes.

Sugar promotes heart disease. A diet high in sugar can change the lipid levels to favor heart disease. This effect is most dramatic in people who respond to sucrose with unusually high insulin secretions, which promote making too much fat.

Sugar leads to malnutrition and cavities. Eating sugar in small amounts is pleasurable, but when the balance is tilted to the other extreme, sugar can lead to becoming malnourished. Sugary foods supply energy without providing nutrients. And since sugar requires the body to utilize B vitamins and other nutrients, this actually causes a deficiency in our system. Also, without fiber and other nutrients in the food, sugar leads to tooth decay.

Linked to behavior disorders. There is a strong link between excessive sugar intakes and ADD. Many children have become sugar-holics. Some authorities have even linked sugar and hypoglycemia (low blood sugar) to violent behavior.

Sugar leads to osteoporosis. Sugar creates an acidic environment that causes your body to cry out for alkaline foods. If you don't get enough calcium in your diet, your body may pull it from your bones and teeth.

Sugar aggravates yeast problems. Yeast loves sugar, but it is kept in check with a balanced immune system. Taking antibiotics and then consuming lots of sugar may cause a person to develop a yeast overgrowth, and the abdomen may swell. This overgrowth also leads to infections. Candida is an example of this problem.

Sugar accelerates the aging process. In 1970, researchers discovered a glucose protein complex forming in collagen, blood vessels, and the heart muscle. They named the complex the "advanced glycation endproducts," or AGE. These molecules interact with neighboring proteins and become destructive free radicals, leading to accelerated aging and disease. This speeds up the aging process and causes wrinkles and age spots to appear on the skin. AGEs are formed naturally through normal life and aging, but they are also formed externally by cooking sugars with fats and proteins. Their studies also found that when we consume these externally formed AGEs, it contributes to atherosclerosis, asthma, arthritis, Alzheimer's, heart disease, stroke, and diabetes-related diseases such as neuropathy, retinopathy, and neuropathy.[174] However, there is great news! We have an answer to this problem. Are you ready? Research at the University of Georgia in Athens has proven the skin and seed of the muscadine grape will reverse the effects of this AGE protein. Their research has proven the muscadine grape—along with its polyphenols and ellagic acid—reverses the aging process, protects and repairs the heart, and reverses type 2 diabetes.[175] Once again God created a solution to our problems in a food!

Lab Sugar

Lab experiments give us artificial sweeteners. Good or bad? Only you can decide this for your family. Many textbooks tout the health benefits of using artificial sweeteners, yet there is growing evidence these products may not be our best choice. Artificial sweeteners are non-nutritive (no nutritional value for your body), non-calorie sweeteners that have been manufactured in a lab. They are intended to help decrease sugar and calorie intake and to be safe for diabetics. However, artificial sweeteners increase appetite in general and interfere with the taste, enjoyment, and satisfaction obtained from eating foods high in complex carbohydrates. They also increase our preference for fat intake and interfere with our body's ability to select foods containing the nutrients it needs.

We will highlight a few of the artificial sweeteners, and if you want to learn about them in more detail you will find the information in the *Treasures of Health Nutrition Manual.*

ASPARATAME(NUTRASWEET)

Aspartame causes some concern for many people. Health complaints from ingesting this lab sugar include: disorientation, difficulty thinking and concentrating, visual blurring (or even monocular blindness), seizures, and heart failure. In the textbook *Clinical Nutrition*, the contributing physicians explain aspartame is well known to have harmful effects on the nervous system and the eyes. It has also been linked to seizures and various forms of brain tumors.[176]

SUCRALOSE(SPLENDA)

One of man's latest lab sugars, Splenda, is a substance called sucralose. This is made from altering sugar into a chlorocarbon. Some of the side effects noticed in animals include shrunken thymus gland, enlarged liver and kidneys, changes in the spleen, reduced growth rate, decrease in red blood cell count, and problems with pregnancy.

HIGH FRUCTOSE CORN SYRUP (HFCS)

High fructose corn syrup is not the same as fructose in fruit. It contains no nutrients and does not nourish the body. HFCS does cause the body to lose minerals, thus causing nutritional deficiencies. In addition, it's associated with various adverse health conditions. It begins as corn grown with genetically modified seeds. From there, the cornstarch is subjected to a complex chemical process with genetically engineered enzymes. The resulting HFCS is far from natural. Cancer, heart disease, diabetes, and obesity have been increasing since the addition of HFCS into processed foods. It's in virtually all processed foods, including beverages, cereals, snacks, and canned and bottled foods. According to Dr. Walter Willet of Harvard Medical School, high fructose corn syrup has no benefits and only adverse metabolic effects.

The Mayo Clinic has this to say about HFCS, ". . . processed foods made with high-fructose corn syrup and other sweeteners are high in calories and low in nutritional value. Regularly including these products in your diet has the potential to promote obesity—which, in turn, promotes conditions such as Type 2 diabetes, high blood pressure, and coronary artery disease.[177]

Common sense says that feeding the brain an unnatural substance may cause it to perform in an unnatural way. Our advice for any artificial substance is: when in doubt, leave it out.

DIGGING DEEPER: In the *Nutrition Manual,* read about diabetes, insulin resistance, and candida. From the Designed Healthy Living website, take the candida quiz. In our class time this week we will be learning more about this health problem that affects a large percentage of people without their even being aware of it. The best way to improve our health is to become knowledgeable. If you miss class this week or are studying individually then you may find it helpful to listen to this talk online.

Taking this treasure to heart: A young man arrived in heaven and Saint Peter was giving him the welcome home tour. They walked along the gold street and saw many mansions, but then they came to a large room. The young man asked Saint Peter what was in this room. Saint Peter cautioned the young man that he might not want to see inside. But the young man insisted. So Saint Peter opened the large oversized doors to reveal a room full of blessings—more than any person could ever imagine. Everything a person could ask for was in this room. The young man, confused about the contents of this room in heaven, asked Saint Peter the meaning of the room. Saint Peter said these were all the blessings God wants to bestow on his children if they would just ask and seek Him with all their heart. Instead they fill their lives with artificial replicas and never get the real deal.

There are many distractions in life that keep us from the best God has to offer. Artificial sweeteners give us fake sweetness instead of the goodness of His foods. What other distractions or artificial substitutes are taking the place of the real blessing God has waiting for you?

Applying this treasure at home: Are artificial sweeteners in your daily list? Do you want to make changes in this area? Take time now to ask God to help you. These sweeteners are addictive, and you will need help. Share this with your foodie friend and pray for each other.

DAY FOUR—OVERCOMING TEMPTATIONS

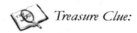 *Treasure Clue:*

No temptation has overtaken you but such as is common to man; and God is faithful, who will not allow you to be tempted beyond what you are able, but with the temptation will provide a way of escape also, so that you will be able to endure it.

—1 Cor. 10:13 NASB

Let's rewrite this verse and personalize it. Fill in the blanks with your name.

No temptation will overtake _____ but only what is common to man; and God is faithful, who will not allow _____ to be tempted beyond what _____ is able, but with the temptation will provide a way of escape also, so that _____ will be able to endure it.

God is there for you no matter what circumstances or doughnuts come your way. Sometimes it may be something as simple as an addiction to sugar, and other times it may be something as exasperating as an addiction to sugar. Last week we journeyed into fasting and the ability to overcome addictions. Now we need to address how we got in this sticky mess.

If we want to make changes, it begins with getting God involved. Read our Treasure Clue again. This time, say it out loud.

Write a prayer of praise for what God can do in your life in view of temptation.

_____

_____

_____

_____

What's Hidden in Your Food?

The stir-fry vegetable dish tasted more enhanced one holiday weekend when we had one of my foodie friends cooking with us. I was doing a quick stir-fry of chicken and assorted vegetables when I let my foodie friend finish it up with spices of her choice. When I took a bite I was amazed that herbs could add such a savory sweet flavor to vegetables. In fact, the vegetables were hardly noticeable due to the new flavor. When I inquired how she was able to come up with this taste, she admitted she had added a couple of tablespoons of sugar to the dish!

Read 1 Corinthians 6:12. This verse could have been written for our sugar habits. Compare the last phrase of the verse in your translation to these two:

". . . I will not be mastered by anything" (NASB).
"I will not be brought under the power of any" (KJV).

Many people are mastered or powered by sugar, but may not even be aware of it. North America has turned into the land of "sugar-holics." We eat huge quantities of sugar, in the form of refined sugars added to foods we choose to eat as well as naturally occurring sugars in fruits and vegetables. Much of the sugar we eat is "hidden" sugar—we are unaware we are consuming it. Foods once unsweetened are now sweetened, and others previously sweet have been elevated to higher levels of sweetness.

Hidden sugars are primarily the result of manufacturers. For example, the sugar content of meat is increased by feeding sugar to animals before slaughter to improve the flavor and color of the meat, and by adding it to the meat itself as it is prepared in packinghouses and restaurants. Any dish prepared with ground meat may contain added syrups to help minimize shrinkage and to improve flavor, juiciness, and texture.[178]

Recognizing foods with sugar is often difficult either because the manufacturers are not required to list the sugar content, or it may be disguised in a product. The following is a list of foods where hidden sugars should be suspected:[179]

Bouillon cubes	Instant coffee or tea
Breading for fried or baked poultry/meats	Iodized salt
Canned and frozen vegetables/fruit	Luncheon meat
Catsup	Peanut butter
Convenience foods	Potato chips
Cottage cheese	Salad dressings
Dry roasted nuts	Soups
Frozen or canned entrees	Hot dogs
Gravies	

The following list contains words that identify that sugar is contained in a product:

Brown sugar	Maltodextrin
Corn syrup	Mannitol
Corn syrup solids	Maple syrup
Dextrose	Molasses
Fructose	Raw sugar
Glucose	Sorbitol
Grain syrups	Sucrose
High fructose corn syrup	Turbinado
Honey	Xylitol
Malt syrup	

How is sugar absorbed in our body? Dr. Krohn, in the book *Allergy Relief and Prevention, A Practical Encyclopedia,* tells us:

Sugar, like alcohol, is rapidly absorbed and floods the system (body), predisposing the sensitive person to severe reactions and addictions. In a study done by Dr. Timothy Jones of Yale University, adults and children were given proportionately equal doses of glucose, the form of sugar to which all carbohydrates in blood are metabolized. The children received twenty teaspoons of glucose, the sugar equivalent of two twelve-ounce colas. The blood glucose levels in both the adults and children recorded similar highs and lows, but the adrenalin levels of the children were twice as high as those of the adults. More of the children felt weak and shaky. As a result of this study, Dr. Jones suggests the increase in adrenalin could be linked to the hyperactivity some children display after eating sweets.[180]

When I was growing up, we always had dessert on Sunday. But when I got married, my husband had other ideas; he wanted sweets after each dinner. That was a new idea I was willing to join with fervor. For the first twenty years of our marriage, we always had sugary treats on hand but we paid the price in our health. Now we have reverted to dessert on Sunday, and we always look forward to it with anticipation.

Review of the Three Principles

Review each principle. Write down how each applies to sugar and what foods we need to avoid and keep in our diet.

Principle I—Eat the foods God designed for us to eat.

_____

_____

Principle II—Eat the foods closest to the way He designed them, before they have been altered.

_____

_____

Principle III—Do not let any food become an addiction.

_____

_____

1 Timothy 4:7 says, "Discipline yourself for the purpose of godliness" (N.ASB). Timothy gives us words we can live with. Sugar is addictive, but discipline will help us overcome this behavior. It will not be easy, but the outcome is, as he says, "for the purpose of godliness." If sugar is more important to you than anything else in life, you have a problem.

Taking this treasure to heart: Let's review the Treasure Clues from this week and pull one truth from each verse you can apply to your life.

"Pleasant words are as a honeycomb, sweet to the soul, and health to the bones" (Prov. 16:24 KJV). Honey in our diet brings healing, just as sweet words renew the soul. If we were to speak sweet words several times a day to the same person, it may become sickening. They may think you are up to something. But the right words at the right time bring comfort. Honey is sweet in the right amounts, but too much can bring discomfort.

Truth from this verse: _____

_____

"Love the Lord your God with all your heart and with all your soul and with all your strength" (Deut. 6:5 NIV). Every part of our being needs to love the Lord. Any distraction from this love leaves us missing in action. God has given us every good gift; no one can take that away. Man may try to alter it or improve on it, but the real stuff is still there for you.

Truth from this verse: _____

_____

"Whether you turn to the right or to the left, your ears will hear a voice behind you, saying, 'This is the way; walk in it'" (Isa. 30:21 NIV). God's ways are clear, but sometimes our minds become foggy with convenience and instant gratification.

Truth from this verse: _____

_____

"No temptation has overtaken you but such as is common to man; and God is faithful, who will not allow you to be tempted beyond what you are able, but with the temptation will provide a way of escape also, so that you will be able to endure it" (1 Cor. 10:13 NASB). This week we have learned all the nutrients God has placed in his gift of sweets. One of the most prevalent problems in our country is too much sugar in our diet. What truth can you find in this verse to help with this problem?

_____

_____

_____

Is sugar a temptation for you? _____ How have you dealt with this in the past?

_____

Did your plan work, or is there still a problem? _____

You are not totally to blame for this problem. Sugar has been increased in processed foods. This increase, along with other chemical reactions in your system, has contributed to this addiction. The question now is how you are going to overcome this problem. Read the Treasure Clue again. What answer to temptation can we find in 1 Corinthians 10:13?

_____

Affirmation: Using one of the Treasure Clues from this week, write out an affirmation. Here is an example: "I will overcome my addiction to sugar because my desire and purpose is for godliness. My life will be filled with a pure joy by following Isaiah's words to walk this way."

_____

_____

Applying this treasure at home: On your Action Plan, write out a plan to incorporate what you have learned this week. Share this with your foodie friend and pray for each other's plans, ask God for a way to overcome temptations.

FABULOUS FOODIE FRIDAY

Grab your sweet foodie friend and start making some changes in your recipes. First, you will need some healthy ingredients. Let's start with some raw honey. If you cannot locate a local source, then find the best health food store around, and most likely it will carry this treat. You will notice the price is a little high. This is actually a good thing—you won't waste it, nor will you encourage your family to eat too much. Once you have found this treasure, always store it in a cool, dry place. Some honeys will crystallize on you, but that can be remedied by placing the container in a pan of water and heating it on the lowest setting until it has liquefied. Sometimes this can take hours if the container is large. Be careful of plastic containers. You don't want to heat them and release plastics into your valuable honey.

Sweet Substitutes[181]

Find a recipe such as cookies, bread, or dressing where you can use honey instead of sugar. I have even used honey in yogurt to make my own "whipped topping." Refer to the _Healthy Treasures Cookbook_ for instructions on cooking with honey.

Then go to the store for these ingredients: vanilla (natural), cinnamon, plain yogurt, organic applesauce, and spices such as mint, anise, cloves, and ginger. All these ingredients are ways for you to create sweet treats without the complications of heavy sugar.

Are you ready to give up the white powder? Here are some suggestions to satisfy your sweet tooth. Remember, moderation is part of discipline.

CINNAMON

Cinnamon is a sweet spice. When used in a recipe, less sugar is needed. A cinnamon stick can also be used as a stir stick in hot chocolate and coffee. Two teaspoons of cinnamon can change a tart apple pie into a sweet one. As an additional perk, one teaspoon of cinnamon contains twenty-eight milligrams of calcium and trace amounts of B vitamins and fiber. It's a divine design!

SWEET SPICES

We already learned that herbs and spices will help us with less salt, but the same is true for sugar. Try these spices to accent the flavors in foods: mint, anise, cloves, and ginger. A sprinkle of nutmeg is an additional sweet complement to cinnamon.

VANILLA

This natural extract helps lessen the amount of sugar needed in a recipe. Other flavorings such as almond, coconut, peppermint, and maple would contribute the same benefit. Try increasing or adding these extracts and lessening the amount of sugar in a recipe. I suggest you do this gradually to avoid an all-out war in your home by cutting out too much sugar at one time. Also try recipes in small batches until you master the taste everyone enjoys. Cutting back sugar a little at a time will gradually help your family become less addicted.

FRUIT CONCENTRATES

Fructose is sweeter than table sugar, and because of its more steady absorption and metabolism in the bloodstream, it doesn't produce the roller coaster effect of refined sugar. Fruit concentrates such as pear and apples are the best. You can buy them in the store already prepared, but the best route to take is to find some ripe pears or apples in the organic aisle. Peel them and throw them in the blender or food processor. The sauce will taste yummy and can be used on ice cream, yogurt, and in recipes to replace sugar and honey.

FRUIT TOPPINGS

Use crushed pineapple, strawberries, blueberries, and applesauce instead of syrup on pancakes and waffles. Sprinkle some cinnamon or nutmeg to bring out the fruits' natural sweetness.

Out With the Old, in With the New

Go through your pantry and refrigerator; remove all foods containing artificial sweeteners. Set them on your counter. Is your draw to any of these foods too strong for you to let go? What will it take for your belief in the foods God designed to help you change this stronghold?

Fanatical Foodist: For those of you who desire a new source of income or just some sweet sticky syrup to call your own, starting your own beehive collection might be the chance you've been waiting for. Look on the Internet for sources to help you get started in the hobby of bees.

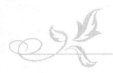

Environment and Toxins

DAY ONE—REMOVING DECAY FROM THE TREASURE

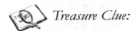 *Treasure Clue:*

*We will stand before this house and before You (for Your name is in this house)
and cry to You in our distress, and You will hear and deliver us.*
—2 Chron. 20:9 NASB

"Don't take another step closer!" Have you ever heard yourself say or think these words? What would the invader look like? Would it be your little three-year-old covered with mud or your husband covered in grease after working on the car? It might even be a stranger. The invaders coming into our homes today are not the unwanted mud, grease, or fear but instead though a Trojan horse. We are actually inviting these enemies inside. Jehoshaphat had the same problem. We can learn a lot from him.

Let's get some background on this king. Read 2 Chronicles 17:1-3.

What did you learn about him?

_____

_____

_____

In chapter 18, verse 4, we see a conversation between Jehoshaphat and King Ahab. King Ahab wants to invade a neighboring country and wants Jehoshaphat to join him. What is Jehoshaphat's recommendation?

_____

Do you see how Jehoshaphat is a man seeking God's guidance in everything he does? This is our model to follow. We are now going to get to the heart of our chapter. Judah is about to be invaded by the armies of Moab, Ammon, and the Meunites.

Treasures of Healthy Living

Read 2 Chronicles 20:1-3. What was Jehoshaphat's first reaction and his response?

_____

_____

_____

Did you notice he proclaimed a fast for everyone—not just himself? How would you feel if our president proclaimed a fast for everyone to partake in?

_____

Find the people's response in verse 4, and record it here. ("Judah" refers to the whole people group.)

_____

_____

_____

Jehoshaphat then stood before the people and gave a mighty prayer. Read this prayer in verses 6-13. Fill in the blanks.

Verse 9 (NASB)—" _____will _____before this house… _____
_____ is in this house."

Verse 12 (NASB)—"Our eyes are on _____"

In verses 14-19, the Lord answers Jehoshaphat's prayer. Fill in the blanks.

Verse 15 (NASB)—"Do not _____or be _____"

Verse 17 (NASB)—"Do not _____ or be _____ …for the
_____ is with _____."

How do those verses make you feel? You see, these verses were not only written for Judah, but also for you and me. We can learn how God works by reading His words from many years ago. Remember, God never changes; if He was there for them, He is here for you today.

More words to treasure:

Verse 20 (NASB)—"Put your trust in the Lord your God and you will be established."
Verse 21 (NASB)—"Give thanks to the Lord, for His loving kindness is everlasting."

The word *established* means "to thrive" or "grow successfully." *Everlasting* means "same as God" and "lasting forever."[182] Take a moment now to really let these words absorb into your heart and mind.

Write out how those verses make you feel.

_____

_____

_____

Jehoshaphat is praying about the evil that is about to come upon his people. This evil might be a sword, judgment, pestilence, or famine. No matter what, the people will stand before this house, and before God, and cry out. We are in a similar situation today and need to stand before our homes and cry out. Our enemy is toxins, and they are coming into our homes in many various ways from our fork to our cleaners instead of a sword; our food is loaded with pesticides (pestilence), and our famine is in the form of disease. We will have to make choices on how to protect our homes and families. Our fast will be from commercials and advertisements. Instead, we will focus on education.

How can we apply Jehoshaphat's situation to our life today?

_____

_____

Our Natural Defense

Our body is designed with an incredible defense system that keeps us healthy even under extreme circumstances, without our having to give it a second thought. God designed our body to handle the trash from our foods and environmental contaminants, and the ability to eliminate and clean at the same time.

Our body contains four main exit points for removing the trash: skin, lungs, colon, and the urinary tract. Before any of those systems work, the liver and the lymph system have already completed the primary work of clean-up in the cells. In a previous week, we discussed the role of fiber and how it helps cleanse the whole digestive system. Our study on water helped us see the benefit of cleansing every cell with the correct fluid balance. But our best defense is the liver.

The liver is the most important organ for detoxification. A properly functioning liver protects you from environmental and metabolic toxins. When it becomes overwhelmed by faulty digestion and an overload of environmental toxins, it stores these toxins in fat cells, much the same way that we put boxes in the garage or basement to deal with later. If the liver has time later, it can deal with the stored toxins, but most commonly it is busy dealing with what is newly coming in and never catches up. As these toxins mount up, they are a continued source of inflammation in the body.[183] This inflammation leads to all the serious health problems listed in this week's study. The liver needs to be fueled properly to perform its detoxification duties and to maintain adequate levels of antioxidants to keep working its job as trash collector and eliminator—or, as I like to call it, the "Toxin Terminator."

Raw foods, especially the cruciferous vegetables, will give the liver enzymes it needs to make its work easier. You may also want to try supplements containing the herbs milk thistle, dandelion, turmeric, reishi mushroom, and artichoke. Research has shown that these herbs will support the body's ability to make proteins to help the liver regenerate liver cells.[184] This means we will increase our Toxin Terminator's army.

DIGGING DEEPER: Read "Functions of the Liver" and "Energizing Enzymes" in the *Nutrition Manual*. Then go to the Designed Healthy Living website to take the Liver Quiz under the Happy and Healthy Tab. These articles and quiz will greatly benefit your understanding of this topic.

From your reading in this study and the *Nutrition Manual* write out three main functions of the liver.

_____

_____

Natural or Synthetics

The use of synthetics—manmade elements—in our purchases has prompted a gold rush among scientists. The first scientist who discovered the ability to make synthetic dyes for clothing in the 1940s earned a fortune. This idea of making chemicals perform like nature—only cheaper, easier to produce, and more permanent—spurred on a new industry. It resulted in the common person being able to afford clothes in a beautiful array of colors and textures. From clothes, to additives to our food, to drugs to keep us going, the lab became the mixing bowl for more and more synthetics. The chemical industry has snowballed into what is now the biggest industry in the world.

This is true of every synthetic created. The chemicals make life easier for the consumer and cheaper for the industry, and there is an unending shelf life to protect the investment. In theory, this is a good business plan with a win-win solution for all. The industry wins with a high-selling product, and the consumer wins with convenience. We are busy families who have less time to cook than previous generations, so we buy processed foods or fast food. We have less time to clean, so we buy cleaners that are guaranteed to make a breeze out of cleaning. We have less time to iron, so we buy clothes that are wrinkle free. And finally, we need drugs to combat all the toxic influences coming into our bodies. But in actuality these choices have cost us our health.

We are ingesting many chemicals such as pesticides, preservatives, additives, pollutants, and contaminants through our foods and food containers. We drink them in tap water, which contains chemicals leached from contaminated soils, environmental pollutants, and even chemicals added deliberately such as fluoride. We absorb them through our skin from cosmetics, toiletries, treated wood, sprayed plants, treated areas of public parks, golf courses, bath water, and swimming pools. We even inhale them in air contaminated with solvents, car fumes, industrial waste, and environmental pollution.

God designed our bodies to have a natural detox (cleansing) system. Without this we would have already lived a short life and would be in heaven enjoying paradise. The problem is that our bodies were never designed to protect themselves against this amount of chemical ambush. As a result, our systems fail to process and remove most of these chemicals once they have entered our bodies, and there is buildup. Consequently, every one of us is now permanently contaminated with these modern synthetic chemicals.

The outcome of this constant poisoning has been linked to the development and triggering of an ever-increasing number of diseases, such as asthma, autoimmune diseases, cancer, cardiovascular disease, diabetes, and thyroid disease. Many leading scientists have hypothesized that these chemicals are now playing a primary role in bringing about an epidemic of these and many other chronic illnesses.[185]

The pace of change has been so remarkable that the number of people affected by many of these diseases appears to be doubling every few decades.[186] The answer to these problems has led to the development of drugs to combat the symptoms. This has worked well for the pharmaceutical companies—better than it has for the average American whose health continues to plummet. We need to get back to the basics and find natural solutions that protect our health and decrease our exposure to the chemicals that are trying to claim our health.

The result from our discovery and application of this knowledge will be truly amazing health benefits when you reduce your chemical toxicity. Not only will you greatly reduce existing disease symptoms, but you may also experience many health side effects such as weight loss, increased energy, less muscular and joint pain, a lower incidence of allergy symptoms, clearer thinking, improved digestion, a more positive outlook, and better skin. These results make it worth it to continue this week's study!

Taking this treasure to heart: Have you made steps to consider the toxins in your environment before this study? Are you ready to guard your treasure chest? Write out one new truth you have learned today.

_____

_____

DAY TWO—BECOME A DETECTIVE ON THE HUNT FOR TOXINS

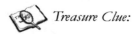 *Treasure Clue:*

How long will you love what is worthless and aim at deception?

—Ps. 4:2 NASB

My son Spencer had just turned three when, one day, I noticed he was coughing a lot. At first, I didn't think anything of it. Kids get sick. I told him to lie down, thinking he'd be fine—it was just a cough. A short time later I realized that his heart was pounding, as if it was trying to beat right out of his chest. Terrified, my husband Roger and I rushed him to the hospital. The emergency room doctors placed our son on oxygen and gave him strong steroids to help clear his airways. We spent the next two nights in the intensive care unit. The doctors told us he had something called reactive airways dysfunction syndrome—a form of asthma.

Asthma? How did our little boy develop asthma? We never heard of asthma coming on so suddenly. We were confused and sick with worry.

We talked to our son's doctor. We talked to other doctors. We asked questions but never got satisfactory answers. Ultimately, we knew our son's condition had to be either genetic or environmental. Neither my husband nor I had any family history of asthma, going back for four generations. So we concluded the cause was environmental.[187]

Sloan Barnett's experience as a consumer reporter helped her investigate the tangled web of information in regard to asthma. She discovered a strong link between the use of certain cleaning products and asthma. "The cause of my son's asthma may have been me. I may have been poisoning my own son."[188]

What Is Clean, and How Does It Affect Our Health?

This week we are going to venture through our homes in detective style. Our quest is to find the villains that are stealing our health. Let's begin with an inventory of your health and see if you are dealing with any toxic problems.

After each health problem below write the name or initial of the family member who is dealing with this difficulty. This does not mean the toxin is the main culprit, but it means we need to address the possibility.

Symptoms from toxins:

Abnormal EEG

Allergies

Asthma

Alzheimer's disease

Anemia

Anorexia

Antisocial behavior

Anxiety

Balance problems

Behavioral problems

Blood clots

Bone damage (including fractures)

Brain damage (particularly children)

Cancer

Coarse tremors

Collapse

Confusion

Convulsions

Deafness and visual problems

Depression

Dizziness

Eczema

Emotional ability

Excessive flow of saliva

Headache

Heart arrhythmias

Heart attack

Hyperactivity in children

Impaired concentration

Increased cholesterol

Infertility

Inflammation of mouth / gums

Irritability

Jerky gait

Kidney damage

Learning disabilities

Lethargy

Loosening of teeth

Loss of concentration

Loss of IQ / thinking

Lowered immune system

Memory loss / difficulties

Mental confusion

Mental status changes

Migraines

Muscle tremors

Nausea

Nervousness

Panic attacks

Paralysis

Personality changes

Problems identifying words, colors, or numbers, and an inability to speak fluently

Reduced energy

Reduced IQ

Seizures

Severe abdominal pain/anemia
Severe fatigue
Skin numbness
Spasm of extremities
Speech disturbances
Stroke
Suicidal tendencies

Swelling of salivary glands
Thin hair and skin
Thyroid disease
Visual disturbances
Vomiting
Weight problems

Does this long list seem overwhelming? Did you make it through without relating to any symptoms? Most of us are dealing with several of them. This was probably a wake-up call, since toxins are not usually considered when dealing with a health problem. Keep in mind Dr. Couey and I are not suggesting you disregard any professional health program as you go through this study. Medications are needed in our society. What we would like for you to do is continue to read, and let's discover together what possibilities are contributing to this trauma and how we can change the environment we live in.

Going Through the Home

Many of us think of our home as a refuge, a place where we know we are safe. When it comes to toxins and carcinogens (chemicals that are known to cause cancer), the Environmental Protection Agency (EPA) has found the home is five times more polluted than outside.[189] In fact, the Center for Disease Control and Prevention conducted a comprehensive study to determine the degree to which Americans are contaminated with specific toxic substances. The result is that most Americans, especially children, have dozens of pesticides and other toxic compounds in their bodies, many of them linking to health threats. The most frequent contributing source for these chemicals is lurking in your home—under your sink and in your cabinets—in typical household cleaners.

These chemicals loiter in our brains, contaminate our immune system, lodge in our fatty tissue, and destroy other vital organs. Dr. Paula Baile Hamilton, in her book *Toxic Overload,* explains our problem: "The problem we now face is from the buildup of toxic effects these chemicals appear to be having on our health. With the average person being contaminated by an average of three hundred to five hundred industrial chemicals, the issue of how to deal with these unwanted invaders has become a problem for each and every one of us whether we like it or not."[190]

Ignoring the problem will not make it go away. If you marked a lot of symptoms on the list, you know we need to do something. Making changes could possibly save your life, and it could be the best investment you will make for your health.

Start in the kitchen by looking under the sink. Take inventory of all the cleaning products you have under the sink or in another cabinet. List them here:

_____

_____

_____

_____

Now let's play a game with the products you wrote down. First, read the chemical names below and the health effects caused from using this ingredient.

SODIUM HYDROXIDE

Take a look at the problems caused by sodium hydroxide:

- Causes 75 percent of all caustic (corrosive) injury to the esophagus of kids under five years old
- Can cause burns in tissues—eyes, skin, mouth, and throat
- Can cause chronic skin irritation
- Can cause irritation to the respiratory tract
- Can cause liver and kidney damage

The following list is a sampling of products that contain sodium hydroxide (the actual brand names have been withheld): drain cleaners, dishwashing liquids, oven cleaners, toilet bowl cleaners, stain pens, kids' toothpaste, adult whitening toothpaste, grease cleaners, deodorants, scrub cleaners, laundry products, laundry soap for whites, and powdered cleansers. Use a red pen to circle the products in your home that might contain sodium hydroxide.

MONOETHANOLAMINE (MEA)

The chemical monoethanolamine has been linked to asthma. It can be found in baby laundry cleaners, liquid laundry cleaners, and floor cleaners. Use an orange pen to mark which of these products you own.

HYDROCHLORIC ACID

Hydrochloric acid can cause the following problems:

- Severe damage to skin and eyes (note: do not inhale)
- Throat irritation, even when exposed briefly and at low levels (note: can be fatal if swallowed)
- Linked to reactive airways dysfunction—asthma

This chemical can be found in toilet bowl cleaners, odor eliminators, and corrosion build-up removers. Mark the products you own with a blue pen.

BUTYL CELLOSOLVE

The following issues are related to the chemical butyl cellosolve:

- Linked to reproductive harm
- Can cause irritation and tissue damage from inhalation
- Fifteen minutes of exposure (such as while cleaning a shower) could cause a person to inhale three times the acute exposure limit

Butyl cellosolve is found in some green building cleaners, all-purpose cleaners, cleaning wipes, floor polish, window cleaners, rug shampoos, electronic cleaners, and degreasers. Mark the products you own with a green pen.

Other toxic ingredients to avoid in your products include: ammonia, formaldehyde, hydrocarbons, petroleum distillates, chlorine bleach, dyes, glycols, and phosphoric and sulfuric acid.

This has been just a preview of chemicals that could be causing harm to you, your family, and your pets. How colorful is your list? When I first did this, mine looked like a rainbow—a deadly rainbow. Every one of my favorite products was harmful. It is time to find safer choices.

What Can You Do?

Though it may seem like every product has harmful toxins, there are many alternatives. The following list will help you replace your toxic products with safer ones.

1. Visit www.householdproducts.nlm.nih.gov/ingredients.htm. This is the National Institutes of Health Household Products Database, where you can find out what toxins you have in your home. Enter the names of chemicals and see which brands contain

them. Then look up "Toxicity Information" or "Health Information" for each chemical. From there you can find safer alternatives. There are only a few good choices, so be
wise in your decision.

2. Replace your toxic cleaners with as little as one natural, nontoxic all-purpose cleaner.
   Our staff was delighted to find a safe, economical, and powerful cleaner for our whole
   home. Contact our office if you want to know our favorite choice.

3. Get clean hands by using pH balanced soap and hot water instead of hand wash with
   alcohol or triclosan. Triclosan increases resistance of bacteria to antibiotics.

4. Accept that real clean has no smell, and get rid of all the phthalates in your air fresheners.
   Phthalates cause reproductive and developmental damage.

5. Replace your laundry detergent with a natural nontoxic one so the clothes you wear
   and the sheets you sleep on have no fumes for you to breathe.

6. Use vinegar, lemon juice, and baking soda to safely clean your home. If you want to
   go this route, you will find many recipes on the Internet. Personally, this is not my
   preference because of the smell and smear.

7. Investigate organics. Organic cleaners are the best choice, but they are not all created
   equal. Choose products from a company that was in the organic cleaning business before it became popular. Many companies are jumping on the bandwagon because of
   profits—not to protect the environment or your health. A "green" product may fit in the
   government guidelines but not be the best for your health. Be smart about your choice.

DIGGING DEEPER: In the *Treasures of Health Nutrition Manual,* read the chapter titled
Healthy Home, including topics such as: "Carcinogens to Avoid," "Chemicals in
Household Products," "Ways to Reduce Chemicals in Your Home and Body,"
"Xenobiotics," and "Plastics—Know Your Numbers."

Other Invaders

The symptoms listed at the beginning of today's lesson are caused not only by the cleaners
in our homes, but also by heavy metals. Heavy metals include aluminum, mercury, lead, fluorine, solvents, and plasticizers. An abbreviated list of sources would include: cooking utensils,
dental amalgam, food additives, food contaminants, tap water, vaccine additives, disinfectants,
gasoline, pesticides, toothpaste, nit shampoo, paints, dyes, flame retardants, rubber adhesives,
mothballs, aftershaves, polystyrene cups, toiletries, and fish.

Basic steps to get rid of these villains in your body:

- Treasures of Health Mediterranean Pyramid
- Exercise
- Healthy supplement program
- Remove all invaders

*We should all be concerned about the future because we
will have to spend the rest of our lives there.*

—Charles Kettering[191]

Taking this treasure to heart: Our Treasure Clue asked us how long we will love what is worthless and aim at deception. Many people love their cleaners so much that change will be difficult. Isn't it funny how we believe commercials? We think that because children on TV are happy from the use of a certain cleaner, we will have a happy home if we use it! Today we learned that there are better options. We can make a difference in our homes.

DAY THREE—LOOKING GOOD ON THE JOURNEY

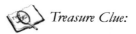 *Treasure Clue:*

The King will desire your beauty. Because He is your Lord, bow down to Him.

—Ps. 45:11 NASB

The King, who sees the inside of us more than the outside, desires our beauty. Everything we have learned from this study (and continue to learn) benefits the whole person. If you want to look beautiful, then follow these teachings.

When you look in the mirror do you "glow"? Is that glow from chemicals or a natural beauty? Some products get really personal. We are attached to these products since they make us smell nice, look pretty, and feel clean. This is an area in which we really need to be on the offensive and get rid of intruders. Let's take a look at our personal care items.

How many personal care items do you use on a normal day? A study done by the Environmental Working Group found that we use an average of nine products daily with a combined total of 126 unique ingredients. This accumulates to more than five pounds of products per year placed on our skin. Sounds heavy to me.

Let's see if your family is any different. Next to each of the following products, write the initials of each family member who uses it at least twice a week. There are spaces for you to add some of your own at the bottom.

Bubble bath	Toner
Cosmetics	Mascara
Eye cream	Shampoo
Conditioner	Shaving cream
Deodorant	Insect repellant
Eyeliner	Mascara
Face cleanser	Shower gel
Lotion	Sunscreen
Powder	Toothpaste
Shaving cream	_____
Soap	_____

 Are you surprised at the number of products used in your household? Did you know there are healthy alternatives for each one of them?

"Look twenty years younger!" "No more wrinkles!" "Have the beauty of a model!" "Have silky, shiny hair!" "Show brilliant white teeth!" The manufacturers of personal care products make promises, and we buy into them. Most of us have assumed that since they are sold to the public they must be safe. However, these products are in the same category as the cleaners—the untested category.

Your skin is your largest organ—and even though it has thirty-two layers it is still the thinnest. Less than one-tenth of an inch separates your body from potential toxins. Worse yet, your skin is highly permeable. Sixty percent of what you put on your skin will end up in your blood stream to be distributed throughout your body. Pharmaceutical companies learned this, and we now have patches to stop smoking, patches for heart disease, and patches for birth control. This is why some people say, "Don't put anything on your body that you wouldn't eat if you had to."

Labels Won't Protect You

When it comes to the beauty industry, anything goes. I find it interesting that the FDA actually has no authority to require the products we use to be tested for safety.[192] A valuable resource is an organization with solid scientific credentials known as the Environmental Working

Group. They maintain a massive database on the ingredients and hazards associated with the vast majority of personal care products sold in this country. It's called Skin Deep and it's easy to check the products you use every day. Just go to www.cosmeticdatabase.com. This database does not list products sold by direct sales or home marketing.

Currently, there are estimated to be more than 10,500 cosmetic and personal care products on the North American market. Of those products, the Environmental Working Group estimates that 98 percent of the products contain one or more ingredients that have never been evaluated for safety.[193]

Some Words to Learn From

The following phrases are often found on cosmetics. It's important to know what they mean. "For Professional Use Only"—This phrase allows cosmetic companies to remove harmful chemicals from their labels.

"Hypoallergenic"—No actual testing is necessary to claim that a product is "hypoallergenic," "allergy-free," or "safe for sensitive skin." Neither the FDA nor any other regulating body requires the companies to prove these claims.

"Harmful Chemicals"—Unless they are intentionally placed in the product, harmful chemicals are not required to be listed.

We are in charge of our family's health, and the solution is to not depend on the FDA since it cannot actively act on a product until after it has already severely injured or killed many people. But we can make a difference by eliminating the ingredients that could possibly cause harm. A number of these potential toxins have estrogen-mimicking effects that can wreak havoc on all your good health intentions. There are other potential problems as well.

The following are some ingredients to avoid:

- Parabens are an ingredient extensively used as preservatives in the cosmetic industry. They can be found in natural foods—and some natural cosmetics may include these ingredients—but they also come from the laboratory in a synthetic form. Parabens may cause cancer due to their hormone disrupting qualities, and they also may have an effect on the endocrine system.[194]
- Mineral oil, paraffin, and petrolatum are all petroleum products and coat the skin like plastic. This will clog pores and create a build up of toxins. They can also slow cellular development and create earlier signs of aging.
- Two common shampoo ingredients, sodium laurel and lauryl sulfate (also known as sodium laureth sulfate), have been found to cause severe epidermal changes in the skin.

These chemicals are not to be confused with the following natural ingredients: sodium lauryl sulfoacetate, disodium laureth sulfosuccinate, or amonium laureth sulfate. As you can see, it is very confusing to determine the natural from the synthetic.

- Acrylamide—found in many facial creams—is linked to mammary tumors.

Besides avoiding these hazards, there are some other steps you can take to create that young-looking skin you *really* want.

Steps to Looking Healthy

It has been said many times, beauty is more than skin deep. Attempting to change your appearance from the outside while neglecting what goes on inside is a temporary fix at best. The steps to looking healthy include the same steps we mentioned yesterday to get rid of toxins: eating the foods you have learned about here in this study, exercising and perspiring, using supplements, and removing all contaminants—especially from your skin. Every day of your life, pollution, grime, and dust attach themselves to the surface of your skin. If you don't take a couple minutes daily to cleanse your face and unclog your pores, your skin may look sluggish, instead of at its bright and shining best. Cleaning your skin is important, just like keeping your internal organs clean and healthy.

It may seem like a cliché, but there are things you can do to prevent damaging your skin. Many of the visible signs of aging are caused by external factors that you can at least partially control.

The following actions may be the easiest and least expensive things you can do to prevent damage to your skin, gain a more youthful appearance, and build a strong foundation for your natural skin care.

- Avoid or minimize damage from hot water and chlorine. Although taking baths and showers may seem like it's health-promoting and relaxing, your skin may disagree. This is especially true if you have chlorinated water, which is almost certainly the case (unless your water comes from a well). Chlorine causes oxidative damage. The hotter the water, the more potential for damage, because the rate of chemical reactions increases with temperature. *Hot water may cause your skin to age faster.* A chlorine filter is a good investment for your showers.
- Use gentle and safe skin care products that are pH balanced. God designed our skin to have an acid mantle. The acid mantle is a very fine, slightly acidic film on the surface of your skin acting as a barrier to bacteria, viruses, and other potential contaminants that may penetrate the skin. Antibacterial cleaners remove the acid mantle and our protection. Choose only products that say "pH balanced" on the label.

- Fragrances were designed to block body odor. Today, body odor is not an issue, so fragrances and perfumes are now used to make a statement. If perfume is on your list of "can't live without" items, apply it to your clothing instead of your skin. Foodie Friday will include a recipe to make your own fragrance.
- Don't smoke. Smoking causes free radical production, which is one cause of the signs of aging in skin.
- If you will be in the sun for extended periods of time, use a natural sunscreen product with safe and effective ingredients.
- Pay attention to the warnings on toothpaste, and avoid fluoride. There are several organic toothpastes that polish your teeth without the toxic chemicals.
- Antiperspirants and deodorants block sweat and cover smell. The jury is still out on conclusively determining the effect of aluminum in deodorants and the link to Alzheimer's, so my decision is to not wait and avoid it as much as possible.
- Nail polish is another product with known toxins such as formaldehyde, toluene, and phthalates. Toluene harms the central nervous system. There are products that are toxin-free, but clean groomed nails are beautiful in themselves.
- Hair color products are among the greatest toxin offenders. A Harvard School of Public Health study found that women using hair dye five or more times a year had twice the risk of ovarian cancer than those who did not.[195] Going gray is the new blond!
- Has your skin taken its vitamins? Whenever you apply skin care products, it is ideal to use products from nature that nourish your skin the same way you nourish your body.
- Look for products that repair cells as well as build healthy new ones. It may take a month, or even two to three months, to notice changes. Plus, it's quite possible that others will notice your increasingly youthful-looking face before you do. Remember: it took years to get where you are today, so show patience when expecting changes and improvements.

DAY FOUR—ALLERGIES—NOT WANTED IN THE TREASURE

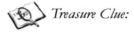 *Treasure Clue:*

Teach me your way, O LORD; lead me in a straight path because of my oppressors.

—Ps. 27:11 NIV

How many times have you been outside on a brisk morning walk when a rock gets in your shoe and starts causing pain? You have two choices: continue in pain or get relief. There are thirty-five million people in the US dealing with diagnosed allergies. The question is how many more would there be if everyone who experienced allergies went to the doctor? My guess is the number would double. That is an alarming number of people either way you look at it. What can be the cause?

What about food intolerances and chemical insensitivities; do they count in the number? They do not. That would be another large group of people who suffer on any given day in America. Those with environmental issues, allergies, and insensitivities are dealing with lots of rocks in their shoes. There are some who walk around without any rocks and are symptom free, enjoying life to the fullest. Are you one of them, or do you want to be?

List the allergies you and the family members living in your home are dealing with.

_____

_____

_____

_____

We need to be on the lookout for the stowaways hitching a ride into our body and causing these allergies. It is time to place a guard on that chest and not allow any invaders. In order to do this we need to be able to identify these villains or pirates. These toxins need to be uncovered for who they really are and how they can steal from our health and longevity. Dr. Jacqueline Krohn comments, "Good health and a strong immune system are our most precious possessions. Allergies are not just a nuisance to be ignored until they can no longer be denied—they constitute a health problem that must be treated. Untreated allergies can lead to more serious difficulties as we get older. Blood pressure problems, diabetes, cardiovascular disorders, arthritis, and other degenerative diseases can develop as a result of untreated allergies."[196]

Our healthy lifestyle is being attacked more each day. More than five thousand new chemicals are being brought into use each year, and only 7 percent of them have been fully studied for toxicity. Our exposure to harmful chemicals is rapidly increasing. Our immune systems are often so overloaded that unless prevention and treatment are practiced, dysfunction and illness may result.

According to the FDA, millions of people suffer from food allergies.[197] Problems with allergies are rampant in our society. Many symptoms that people take for granted as a condition of life are actually symptoms of an allergic reaction. If your family is not yet plagued by food allergies, you are in a great position to prevent it by making changes now. If you already have these allergies, you can still make a difference. Start by going through your pantry and cupboards. What foods are you willing to remove for the sake of your family's health?

Understand Allergies and Testing

There are numerous methods of testing for allergies. In week seven of this study we learned the benefits of fasting. One type of fast is the removal of a certain food or food group. Doing this method for four to seven days and then reintroducing the foods one at a time and observing the symptoms is a simple way to find an allergen. The problem is our addiction to the foods we are allergic to. This means the withdrawal symptoms may be severe. In the *Nutrition Manual* you will find an article titled "The Healing Crises." This article simplifies the process of healing when we start to make changes in our diet and nutritional products. The same crises will happen when we work to eliminate the foods that cause allergies. Other than fasting, there are dozens of other methods to determine allergies. It is best to work with a physician who specializes in environmental medicine. The book *Allergy Relief and Prevention* by Dr. Jacqueline Krohn goes into explicit detail regarding allergies, testing, and how to get relief. We are going to learn a few of these important details today in our study, but I encourage you to read the whole book if you want a thorough understanding of this topic.

Types of Food Allergies and Reactions

Food allergies may be classified in different ways. Immediate reaction allergies are those where symptoms are obvious within minutes. The symptoms may include wheezing, hives, eczema, rhinitis (ringing in the ears), swelling of the lips and face, or anaphylactic shock. A delayed reaction allergy has symptoms that may not appear until the next day or several days later. Symptoms would include headaches (frequently migraines), chronic indigestion or heartburn, fatigue, depression, failure to thrive, joint pain, recurrent abdominal pain, canker sores, bronchitis, and bowel problems such as colitis, diarrhea, or constipation. This type of food allergy is typically misdiagnosed.

In our fasting study I shared with you the story of my husband, who eliminated all animal products including dairy for one month. On day three of this fast he no longer needed his Prevacid™ and was sleeping through the night without any problems. Our further investigation led us to discover he was allergic to milk products, specifically ice cream. Before this discovery he enjoyed ice cream in the evening with lots of chocolate syrup. His physician had him on two prescriptions for the symptoms of this unknown allergy. By eliminating this food, he was able to get off the prescriptions and be pain free! This is why it is important to find a physician who specializes in environmental medicine. They have the added training to help diagnose allergies. Let me truthfully tell you, Steve did not remove *all* the ice cream from his diet, only enough to not have problems. We still enjoy it on special occasions.

Disease Symptoms Associated with Foods

Not everyone realizes that many diseases could be caused by various foods. The following list outlines some of these diseases:

- Arthritis—This disease is linked to sugar, pork, processed wheat, and nightshade vegetables including tomatoes, potatoes, bell peppers, eggplant, chili peppers, tobacco, and pimentos. The nightshade vegetables must be avoided for six to nine months in order to determine the role of these foods in arthritis.
- Asthma—This has links to eggs, milk, seafood, peanuts, chocolate, corn, and nuts.
- Bad breath—This can be caused by any food. Take the Candida Test in the *Nutrition Manual* to determine if candida is the reason for the bad breath.
- Colitis—This disease is most frequently linked to milk and meat, although it can be caused by wheat, corn, eggs, chocolate, and nuts.
- Eczema—This problem is frequently due to a food allergy. In children, suspect milk first, although other contributors would be fruits, chocolate, peas, beans, peaches, grains, and eggs.
- Headaches and migraines—These two may be triggered by food or chemicals. Any food can cause a migraine. Eggs, wheat, milk, chocolate, corn, cinnamon, wine, pork, and nuts are common offenders.
- Bedwetting—Milk is the most frequent offender of bedwetting, followed by wheat, corn, eggs, orange, and chocolate. Constipation also plays a role in bedwetting.
- Recurrent ear infections—Many children suffer from this problem. Almost any frequently eaten food or exposure to natural gas can trigger this reaction, but milk is the primary culprit.

There are many other symptoms of food allergies, including acne, restless leg, fatigue, body odor, and depression. I have only included a few to help you see the connection. The foods listed are the primary ones, but any food digested incorrectly can become an allergy. Sometimes it is the handling and processing that causes the reaction and eating organically grown foods or whole foods from the garden will not present the same problems.

Pork was noted in several of these symptoms. It is the most frequently processed of all meats. Organic pork is safer than conventional pork (if you choose to eat this unclean meat), but it comes from pigs that are fed a corn diet, which is contrary to the design of the animal. This is also true of most other animals. Remember back to the meat chapter and your visit to a farm. Animals fed on natural grasses—the way they were designed—will give us less problems with allergies.

Reading Labels

From what you have been reading, you may feel all your favorite foods have been eliminated. Take heart; there are some simple plans to follow. But first we must learn how to read labels.

The safest foods for people with allergies continue to be the foods we have studied: fresh, organic fruits, vegetables, and meats. However, because many of us are unable to grow our own food and because top-quality food is not always available, we are forced to buy commercial and some processed foods. It is important to learn to read food labels intelligently in order to recognize food additives and to make wise food purchases.

ADDITIVES

A food additive is a substance or mixture that has been added to aid in production, processing, packaging, or storing a food. Additives began thousands of years ago when people discovered that salted meat would store longer.

More than ten thousand intentional additives are currently used in foods. While not all of them are harmful, many of them do cause problems. For example, the common additives tartrazine and benzoic acid can increase hyperactivity in children.

PRESERVATIVES

Preservatives prevent changes affecting color, flavor, texture, or appearance. Traditional preservatives include salt, sugar, vinegar, spices, and wood smoke. Wood smoke is no longer considered safe. Other preservatives include BHA, BHT, and benzoic acid. BHA affects the liver and kidneys. BHT affects the kidneys and is prohibited as a food additive in England. Benzoic acid can cause allergic reactions including asthma, red eyes, and skin rashes.

COLORING AGENTS

Both natural and synthetic food colorings are used in processed foods to heighten taste and attractiveness. Color can also be used to conceal damage or inferior quality. Synthetic coloring is typically a petroleum byproduct.

FLAVORINGS

There are more than two thousand flavoring agents in use, of which only five hundred are natural. Flavorings are used to modify the flavors of foods that lose their original flavor as a result of processing. If a food tasted processed, you would not want to eat it. Therefore, we have flavorings.

PHYSIOLOGICAL ACTIVITY CONTROLS

This is a long title for something I had never considered before. Have you ever stored potatoes in your pantry only to have them sprout? Why do they never sprout at the store? These controls are the reason. These controls involve chemicals that serve as ripeners (such as ethylene gas) to speed the ripening of bananas or as anti-metabolic agents to keep potatoes from sprouting. Maleis hydrazinde used with potatoes is highly toxic to humans and has caused genetic damage to plant and animal systems. The FDA has allowed a residue tolerance for potato chips to be no more than 160 ppm (parts per million). Did you want this residue on your potato chips? Natural enzymes can also be used as controls, and people with allergies do not usually react to these enzymes.

BLEACHING AND MATURING AGENTS

These agents are used to improve the appearance of food products. Both of them are applied to flour to accelerate its aging process in order to improve its baking qualities and reduce storage costs, spoilage, and the possibility of insects. These agents also reduce the nutrients in food.

PROCESSING AIDS

Processing aids include sanitizing agents that remove bacteria and debris from products. This includes sodium nitrate and nitrite, which are used to develop and stabilize the pink color of meats. Many people are allergic to these meat-processing aids, and some aids are known carcinogens.

OLESTRA

Olestra is a new food additive and is an indigestible fat substitute. Olestra contains no fat or calories and is made from sugar and vegetable oil. The body is unable to break down the structure so it absorbs neither the fat nor the sugar. However, it causes unpleasant side effects including bowel urgency, diarrhea, and cramps.

Managing Our Food

Once again, we are faced with choices—to make changes and reap rewards or stay on the same diet and program and keep getting the same results. Have you noticed that with each health issue we cover the answer is the same? The foods God gave us will build health, and the ones that have been altered may cause problems.

Let's review the Three Principles again. Write out the principle and then apply what you have learned about allergies.

Principle I

_____

_____

_____

Principle II

_____

_____

_____

Principle III

_____

_____

_____

God has given us the best to help heal our body. But we must decide whether or not to make changes. Even with allergies, if we maintain the same unhealthy diet there is no chance for the body to repair itself, which leads to gradual decline of health. Continued reactions over a period of time will weaken the immune system, which can ultimately lead to degenerative (gradual deterioration in the body) diseases and increased infections.

DIGGING DEEPER: We have very briefly covered the subject of allergies. This subject fills volumes of textbooks and reference manuals. Let me encourage you again to check out Dr. Jacqueline Krohn's book, *Allergy Relief and Prevention: A Practical Encyclopedia*. We have only hit the highlights from this book, and reading the whole thing will give you a more complete guide to making changes in your diet, health, and life.

Human nature defends who we are and expects others to change.
God's nature accepts others as they are and through Him we change.

—Marita Littauer

Taking this treasure to heart: It is easy to want a better life and add convenience, but sometimes convenience costs us too much. Consider in what areas you can make changes this week in your home or diet. Pray for guidance and wisdom when making those changes.

Applying this treasure at home: What steps are you going to make this week based on what you have learned? Record them on the Action Plan and share them with your foodie friend.

FABULOUS FOODIE FRIDAY

Foodie Ideas

Create a spa atmosphere in your home for you and your foodie friends. Have fun with this and see how many ideas you can come up with. Here are a few to get you started:

PERSONALIZE YOUR OWN PERFUME

To make your own perfume, you will need:

1 tablespoon beeswax—found in health food stores
1 tablespoon almond oil or jojoba oil
8-15 drops essential oil—your choice (found in many health food stores)
1 container (small sealable case made of glass, ceramic, or sterling silver)

Pour about an inch of water into a small saucepan; then put a small glass jar or Pyrex bowl in the water. Measure out the beeswax and almond oil into the jar. Then bring the water around it to a boil. The wax will melt gradually. When it is 100 percent liquid, remove from heat and stir in essential oil (a straw works best and can be thrown away when finished). When everything is thoroughly mixed, pour the liquid wax immediately into your final container. In about thirty minutes, it will be cooled, solid and ready to use. Keep sealed to store.[198]

PURIFY WITH PLANTS

Enliven your home with the air-cleansing properties of plants. Varieties such as Boston ferns, English ivy, philodendrons, and spider plants are all excellent air purifiers. They have the ability to increase oxygen, remove pollutants, reduce stress on the job, and keep blood pressure under control—possibly due to the soothing effect.

PREPARE A PEDICURE BAR

Invite your foodie friends to join you at the pedicure bar, where they can enjoy a relaxing soak. Shelly Ballestero gives us some pointers in her book *Beauty By God*.[199] Most of the ingredients for this fabulous soak are already in your pantry:

1 teaspoon honey
1 sprig rosemary
½ cup coconut milk
2 ounces olive oil
¼ cup Epsom salt
½ cup cornmeal

Mix the ingredients in a small bowl. Pour the mixture into a foot bath or salad bowl filled with filtered hot water. Soak feet for a few minutes. Use some undissolved mixture to exfoliate rough spots.

Treat yourself and your friends to tea and cookies during your soak. Have fun, keep the joy in your friendships, and embrace life. Remember, the best makeup of all is joy!

PLAN AN ORGANIC DINNER

Go all out and plan an elaborate dinner with your foodie friends. The trick is that the entire menu and setting must be organic. Depending on the season, your menu may be easy or it may require a little more persistence to find the right treasure. Decorate your table with organic candles, organic place mats, napkins, and flowers or a container of herbs to add the finishing touch.

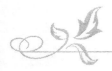

Stress and Forgiveness

Day One—Turning Stress into a Treasure

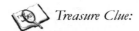 *Treasure Clue:*

*He gives strength to the weary, and to him who lacks might He increases power. Though youths grow weary and tired, and vigorous young men stumble badly, Yet those who wait for the L*ORD *will gain new strength; They will mount up with wings like eagles, They will run and not get tired, They will walk and not become weary.*
—Isa. 40:29-31 NASB

Cold winter mornings would find us packing for a favorite field trip. We would get up very early, layer ourselves with warm clothes, pack our breakfast with lots of hot chocolate, and then drive from Imperial, Missouri, to Alton, Illinois. The drive along the bluffs of the Mississippi would take us closer to our destination. Straining our necks to look high in the trees and sky, we saw eagles that came to roost. This was a time when we could slip away from homeschool assignments, never-ending housework, and the general stress of being overcommitted in life.

The eagles would soar above the highest clouds and then come down into the icy river waters to get their catch of fresh fish. Some days we would see up to twenty of these magnificent birds gliding through the air as if there was no worry in the world. Their wings would catch the wind and they would freely soar. Watching them in their splendor helped us forget about the stress waiting back home. And while we knew it would be there when we returned, we always came back more refreshed with one more memory to treasure in our minds.

When you get a chance, find a place where you can view eagles in the wild, especially in the winter. As you watch them glide up in the skies you will understand what Isaiah means when he tells us that God wants us to mount up like wings of eagles, to walk and not grow weary. It is hard for me to feel stressed when I see God's handiwork in action. Watching the eagles is one way I can turn stress into a treasure.

Poet Stacy Smith has captured this idea in her poem *From an Eagle's View.* Make a copy of this poem and keep it at your desk or workstation and just relax for thirty seconds while reading it and envisioning the eagle. Take a deep breath and fill your lungs, then exhale all the air.

Then stretch your arms out as far as they can go in front of you. Stretching, breathing, relaxing, and reflecting will give your cells a burst of energy and relief from constant pressure.

From an Eagle's View

Have you ever wondered what it's like to fly free,
To see the world as far as the eye can see,
To view the surroundings from high and from low,
To hear only the sound of a distant echo,
To float in the air with the wind being your guide,
To admire many rainbows that the trees tend to hide,
To see the misty mornings over a beautiful mountaintop,
To glide over a flowing river that never seems to stop,
To watch the animals from over a mile away,
Or to rise above the treetops that glisten in the day?
If you were an eagle you would wonder no more,
For it can see things you have never seen before.
Next time you look into the sky of blue,
Think of what it's like from an eagle's view.

Is Stress Good or Bad?

"Do not be anxious about your life" (Matt. 6:25 ESV). Stress has been called the fastest-growing disease in the Western world. It is all around us; it begins with our first breath and ends with our last. Our daily lives offer us many challenges and opportunities. These situations show up in various ways, but how we respond determines if the stress created by these challenges is good or bad. A positive (good) stress is a challenge or opportunity that typically requires us to stretch ourselves; a negative one is overload and the stretch may cancel any pleasure. We define our reaction to negative stress with words like: fear, anxiety, frustration, anger, and depression. Often we are unaware of how much these feelings affect both our short- and long-term health.

Examples of positive stress situations include: the announcement that you are going to be parents or grandparents, a promotion at work, completion of a difficult project, shopping a great sale at your favorite store, moving into the house of your dreams, or reaping a bountiful harvest in your own garden. Examples of negative stress could include: the challenges of a bad health report from the doctor, losing a job, getting a speeding ticket, any number of family issues, and the many other problems facing us today. Stress means opportunity, and how we accept and handle that opportunity will determine if it is a negative or positive event in our lives.

Recognize that stress is all around us and affects every area of life: emotional (soul), physical (body), and spiritual. No matter what type of stress we encounter, knowing how to recognize it and handle it efficiently will make the difference between a healthy life and one that is destined for problems.

So is stress good or bad? Read James 1:2 and write it out here.

_____

_____

Everyone experiences stress, both good and bad. As we look deeper into God's Word, we can count it all joy when it arrives as an unwanted guest and overstays its welcome, or we can count it all trouble when we are unable to handle it. We need to learn to recognize the warning signs of stress and learn how to handle it in order to turn it into a treasure.

What Is Stress?

Stress is the gap between the demands that are placed on us and the strength we have to meet those demands. In Part I of our study we learned about the health bank account. Our account will play a major role in our ability to handle stress. The same situation can happen to us at different times in our lives, and we can respond completely different each time. What is the reason for our varying actions? It is our health bank account. Remember that our bank account has deposits and withdrawals with daily decisions about whether or not to exercise, eat healthy foods, have an attitude of thankfulness, or spend time in prayer and Bible study. These factors will greatly affect how you respond to the demands placed on you.

Some people believe that Christians shouldn't have problems or stress and that if you are encountering problems, you are not spiritually mature, don't have enough faith, or are not praying and working hard enough. Others believe God punishes you for past failures. Don't believe these lies. Christians need to learn to expect stress in their lives. Stress will help you to grow stronger, draw closer to God, and seek His invitations to totally rely on Him. Stress is an opportunity to experience God's sufficiency. Stress can be an opportunity, but that does not mean we don't need to make changes in our lives to decrease the overbearing load. Learning to handle stress will keep us balanced in life and in health.

What Causes Stress?

Stress comes into our lives with and without an invitation. Examples might be a death in the family or pollution in the environment. Stress affects both our emotional and physical health. Emotionally, stress can be caused by adversity, opportunity, and necessity. Adversities are those things that come upon us unexpectedly and are sometimes referred to as the "storms of life." Opportunities are the things we want to do. Necessities are the things we must do. Any one or all three of these can cause us to be out of balance, and this can lead to stress.

There are four main causes of stress:

- Environment (external)—noise, heat and cold, toxins, travel, jobs, family
- Diet—malnutrition, illness, weight problems, drugs, processed foods, medicine
- Exercise—lack of exercise can cause small amounts of stress to seem monumental
- Attitude—anger, resentment, envy, guilt, revenge, tension, anxiety, unforgiveness, fear of change, rejection, job loss, finances, home life, depression, love, joy, unrealistic expectations, low self-esteem, self-criticism, perfectionism, and worry

List some of the causes for the emotional or physical stress you are experiencing right now.

_____

_____

_____

In the list you have just written, write a "P" after a cause if it is positive and an "N" if it is negative. Which negative ones are you ready to get rid of? Circle them. Keep reading, and you will learn how either to remove them from your life entirely or learn to handle these stresses better.

As we have discussed stress and its effects on us, perhaps you noticed that you cannot control much of what causes stress. So it is of utmost importance to follow a healthy diet and maintain a close relationship with God. We will look at diet later.

Symptoms of Stress

How does the body respond to stress? Stress creates upset stomachs, splitting headaches, intense grief, ministerial burn-out, and violent arguments. Stress dulls our memories, cripples our thinking, weakens our bodies, upsets our plans, stirs up our emotions, and reduces our efficiency. But stress also motivates us to work, encourages us to keep going when life gets difficult, spurs us to action in the midst of crises, helps us to mature, and, at times, makes life exciting.

The following chemical and physical changes accompany stress:

- Stress increases the production of adrenaline and stress hormones, which in turn causes a depletion of vitamins B and C.

- Stress can cause blood sugar to rise. With depleted stores of Vitamin B, the body is unable to convert sugar to energy, so the pancreas becomes overworked in producing insulin to control the sugar. The pancreas then collapses, which leads to hypoglycemia and diabetes.
- Stress causes the heart to pound and the lungs to breathe faster. Vitamin E is depleted, bringing more oxygen to the cells.
- Stress causes muscles to tense. A depletion of calcium/magnesium means difficulty in handling stress.
- Stress can cause the digestive and reproductive systems to shut down. Food is only partially digested, enzymes slow down, food putrefies, and the colon becomes sluggish, possibly leading to ulcers and cancer. Prostate problems, impotency, PMS, endometriosis, fibroid tumors, menstrual problems, and much more can result.

It is important not to remain in a state of stress. Some people work better under stress. Our bodies are designed to work harder under stress, but in our society many never get to escape. When our hormones are stressed and working nonstop, they are not available to follow daily routines. For some of us that routine may be preventing PMS or blood pressure problems. When we are constantly under stress with no relief in sight, certain signs and symptoms present themselves and can lead to more serious health problems if the stress is not alleviated even for short periods of time. Our response to stress determines its effect on our bodies, so we must learn how to deal with stress appropriately.

Read Jonah 2:2 in your Bible. What did Jonah do in his time of stress?

_____

How did God respond? _____

Jonah's body was definitely reacting to stress. He ran away, was thrown overboard from a ship during a mighty storm, was swallowed by a great fish, and he thought he was at the point of death. The natural chemical changes from being under stress were probably causing Jonah digestive disorders, heart problems, and muscle tension. Just when he had reached the end of his rope, he cried out to the Lord, and God answered him! Don't you just love those words, "God answered him"? The Lord will also answer us when we cry out to Him.

Has there been a time in your life where you felt trapped, like Jonah in the belly of that great fish? Did you cry out to God? How did He respond?

_____

_____

_____

Warning Signs of Stress

In Jonah 2:7, Jonah recounts, "I was fainting away" (NASB). We want to be able to recognize the stress in our life before we get to the point of "fainting away." Life is full of distractions and it is important to recognize stress before it has manifested itself as disease.

In our country we are not dying of infectious diseases anymore. Instead we are dying of lifestyle and degenerative diseases such as heart disease, cancer, and diabetes. Stress can bring about any one of these three diseases in spite of eating the right foods, exercising, and supplementing correctly. Stress creates an excellent breeding ground for illness. It is estimated that stress contributes to 75-100 percent of all major illnesses, along with the majority of back problems. It can also lead to emotional difficulties such as depression and anxiety.

In recognizing the danger, it would be helpful for us to look at the warning signs of stress. Here is a brief summary of some of the symptoms a person may experience.

Use a marker to highlight any symptoms on the list below that you are currently experiencing; then make each one a matter of prayer.

Moodiness	Diarrhea or constipation
Agitation	Nausea, dizziness
Restlessness	Insomnia
Short temper	Chest pain, rapid heartbeat
Irritability, impatience	Weight gain or loss
Inability to relax	Skin breakouts (hives, eczema)
Memory problems	Sleeping too much or too little
Indecisiveness	Isolating yourself from others
Inability to concentrate	Procrastination, neglecting responsibilities
Trouble thinking clearly	Using alcohol, cigarettes, or drugs to relax
Poor judgment	Nervous habits (e.g. nail biting, pacing)
Seeing only the negative	Teeth grinding or jaw clenching
Headaches or backaches	Feeling tense and "on edge"
Muscle tension and stiffness	

Stress leads to distress, and unmanaged distress leads to disease. The following is a list of medical conditions that are caused or made worse by stress:

Chronic pain	Heartburn
Migraines	High blood pressure
Ulcers	Heart disease

Diabetes

Infertility

Asthma

Autoimmune diseases

PMS

Irritable bowel syndrome

Obesity

Skin problems

What is your first impression of the symptoms that you highlighted?

_____

_____

_____

_____

How many items did you highlight? _____

DIGGING DEEPER: Read "Solutions for Stress in Children" in the *Nutrition Manual.*

Taking this treasure to heart: Stress is very underrated and ignored, for the most part. Yet as you read the list of illnesses and health problems, it is obvious we need to address it. What is one nugget of truth you have learned today to help you address the stress in your life?

_____

_____

Applying this treasure at home: Is there someone in your family who needs your prayers regarding the stress in his or her life? _____

Day Two—Stress in the Bible

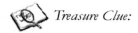 *Treasure Clue:*

And which of you by being worried can add a single hour to his life?

—Matt. 6:27 NASB

Yesterday we learned how the body is greatly affected by stress. Now take in a deep breath, grab a cup of herbal tea, and let's unveil the answer God has for you.

First, if you are a Christian, remember it is not a sin to be stressed or weary. Even Jesus was weary; He was tired. Jesus set us an example of spending time in prayer with His Father.

Second, many people in the Bible dealt with stressful situations: Ruth traveled with her mother-in-law to a foreign land, Daniel was thrown into the lions' den, Jonah was sitting in the huge garbage pit of a large fish's stomach, Moses cared for two million people who whined and wailed over every little inconvenience, Hannah experienced infertility, David fled from Saul in fear of his life, Samson defeated the Philistines, Peter denied Christ three times, Joseph learned about Mary's pregnancy out of wedlock, and Christ wrestled in prayer in the Garden of Gethsemane.

The Bible does not specifically use the word *stress* but it does address the idea of stress. Scripture uses words like *distress, tribulations, trials, ordeals, hardship, trouble, difficulties, persecution, affliction, suffering, adversity, pressure, disaster, discipline,* and *circumstances.* Then Scripture gives us a plan for stress using words like *grace, peace, love, joy, content, strength, encourage, abundant, courage, perseverance, acceptance,* and *faith,* and commands like *rejoice, rest,* and *trust.*

Let's look as some of these treasures in God's Word. Read each scripture and mark the ones that you can relate to today. Then circle the promises from God found in the middle of the verse to help in your situation. This is your opportunity to turn stress into a treasure and give God the glory. Don't rush; take your time, reflecting on each verse independently. Stress does not have to defeat us.

Philippians 4:6-7 (NIV)—"Do not be anxious about anything, but in everything, by prayer and petition, with thanksgiving, present your requests to God. And the peace of God, which transcends all understanding, will guard your hearts and your minds in Christ Jesus."

Psalm 29:11 (NIV)—"The Lord gives strength to his people; the Lord blesses his people with peace."

Psalm 55:22 (NIV)—"Cast your cares on the Lord and he will sustain you; he will never let the righteous fall."

Jeremiah 17:7-8 (NIV)—"But blessed is the man who trusts in the Lord, whose confidence is in him. He will be like a tree planted by the water that sends out its roots by the stream. It does not fear when heat comes; its leaves are always green. It has no worries in a year of drought and never fails to bear fruit."

Matthew 11:28-30 (NIV)—"Come to me, all you who are weary and burdened, and I will give you rest. Take my yoke upon you and learn from me, for I am gentle and humble in heart, and you will find rest for your souls. For my yoke is easy and my burden is light."

John 14:27 (NIV)—"Peace I leave with you; my peace I give you. I do not give to you as the world gives. Do not let your hearts be troubled and do not be afraid."

Proverbs 3:24 (NIV)—"When you lie down, you will not be afraid; when you lie down, your sleep will be sweet."

Philippians 4:11 (NASB)—"Not that I speak from want; for I have learned to be content in whatever circumstances I am."

James 1:2 (NASB)—"Consider it all joy, my brethren, when you encounter various trials."

1 Peter 1:6 (NASB)—"In this you greatly rejoice, even though now for a little while, if necessary, you have been distressed by various trials."

John 16:33 (NASB)—"These things I have spoken to you, that in Me you may have peace. In the world you have tribulation, but take courage; *I have overcome the world*" (emphasis added).

Acts 14:22 (NASB)—"Strengthening the souls of the disciples, encouraging them to continue in the faith, and saying, 'Through many tribulations we must enter the kingdom of God.'"

Romans 5:3 (NASB)—"And not only this, but we also exult in our tribulations, knowing that tribulation brings about perseverance."

Romans 8:35 (KJV)—"Who shall separate us from the love of Christ? Shall tribulation, or distress, or persecution, or famine, or nakedness, or peril, or sword?"

Psalm 86:7 (KJV)—"In the day of my trouble I will call upon Thee: for *thou wilt answer me*" (emphasis added).

2 Corinthians 8:2 (NASB)—". . . that in a great ordeal of affliction their abundance of joy and their deep poverty overflowed in the wealth of their liberality."

1 Peter 4:12 (NASB)—"Beloved, do not be surprised at the fiery ordeal among you, which comes upon you for your testing, as though some strange thing were happening to you."

2 Corinthians 3:5 (NASB)—"Not that we are adequate in ourselves to consider anything as coming from ourselves, but our adequacy is from God."

2 Corinthians 12:9 (NASB)—"My grace is sufficient for you, for power is perfected in weakness."

Romans 12:12 (NASB)—"...rejoicing in hope, persevering in tribulation, devoted to prayer."

James 1:12 (NASB)—"Blessed is the man who perseveres under trial; for once he has been approved, he will receive the crown of life which the Lord has promised to those who love Him."

Galatians 6:9 (NASB)—"Let us not lose heart in doing good, for in due time we will reap if we do not grow weary."

Write out 1 Peter 5:7 here.

_____

_____

_____

Paraphrase this verse in your own words as a personal prayer to God.

_____

_____

_____

Many times, in our stress, we just want someone to come in and take over for us so that we don't have to deal with the problems. This is exactly what Peter is teaching us in this verse. He is telling us to cast our anxieties and cares upon the Lord because He will take care of us.

Write 1 Peter 5:7 again, only make it into an affirmation of God's promise to you.

_____

_____

_____

DAY THREE—OVERCOMING STRESS

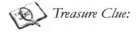 *Treasure Clue:*

Rejoicing in hope, persevering in tribulation, devoted to prayer.

—Rom. 12:12 NASB

Here are some fun sayings that my foodie friends came up with.
You know you are under stress when you . . .

- . . . put the milk in the cupboard and the cereal in the refrigerator.
- . . . arrive at work and notice you have on different shoes.
- . . . realize there is only one brownie left from the pan you baked an hour ago when you were home alone.
- . . . arrive at work and wonder why everyone is late, until you realize it is Saturday.
- . . . kiss the dog and pet the wife.
- . . . write a check to pay a bill, then sign the back of it like you're going to deposit it.
- . . . leave your keys in the fridge.
- . . . answer the phone with, "What now?!"
- . . . wish you had one of those "clap on, clap off" gizmos attached to your keys because you can never remember where you put them.
- . . . consume all of the chocolate in your house!

How can you and your foodie friends complete the same sentence? You know you are stressed when you...

_____

_____

_____

The final phase of turning stress into a treasure is following a plan to help you cope with the stress. This includes five areas: developing a positive mental attitude, practicing good nutrition, making lifestyle changes, adding supplements, and getting proper rest.

Developing an "I Can Handle It" Attitude

Positive self-talk will take us a long way toward successfully coping and being able to handle difficulties. Many situations can be turned into a funny story later, so look for the positive side of your circumstances.

Recently I was getting adventurous with my daughter's bike. I needed a few groceries, so I decided to ride it to the store a few miles down the road—in the heat of summer. I completed my shopping, only to come out and find both tires flat! No problem, right? I could handle it! Well, I felt a little silly walking the bike home but it was that or sit and wait for hours for someone to pick me up.

Later this week we will talk about forgiveness. This is one situation where the "I can handle it" attitude will greatly help. Wrongs will be done to you—there is no escaping—but you can handle it and forgive.

We need to establish priorities to put our problems in perspective. If we feel overworked and there are not enough hours in a day, we should set schedules based on what can be achieved realistically.

Conflict and pressure will always exist. It may be in our personal or professional life. There is nothing wrong with feeling angry and frustrated if it is properly expressed. To maintain harmony with others and within yourself, keep communication lines open. Do not be afraid to let people know when you need help or support. They are not mind readers.

When you feel yourself becoming tense, slow down and try to be rational. You may find that some of the things that are most annoying or frustrating are not worth getting worked up over. It is important to be healthy and happy—at the same time! You can do it!

Diet and Stress

The same foods filling our treasure will prepare us for stressful situations before they arise. When stress comes along and our eating is atrocious, we need answers quick. The diet for stress is no different than the diet we continue to study throughout this entire book. When we give our bodies a smorgasbord of high quality protein, whole grains, and raw fruits and veggies, our bodies are better prepared to handle stress and recover quickly.

I know you want me to include chocolate in this list of foods to eat and, honestly, I did numerous hours of research hoping I could give you a definitive answer that chocolate is good for you. According to Dr. Steve Parker, author of *The Advanced Mediterranean Diet*, dark organic chocolate with 65 percent cocoa may contain flavonoids to give your body wonderful antioxidants.[200] These antioxidants can lead to a relaxation of the heart muscle, thereby reducing high blood pressure and working as an antidepressant. Most studies conclude that the magnesium found in the cocoa plant can have a calming effect on your body, but the adverse affects of the sugar negate much of that benefit. Milk chocolate does not list the same benefits because it is made with dairy. The decision is yours. Personally, I believe that a small bite of organic dark chocolate is beneficial, but a handful of M&M's is not a good choice.

Meal Management

A meal management plan to tackle stress should include:

- A heavier meal in the morning
- A lighter meal at night
- Salads before the meals
- Fruits as desserts at the ends of the meals

Follow these tips for your overall diet:

- Eat a diet with at least 50 percent raw fruits and vegetables.
- Avoid processed foods, artificial sweeteners, soda, fried foods, pork, white flour products, foods containing preservatives, chips, and "junk" food.
- Eliminate dairy for three weeks; the allergic affect to some people contributes to stress. Reintroduce it slowly and watch for symptoms or allergic reactions.
- Limit intake of caffeine, remembering that caffeine whips your adrenals into a frenzy. Avoiding it altogether is better.
- Eliminate alcohol, tobacco, and mood-altering drugs as these only mask the problem and do not solve it.
- Fast one day a month for six months. This discipline will help you to rely on God's mercies.

Follow these lifestyle choices:

- Get regular exercise—1 Corinthians 9:27.
- Sleep – Psalm 4:8, Sleeplessness can be one of the many signs that your body is under stress. Train your body to get at least eight hours of sleep. Proverbs 3:24
- Make a list of what is important in life and eliminate everything else either temporarily or permanently. Let the Holy Spirit guide you.
- Schedule your day wisely, Psalm 37:23

- Master your money and tithe. Budget problems are high on the list for causing stress. Bottom line – pray about every purchase. Luke 16:11
- Enjoy today. Matthew 6:34, "Yesterday is over and tomorrow will come later." Enjoy the present and all that God has given you.
- Resolve conflicts, Matthew 18:15, "Pray about issues that concern you and resolve one issue at a time."
- Limit contact with stress-producing people. Romans 12:18
- Laugh. Proverbs 17:22, "A merry heart does good, like medicine."
- Love your family and the people God has brought into your life.
- Continue in your faith and belief in God's promises. Romans 4:20

DIGGING DEEPER: Read "Stretching Exercise to Relieve Muscle Tension": in the *Nutrition Manual.*

He who rides tiger is afraid of dismount.

—Chinese Proverb

Supplements for Extra Help With Stress

Symptoms can still persist, even with the Treasures of Healthy Living diet. If that is the case, supplements may be necessary to allow the body to be prepared and recover quickly from stress. When referring to supplements, remember to consult the *Nutrition Manual* or the Designed Healthy Living web site for guidelines on how to make the wisest choices. Not all supplements are the same, and they never will be. Be a smart consumer. Suggested supplements for stress would include: B-Complex, Multi-Vitamin, Protein (such as high quality soy protein—these vary greatly), Vitamin E, Vitamin C, calcium/magnesium, enzymes, zinc (for skin problems), and herbs (ashwaganda, beta-sitosterol). Beware of products that contain kava, because it is associated with severe liver damage.

Rest and Relaxation

The final prescription for stress is to allow time for adequate rest and relaxation. We all need sleep time, but we also need time for just plain relaxing, time to write an overdue letter, or time to put our feet up and let our minds wander.

Read Mark 6:31. What does Jesus say about rest?

_____

_____

Dr. Couey has given us some guidelines on how to really relax our bodies.

Research has shown that the best way to relax muscles and nerves is through a progressive relaxation program. This program consists of lying on a firm mat on the floor in a dimly lit room with soft music playing. Lie flat on your back with arms to your side, close your eyes, take deep breaths, and allow your mind to relax all your muscles to the extent there is no movement in your body. After you have achieved silence in your nerves and muscles, you are ready to progressively relax each group of muscles in your body. Begin by contracting all the muscles in your legs and arms for five seconds. After the five seconds are over, allow your mind to concentrate on relaxing those muscles. After achieving relaxation in your upper and lower extremities, contract the muscles in your jaw, eyes, and forehead for five seconds. Then achieve complete relaxation in your head muscles. After this, concentrate on relaxing the whole body for five minutes. Don't allow movement to occur in any part of your body. After approximately five minutes, stretch your muscles and experience how much better you feel.

> *Do not fear, for I am with you; Do not anxiously look about you, for I am your God. I will strengthen you, surely I will help you, surely I will uphold you with My righteous right hand....I am the LORD your God, who upholds your right hand, who says to you, "Do not fear, I will help you."*
>
> —Isa. 41:10, 13

It is clear that stress affects the body, soul, and spirit. We have looked at the warning signs to help us recognize stress in our lives and the many ways we can better handle stress to persevere in our treasure hunt for great health. Remember, God has a plan for our individual lives and any deterrent from that plan is a distraction that Satan prefers. In all we do we must lean not on our own understanding but instead must acknowledge God in everything we do, and He will direct our ways, turning our stress into a treasure (Prov. 3:5-6).

Taking this treasure to heart: Take a moment to write out what God has taught you in this lesson.

_____

_____

_____

Applying this treasure at home: What commitment are you going to make to improve your own health? What steps can you make this week to reduce or handle your stress better? Record your answers on the Action Plan and share them with your foodie friend.

Day Four—Treasure of Freedom in Forgiveness

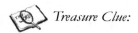 *Treasure Clue:*

Forgive us our debts, as we also have forgiven our debtors.

—Matt. 6:12 NIV

Is bitterness in the treasure chest? Not if you want optimal health. Bitterness is like a murky swamp blocking us from the treasure. In the past, I tried to wade through this dark, infectious water not realizing the power of hope that was dangling from a rope that could pull me from the entangled marsh to freedom. This rope would allow me to swing like Tarzan (or in my case, Jane) across the swamp and land gracefully, clean, and dry on the other side. But what kept me from taking hold of that rope?

The entanglement of bitterness affected my physical, mental, and spiritual outlook on life. At times I would try to pull others down into my swamp by transferring blame. This benefited no one. I then shifted my focus, changed my plan, and made a list of people I needed to forgive. The list stared back at me and revealed how out of control this area in my life had become. It was time to change. I was ready to reach for the rope. The decision to get relief from the murky waters was mine all along. Don't misunderstand me, some of the people I needed to forgive had also wronged me or my family, but it was still my lack of forgiveness that held me in the swamp.

Read 2 Corinthians 2:10-11. What truth can you learn from these verses? How can you apply it to those you need to forgive?

_____

_____

_____

Stress and Forgiveness

In the book *The Healing Power of Forgiveness*, Ray Pritchard, pastor of Calvary Memorial Church in Oak Park, Illinois, explains how the way we treat others directly affects our relationship with God.

As long as we harbor relational sins and wrong attitudes, we will never grow spiritually. These relational sins are like junk food of the soul. They choke off our craving for the Word so that instead of growing, we stay just as we are. As long as you treat people unkindly and gossip about them and harbor bitterness, you will never grow spiritually—even if you come to church four times a week and go to Bible study every other day. Your relational sins will choke off God's Word in your life. That explains why some people come to church for years and never get better. They're harboring a relational garbage pit on the inside. They make excuses for their envy, they ignore their gossip, they make light of their cutting comments, and they justify their meanness toward others. And they don't grow because they can't grow. When your horizontal relationships with others are messed up, your vertical relationship with God will never be right. God has wired us up so that the horizontal and the vertical go together. John says it very plainly: "If anyone says 'I love God,' yet hates his brother, he is a liar. For anyone who does not love his brother, whom he has seen, cannot love God, whom he has not seen" (1 John 4:20 NIV). We cannot say, "I hate you" to a friend or family member and then say, "Lord, I love You. Please bless me right now." God says, "No deal. It doesn't work that way."[201]

A dear friend of mine wrote a testimony to share in this book with the hope that someone may recognize himself or herself in this story.

Bitterness was poisoning my life for over twenty years and I did not know it. Finally it came to a standoff in my relationship with God, and I knew I needed to do something. The pastor I decided to meet with suspected I was bitter, but I was not convinced. So he gave me an assignment to do. Every day I was to confess my sins, ask God's forgiveness, and then tell God that I trusted Him. Being a Christian since childhood, I could easily confess the bad things I had done, but I could not say, "I trust You, God." I did not trust God to do what was best. What kind of God would allow some of the extremely painful things in my life and say in the Bible He works all things out for good? How could these things be for my good? So I searched the Bible and talked with the pastor. In order to trust God, I had to accept that He was in charge and that He was going to make things right in the end ("vengeance is mine, says the Lord"). My resentment toward my parents was hurting me far more than them and I had to let it go to really believe what God says in the Bible, that He will take care of things and that He wants good for me. It was hard to get to that point, especially since my parents are not sorry for the cruel things they have done and continue to do.

The bitterness toward my parents was unveiled, and I was able to be released from it with God's help. Since then my life has been transformed in ways I never would have guessed. Strong cravings for sweet foods for over twenty years were almost totally gone. Because of that I have lost over twenty-five pounds in eight months without being on a diet. My new relationship with my parents is almost easy, instead of the chore it has been all those years. Relationships with my spouse, children, and even in-laws are better. I can think more clearly and make decisions better. It seems I have more time, though my responsibilities are the same. My unhappiness was getting worse, even though I had a very good life outwardly. Now joy and peace, for the first time in many years, fills my days. My life is not perfect, and I lose my joy and peace at times, but they return with prayer and biblical thinking about whatever issue is stressing me. My life is so different that it cannot be compared to before—and the key was getting rid of bitterness. I feel so free![202]

Revealing the Bounty of Forgiveness

"Forgive us our debts, as we also have forgiven our debtors" (Matt. 6:12 NIV). The command to forgive people who've wronged us is centuries old. We've heard it from parents, pastors, and teachers. C. S. Lewis says, "Everyone says forgiveness is a lovely idea until they have something to forgive." We have even been told forgiveness is good for us. Generally, forgiveness is not a problem as long as we haven't been hurt too deeply. Minor offenses are a good place to start and we're content to get that far. However, the real issue comes when a person crosses that invisible line called "too far." A coworker disrespects you, a criminal kills someone you love, a thief takes some of your possessions. Whether friend or foe, that person has stepped over the line where you're not able or willing to forgive. The deeper the hurt, the harder it becomes to apply the balm of forgiveness both to your heart and theirs.

Why is it so difficult for us to forgive? It seems normal that we'd have difficulty forgiving enemies, but we appear to have an equally hard time or even harder time letting go of offenses committed by family members, loved ones, or even God. For many people, the hardest person to forgive is themselves. The reason forgiveness is such a challenge for our hearts and minds is that there exists a genuine debt. If a person has wronged you, he has taken something precious from you. He has stolen a person, an object, or your reputation. The result is an outstanding balance, a debt that the person owes you. And this debt is not just in your mind. It is real. "And forgive us our sins, for we also forgive everyone who is indebted to us" (Luke 11:4, NKJV).

Think of the people around you. Has anyone taken something from you? Are you aware of a debt (wrong done), or multiple debts, existing in your heart? Write those debts here, along with the name of the person who owes it to you.

_____

_____

_____

With regard to these debts, we have some choices. We can continue living our daily lives, acting as if nothing bothers us. No one can see these offenses, and they appear invisible. So we can go on with our game of pretend—even to ourselves—hoping that our pain will eventually evaporate and disappear. We can go for years, falsely believing that we have dealt with the issues of the past. However, the debts that people owe you, even though they appear undetected, still have a profound effect. Those owed debts actually have weight. The greater your loss, the more it weighs on you. And the cumulative total of these debts toward you weighs down on your mind and body. The weight acts like a wooden yoke that binds two oxen together. Both the offender (person who has wronged you) and the offended (you) feel the load.

Mark 11:25-26 says, "And when ye stand praying, forgive, if ye have ought against any: that your Father also which in heaven may forgive you your trespasses. But if ye do not forgive, neither will your Father which is in heaven forgive your trespasses" (KJV). Jesus showed that we cannot hold anything against anyone. Not only do we hold on to the debt, but we also hold it against the one who wronged us.

When I learned to forgive, it was like a million pounds lifted from me.
—Reba McEntire

Carrying this weight around on your inside is like lugging around a physical load. It will literally wear you down. Imagine if you had to drag around a one-hundred-pound bag of sand everywhere you went. You would eventually feel achy joint pain, and your heart rate would climb. After days, weeks, or even months of this labor, you would start feeling depressed. The stress of dealing with this burden promises only anxiety. This is precisely what occurs when you insist on unforgiveness. You clutch to your heart and drag around a massive weight that is dangerous for your health.

Right now, is a weight weighing down your mind, crippling your feelings or even adversely affecting your body? Write down some of the symptoms you're experiencing that could be attributed to an unresolved grudge.

_____

_____

_____

It is by forgiving that one is forgiven.
—Mother Teresa

Begin Forgiveness

In order to eliminate these negative effects and to begin experiencing renewed health, you need to forgive those who are indebted to you. As long as you focus on the wrongs people have done to you, forgiveness is impossible. As stated earlier, forgiveness is not a synonym for repression. You can't just ignore these debts, because they truly exist. However, it is also important to know that forgiveness is not a release from legal or spiritual obligations. If someone's debt toward you is also a debt toward society, then that person still has to be brought to justice. For example, if someone has stolen your car, you can forgive the perpetrator, but if he gets caught, he still will have to go to jail. From a biblical standpoint, every sinner's offenses are ultimately against God and His righteousness. And, at the end of time, every person will still have to pay for his wrongdoing. The only exception to this rule is if the person repents before God and trusts Jesus Christ to have paid that debt in full at the cross at Calvary. In any event, the debt must be paid.

Forgiveness is setting a prisoner free and then realizing the prisoner was you.

—Lewis Smedes

If forgiveness is not suppressing memories or releasing to justice, then what specifically does Jesus call us to do? Throughout the Bible, sins and offenses are viewed as burdens or weights. The Hebrew term used in the Old Testament for "forgive" is rooted in the concept of "lifting up" the weight, taking it off the shoulders of yourself and the one who has wronged you. "Thus you shall say to Joseph: 'I beg you, please forgive [lift up] the trespass of your brothers and their sin; for they did evil to you'" (Gen. 50:17 NKJV). In the Greek background of the New Testament, the basic meaning of the word translated "forgive" is "to send away." You would take the offense that is pulling you down and get rid of it.

"If we confess our sins, He is faithful and just to forgive us [send away] our sins and to cleanse us from all unrighteousness" (1 John 1:9 NKJV). The Bible teaches from beginning to end that in forgiveness, we need to lift off the burden, like that yoke that pulls us down.

Perhaps you have attempted to forgive others or forgive yourself, but you weren't able to totally throw off the weight. You're trying, but the offense just won't budge. The problem is that there is a lock on the yoke. Something in the situation is binding the debt to you. That lock comes from a sense of unworthiness. For example, you may be endeavoring to forgive someone else, but deep down you don't genuinely believe that he or she is really worthy of your forgiveness. They have been devalued in your eyes. And if you're trying to forgive yourself, you don't feel worthy yourself of being released from the debt.

Stress and Forgiveness

As costly as it is to forgive, there is only one consolation—unforgiveness costs far more.
—Ray Pritchard

Why don't you feel worthy of forgiveness? Write down what you've been telling yourself about your lack of worthiness.

_____

_____

Why do you think others aren't worthy? List a few reasons.

_____

_____

For true release, you must give up trying to force people to understand how much they have hurt you. Regardless of how you feel, every person is worth being forgiven. Yet their worthiness is not based on any past track record or how well they've done in life. Rather, their worthiness flows out of who they are as created beings. All individuals have been made in the image of God. As such, they hold a genuine value. It's just like a gold wedding ring that got misplaced. It has perhaps been bent, marred, and dirtied. But it still holds great value, not only because it's gold, but also because it has sentimental significance to someone. In the same way, people can tarnish the image of God He created in them, but He still loves them. That's the basic message of John 3:16.

Put your name in the blank lines to remind yourself of how much God loves you.

"For God so loved _____ that He gave His only begotten Son, so that if _____ believes in Him, _____ will have everlasting life" (John 3:16, paraphrased).

In order to forgive anyone—God, yourself, family, a friend, or an enemy—there are three steps you need to take to successfully remove this burden.

1. Identify the debt or wrongdoing. Make sure you know all that has been taken from you.
2. Acknowledge the worthiness of the person you are to forgive. You may not feel that he or she is worthy, but God's Word tells us he or she is.

3. Ask God to help you lift the weight and send it away. If the burden is especially heavy, you don't possess the strength to hoist it up and off your shoulders. Invite the Lord to assist you.

Read Numbers 12. In this chapter Miriam sins against Moses and ultimately against God. She sullied Moses' reputation and questioned his authority. Suddenly, she was stricken with leprosy. Aaron was also a part of this mutiny, but when he realized his error, he asked for forgiveness. Moses considered Miriam worthy of forgiveness, for she was his sister. So he asked God to remove that burden of guilt from her. True to His character, God forgave her, but she still had to pay the price for her act of rebellion and make the required sacrifices.

Are you ready to apply Scripture to this area of your life? Read Matthew 6:9, 12.

According to verse 9, why is another person worthy of our forgiveness?

_____

_____

_____

This scripture begins with "Our Father in heaven." We all belong to Him and He forgives. Since He forgives us, we can then forgive others. Since God finds us worthy to forgive, others are worthy of our forgiveness.

Do we all have debts that need to be forgiven?

_____

Is it possible to have your debts forgiven and yet not forgive others?

_____

Is there anyone you need to forgive right now? I pray your list will not be as long as mine was when the Lord helped me through this.

_____

_____

_____

If you live a life characterized by the regular forgiveness of others and of yourself, your health will benefit in ways such as the following:[203]

- lower blood pressure
- reduction of stress
- lower heart rate
- fewer symptoms of depression
- fewer symptoms of anxiety
- reduction in chronic pain
- improved psychological well-being

A True Act of Forgiveness

On the morning of November 21, 2002, as the sun rose over the horizon in the port city of Sidon in southern Lebanon, Bonnie Witherall was up early. That day she was going to work at the prenatal clinic that offers medical services to the Muslim women from a nearby refugee camp. Tensions were running high because of events elsewhere in the Middle East, and Americans in general and missionaries in particular had been warned of potential danger. Bonnie and her husband, Gary, both had come to Lebanon with a burden to share Christ in the Muslim world. For several years they had studied Arabic so they could communicate with the people they hoped to reach with the gospel.

At approximately eight a.m., Bonnie answered a knock at the clinic door. Authorities can only surmise what happened next. Evidently a man hit her in the face and chest, and then he shot her three times in the head, killing her instantly. When Gary heard the news, he ran to the clinic. By that time the police had come and the gunman was nowhere to be found. Gary tried to fight his way into the room where his wife lay in a pool of blood, but the police wouldn't let him enter. In one of the cruel ironies of our modern world, someone took a picture of Bonnie after she died, and that gruesome picture somehow ended up on the Internet.

The next day, the London *Times* carried a report on the murder of Bonnie Witherall. It quoted Gary as saying he had forgiven his wife's killers. "God led us to Lebanon and we knew that we might die....It's a costly forgiveness....It cost my wife." On the long flight while accompanying his wife's body home to America, Gary came to a simple conclusion: "God said there's a seed that's been planted in your heart. You either hate and be angry, or you forgive. I said I have to forgive."[204]

In the end, forgiveness is not about us or about those who have hurt us. Forgiveness is all about God. Until we grasp this, unforgiveness will remain a terrible burden we cannot bear. The treasure of health that is found in forgiveness comes from the One who gave us abundant life. In forgiveness of others, ourselves, and God, we find a great piece to the treasure map, one of the key ingredients to having a life full of health and vitality.

Taking this treasure to heart: Take a moment to write out what God has taught you in this lesson.

_____

_____

Applying this treasure at home: What commitment are you going to make to improve your health? What steps can you make to work toward forgiveness? Record this on your Action Plan.

Suggested Further Reading:

Ray Pritchard. *The Healing Power of Forgiveness.* Eugene, OR: Harvest House, 2005.
Stephen and Alex Kendrick. *The Love Dare.* Nashville: B&H, 2008.
Kent Whitaker. *Murder by Family.* West Monroe, LA: Howard Books, 2009.

FABULOUS FOODIE FRIDAY

Foodie Time

It's time for a Chocolate Extravaganza! Stress and forgiveness may lead some of you straight to the chocolate bar. Let's explore the world of chocolate. Join your foodie friend and see how many different foods you can make with this delicacy. Experiment with the various flavors of chocolate and the different manufacturers.

Experiment with the following recipes from the *Healthy Treasures Cookbook:*

Impossible Pie—adding chocolate makes this an even better treat
Granola—any recipe can have chocolate chips added (chop the chips up first so they are small, otherwise they are overpowering)
Fresh Fruit Ice Cream—add chocolate to this to make it unique
Chocolate Cloud—a light, low calorie treat (a *must* on the foodie list!)

I am sure you have found other chocolate recipes that give you delight in being a foodie. When you make a great recipe discovery, send it to Designed Healthy Living to post on the website for other foodies to try.

Here's one more fact regarding chocolate so you won't feel guilty. Men and women everywhere have always known of the benefits of chocolate. Now the world knows of its health benefits as well, not to mention the fact that organic chocolate helps our environment. The phenols in chocolate are known to help the immune system, reduce the risk of cancer, and promote heart health. Dark chocolate, pound for pound, has higher levels of antioxidants than blueberries! Dark chocolate also contains more flavonoids than green tea.[205]

Don't forget Principle III!

Chocolate is good by yourself, but better when shared with friends.

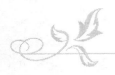

Exercise

DAY ONE—THE GLORY OF THE TEMPLE

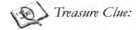 *Treasure Clue:*

I will praise You, for I am fearfully and wonderfully made; Marvelous are
Your works, and that my soul knows very well.

—Ps. 139:14 NKJV

At the airport for a business trip, I settled down to wait for the boarding announcement at Gate 35. Then I heard an announcement: "We apologize for the inconvenience, but Delta Flight 570 will board from Gate 41."

So I hurried over to Gate 41. Not ten minutes later, another announcement: "Delta Flight 570 is indeed boarding at Gate 35. Sorry for the inconvenience." So I hurried back to Gate 35.

Soon I again heard the public address system say, "Thank you for participating in Delta's physical fitness program."[206]

Are you ready for a fitness program? How do you view your body? Is it something that you treasure as a gift? Or is it just available to use at your disposal? How we take care of our body reflects on how we view God.

God has gifted us with a "fearfully and wonderfully made" temple designed to perfectly glorify Him. In the ancient days, the glory of the God of Israel dwelt within the sanctuary of the temple, and meticulous care was taken to honor His throne. Do we take that same care of our physical temple today? There is a holy call to worship our Creator by offering our bodies as a living sacrifice in gratitude for the price He paid for us.

God created us for His glory as complete, synchronized beings. Just like the temple, we have a foundation that is based upon cells that are responsible for efficiently performing every function of our bodies. Our bones provide a structural support system and framework to support the bodily temple. And the skin provides efficient protection, communication, and sensation as an exterior covering.

Read Romans 12:1 and write it out here.

_____

Does God care about how we treat our bodies? He created us in His image, sent His Son to die for us, and because He gave His life, we worship Him by surrendering our lives. As Christians we cannot fulfill the planned purpose of God if we are unhealthy due to neglecting our bodies. God has ordained us as stewards, and we cannot fully develop spiritually until we have developed physically.

So how do we develop physically? We've learned about eating and resting properly, but the other component to a healthy lifestyle involves exercise and movement. Exercise is important for the following reasons:

- An increased general feeling of health and well being
- Getting tired less easily
- Prevention, delay, or a great ability to withstand and recover from heart problems and other degenerative diseases
- Controlled body weight
- Improved posture and appearance
- Relief of tension and/or stress
- Prevention of lower back pain
- Delayed aging process
- Delayed aging of brain cells
- Improved neuromuscular skill and physical performance
- Clearer thinking
- Better digestion and bowel movement
- Improved functioning of the internal organs

He who does not take time for exercise will take equal time for illness.
—Dr. Richard Brouse

Take a look at the following story, "A Personal Journey into Fitness," by Pastor Jeff Brauer.

Though I came from a family that practiced many aspects of good nutrition and exercise, I was doing neither when in my early twenties I developed symptoms generally diagnosed as fibromyalgia. My doctor recommended exercise as the cornerstone of my strategy for diminishing the impact my malady would have on my life. He believed in it so much he actually gave me a prescription for an indoor bike so that I would be exempted from paying sales tax.

I began to use it at a low level for twenty minutes three times a week. That was over twenty years ago. I eventually put over 10,000 miles on that indoor bike. Now I exercise a couple hours a day, six days a week. I have ridden a century (one hundred miles in a day) on my outdoor bike, run a 10k race, a half-marathon (13.1 miles), and have completed a 70.3 mile triathlon.

When I saw the benefits I was gaining from exercise, I followed the advice given in Proverbs 18:15, "The heart of the prudent acquires knowledge, and the ear of the wise seeks knowledge" (NKJV). I began to "acquire knowledge" concerning exercise and its worthy sibling, nutrition. So while I have never been formally trained in the field of exercise, for over twenty years I have experienced the immense benefits derived from it and learned all I could pertaining to this discipline.[207]

The improvements to our health and the personal testimony give us an insight to the power of this discipline of exercise. Whom do you know who could benefit from adding five minutes of exercise or stretching into his or her daily life?

"Or do you not know that your body is a temple of the Holy Spirit within you, who you have from God? You are not your own, for you were bought with a price. So glorify God in your body" (1 Cor. 6:19-20 ESV). This verse tells us three things about our bodies:

- **Occupancy**—The Holy Spirit dwells within us. When I realize the very presence of God is living inside me, it changes what I do with my body and where I take it. When I defile or neglect my temple, it's as if I'm destroying the very resting place of the most Holy God.
- **Ownership**—Our bodies do not belong to us, but to the one who has purchased us with His blood. We have been given stewardship of these earthly bodies, so we must honor God by taking care of what we've been given. If someone offered you a really nice car and said you could keep the car only if you kept it in good condition, you would do everything in your power to take care of that car, right? It's the same with our bodies: we can only keep them if they stay in a healthy condition.
- **Obedience**—We have been given a free will to choose, but we also have personal responsibility to eat, rest, and exercise properly. As we practice self-discipline, our good health will enhance our service to God. As 2 Timothy 1:7 says, "For God gave us a spirit not of fear butof power and love and self-control" (ESV).

What does the Bible say about our bodies?

_____

_____

Why is it important to protect and preserve our temples?

_____

_____

_____

The Mind of Christ

Read Philippians 2:1-18. What is our attitude supposed to be?

_____

_____

No matter what we do, we are not supposed to grumble or complain! That's especially hard to remember whether it's your first week of exercising or whether you're at miles nine or ten of a twelve-mile run. And it's even easier to forget not to grumble in reference to most exercise. But we are called to be lights in a dark world, to display Christ to others, and I believe that means taking care of our gift of life. It's imperative that we don't destroy our temple with drugs, alcohol, nicotine, processed foods, and neglecting to exercise. The world is watching us; will they see Christ in our actions?

Sometimes it's difficult to find motivation to exercise. But changing our attitudes and mindsets is essential in order to find inspiration. Some ways to think positively:

- Focus on the benefits of exercise: increased energy, mental focus, and self-esteem; weight loss, staving off disease, and longer life
- Set goals
- Look for improvements: a faster mile, a few more reps, or one less dress size
- Join your foodie friend or find a buddy
- Do something you like
- Spend time with God on a run, bike ride, etc

Think of some ways to be motivated to get up and move! List three things that will help motivate you to move purposefully and intensely every day:

1.
2.
3.

It always helps to get inspiration from others. Read Hunter Stoner's testimony about changing focus.

A few years ago I never could have encouraged people to exercise. I boasted skills in computer games and TV trivia, laughed at runners with no destination, and thought that the five o'clock gym-goers were insane. As of now, I can boast of my skills in Irish dance (a highly athletic and demanding dance that I compete in at the highest level), I ran a half marathon (preparing for my second, as well as training for Division 1 college cross country), and I wake up as early as possible to fit my exercise in.

What changed? I wish there was a magic formula. I found things that I loved—for a few years it was dance, now it's swimming and running—that kept me motivated and focused. When I have goals, whether it's a faster mile or to move up a level in dance, all of my determination and energy is spent trying to accomplish that goal. I also began to learn about exercise science, and when I discovered the benefits of what I was doing it only made me want to work harder, not to mention I felt better about myself after I became lean and strong.

There are times I still find getting out the door at six a.m. for a long run difficult; we're all human. I remind myself that Christ is the only one who strengthens me; He provides every breath and in all I do I glorify Him. By preserving and protecting my temple I am a witness to the world of what active worship looks like.[208]

Taking this treasure to heart: Think about your view of exercise. If you were in the airport when the departure gate was changed, would you be disgruntled or chuckling at the unexpected chance to get a workout?

Are you ready to look at ways to introduce exercise into your health program?

How will you need to change your focus to make exercise important?

_____

_____

Applying this treasure at home: Take a moment to pray about how God would have you implement the discipline of exercise into your daily activities.

Day Two—Pressing on in the Race with Exercise

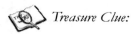 *Treasure Clue:*

Therefore, since we are surrounded by so great a cloud of witnesses, let us also lay aside every weight, and sin which clings so closely, and let us run with endurance the race that is set before us, looking to Jesus, the founder and perfecter of our faith, who for the joy that was set before him endured the cross, despising the shame, and is seated at the right hand of the throne of God.
—Heb. 12:1-2 ESV

Hebrews talks about a race that is set before us. When did this race begin? A compelling verse that answers this question in regard to the importance of physical exercise and how it ties into our complete well-being is Genesis 2:15. It says, "Then the Lord God took the man and put him in the Garden of Eden to tend and keep it" (NKJV). This, of course, was before sin came into the world and while everything was still perfect. So even before the ravages of sin began to take their toll, it was beneficial for man to have work—or a hobby—to do. He would not be working himself to death as has often happened since the fall, nor would he live a subtly destructive sedentary life as, again, so many have done. God made us and knew that exercise would benefit us in so many ways! He knew we would have a race to finish.

As we continue through the expedition of health, Jesus will carry us through the trials, roadblocks, and tears, imparting joy and peace for the journey. Pressing on toward the mark, we will keep our eyes fixed on the One who guides our steps and enables us to proclaim that we have kept the faith and fought the good fight. Make it a daily passion to run with Christ, and He will carry you across the finish line of your faith. Because He defeated death, we have the victory in Christ Jesus: we are destined to win. We do not run aimlessly, but with purpose in every step.

1 Corinthians 9:24-27 tells us, "So run that you may obtain [the prize]. Every athlete exercises self-control in all things....I discipline my body and keep it under control, lest after preaching to others I myself should be disqualified" (ESV). Our God requires us to practice self-control in all aspects of life. We do this not only in obedience, but to display to the world the difference that Christ makes in us. Exercise is a discipline: a training that develops and molds who we are physically, mentally, and spiritually.

Read Philippians 3:14 and write it out.

_____

_____

_____

Are you pressing on? Or does it seem like the goal is just too far away? The finish line is not yet in sight, but our Father provides mile-markers to inform us that He is still pacing us. Sometimes it's easy to forget why we are here and what our calling is while we're on Earth. As we forge on ahead in the race, let us keep our gaze focused on that day when we will meet our Savior, the Lord Jesus Christ, who will transform our lowly bodies to be like His glorious body. Let us throw off every weight and sin, so that we may run freely without fainting and rise up on eagle's wings.

Getting Started

There are many different ways to exercise, and a great variety of goals can be achieved. The most important forms of exercise are those targeting the cardiovascular system, which refers specifically to the heart and blood vessels but benefits every system in the body. You can do other forms of exercise after you are fit from a cardiovascular standpoint, but it would be foolish to do them in lieu of other exercises. If your goal is to lose weight, the same exercises that bring cardiovascular fitness also are best for weight loss. Some people think to lose fat from a certain part of the body, you exercise that part. For instance, if someone wants to lose belly fat, they do crunches. The fact is your body has a blueprint it follows on where to store fat. Unfortunately, we can't change! The only way to get rid of fat is to burn more calories than you consume. Usually a one-two punch of restricting intake and increasing the burn rate through exercise works the best. If we want to burn more calories, we exercise the biggest muscles in our body, which are in our legs, not the tiny muscles that are found around our abdomen. As you burn calories through exercise, your body takes off fat according to the blueprint.

It is helpful to understand cardiovascular health and target heart rate. No one is excused from exercising. Even those who are unable to walk can exercise their arms and chest muscles. If you have not exercised in the last several years, there are several tips for getting started. But the most important thing to remember is the need to move.

Cardiovascular and Aerobic Fitness

Cardiovascular workouts are the most important of any fitness regime because they strengthen the heart, blood, blood vessels, and lungs. Circulatory disease affects the heart and lungs and is the leading cause of death in the world. Maintaining cardiovascular fitness prevents these diseases in most cases.

Cardio workouts are intense sessions that raise your heart rate to receive training benefits. You can elevate heart rate by walking briskly, running, swimming, cycling, and playing vigorous sports. To determine your target heart rate to set as your goal during exercise:

- Subtract your age from 220. This is your maximum heart rate.
- Prior to exercise, count your heart rate (pulse) for one minute (this will be your resting heart rate) and subtract that number from your maximum heart rate.
- Multiply the difference by .7 if you have been exercising consistently, and by .6 if you haven't exercised in months or are over fifty years old
- Add your resting heart rate again to get your aerobic threshold

220 - _____ age= _____ (maximum heart rate)

-_____ (resting heart rate)

=_____ x .7 (or .6)

=_____ + resting heart rate

=_____ desired working heart rate or aerobic threshold

If you are just starting an exercise program, start slowly and train at around 70 to 60 percent of your aerobic threshold. Duration of exercise should mirror what your fitness level is. If you can only do five or ten minutes of exercise at first, that's all right. Do what you can. Your body will adjust as you get stronger and you will be able to handle more in a few weeks. If you are fit, you should be exercising longer. The key is consistency; make an effort to exercise at least three times a week, preferably four to six times. Once five minutes is no longer a struggle, increase your time by five minutes every week until you are up to twenty minutes. Set aside a time of day that you prefer, and stick to your schedule.

If you have been inactive for four weeks or longer, start a walking program to slowly develop your leg muscles. For older adults or those with a low level of cardiovascular fitness, walking provides enough physical stress to increase cardiovascular fitness.

Check out these important things to remember:

- Get a medical examination before starting an exercise program
- Always warm up before exercising
- Cool down after exercising
- Exercise within your tolerance
- Progress slowly
- Get adequate rest and nutrition
- Exercise regularly
- Wear proper shoes
- Exercise cautiously in hot weather
- Dress appropriately in cold conditions

Strength Training

"Strengthen the weak hands, and make firm the feeble knees" (Isa. 35:3 RSV). Weight training, if done properly, will not make you look like Arnold Schwarzenegger or break feeble bones. There are more than six hundred muscles, and research has shown that muscles will degenerate if they are not constantly used and strengthened. Training the muscles will help correct posture, lower back pain, and neck joint disorders; build muscular balance, endurance, and strength; and prevent injuries when exercising. Two thirty-sixty minute workouts per week should be sufficient for building the muscles.

Don't forget to build your abdominals. Our core muscles protect our lower back and are the stabilization to every movement we make. It's important to build these muscles in order to increase strength, agility, power, and speed.

If you've never done weight training before, I suggest finding a book at the library that will show you different exercises for specific muscles and the proper form to do them. It may also be helpful to find a personal trainer who will supervise your workout sessions. When developing a program, you want to include all five types of muscular contractions and movements:

1. Flexion—Bending or decreasing the angle between two bones; for example, bringing the forearm to the shoulder
2. Extension—Increasing the angle between two bones; for example, returning the forearm to its original straight position

3. Abduction—Moving the bone away from the midline of the body (the invisible line that divides the body into right and left halves); for example, raising the arm out to the side of the body
4. Adduction—Moving the bone towards the midline of the body; for example, returning the arm to the side
5. Circumduction—Moving in all planes; for example, rotating the arms in circles

Stretching

Stretching is essential for maintaining flexibility, reducing muscle soreness, and preventing injury. Take at least ten minutes each day to stretch out all of your main muscle groups; this will help keep you relaxed and limber. Stretching in the morning will make you ready for the day. Some of these stretches can be done while sitting at a desk. Here is an example of an easy stretching routine:

- Head—Gently roll your neck in a circle several times. Switch directions.
- Neck—Place your right hand over your head and onto the left ear. Gently pull with your hand and tilt your head towards the right. Repeat on the opposite side.
- Triceps—Lift one arm in the air, bend your elbow, and place the arm behind your head. Place the other hand on the bent elbow, stretching out the back of the arm. Repeat on the opposite side.
- Shoulders—Clasp your hands together, out in front of you. Roll the palms outward while hunching over to stretch out the shoulders.
- Sides—Lift your right arm in the air, place your left hand on your hip. Bend over to your left, stretching out the right side. Repeat on the left side.
- Hips—Stand with your feet farther than shoulder width apart. Bend at the knees into a deep plié, placing your hands on the tops of the thighs for support. Feel the stretch in the inner thigh and groin area.
- Hamstrings—With your feet together, step the right foot out about two feet. Lean forward at the waist, keeping the back straight. Feel the back of the leg stretch. Repeat on the left side.
- Quadriceps—Bend your right leg back behind you and grab the foot with your right hand. Feel the front of the thigh stretch. Repeat on the other side.
- Calf—Standing on the edge of a stair, place your foot so your heel is off of the stair. Gently push your heel down to stretch the back of the calf. Repeat on the other side.

Keep in mind that whatever exercise you choose to do, it will only be effective if you stick with it! The first couple of months are the most crucial. Especially at the very beginning, your body will complain, your schedule will resist, and you will think of a thousand reasons not to continue. If you persevere, the reward of a gift of better health awaits you. You will sleep better. You will look better and feel better—not just physically, but emotionally as well. Exercise not only puts the physical benefits back into our lives, but the emotional benefits as well. Exercise gives us time to think. If we do it with a spouse or friend, it gives us a time for healthy, informal interaction with others.

Make every day an opportunity to move purposefully and intensely. We draw close to Jesus by appreciating who He has created us to be and discovering the unique capabilities of our bodies. Remember that we are accountable to God for the way we control our bodies under His authority.

Read 1 Timothy 4:8. What is more valuable than physical exercise?

_____

_____

What is the promise that we have?

_____

_____

We must also train ourselves for godliness: "For while bodily training is of some value, godlinessis of value in every way, asit holds promise for the present life and also for the life to come" (1 Tim. 4:8 ESV). We toil and strive because our hope is in the living God, our Savior. Being physically fit enables us to live up to our potential as whole human beings in God's service, which will bring us joy and peace.

YOU CAN (words of Dr. Couey)

I once shared an office with a colleague and friend who had a sign displayed on our office wall that read in large letters "You Can." I can't begin to tell you how that sign has changed many facets of my life. Every time I'm faced with a new challenge in my busy schedule, I immediately respond with excuses and rationalizations that I cannot possibly accept this new challenge. Then I look at that sign hanging on the wall and confidence overshadows my laziness. The point is, "You Can."

You can start an exercise program at any age and any weight. There are thousands of senior adults who can testify to that statement. Recently a senior adult woman came up to me after a fitness seminar and remarked: "Look at me, I'm so old I can barely walk. How can I start exercising?" My response to her question was, "Then start barely walking." Two years later I received a letter from her with these responses: "I took your advice about walking. I'm now walking three miles a day. I feel better, my body is stronger, and I can do more work for God. By the way, I won three people to Christ on my eighty-eighth birthday."

Many Christians use excuses such as "I'm too handicapped by some physical malady to begin an exercise program." Let me share an experience of the most courageous accomplishment I have ever witnessed in a sporting event. After completing a marathon run of twenty-six miles I decided to watch other runners finish the marathon course. After watching for about five minutes, I saw the crowd giving a standing ovation to a pair of runners and sensed an emotion so strong that chill bumps covered my body and tears came to my eyes. For you see, these runners had run stride for stride twenty-six miles together with unbelievable handicaps. The lead runner's feet were amputated at the ankle joints and he had run on a wooden prosthesis. He held a rope in his hand and running behind him was the other runner holding the rope, who was completely blind. I looked at the pride of those runners crossing that finish line and again the words of that sign in my office entered my mind.

Taking this treasure to heart: Many days will come when exercise will not be on the list of things you want to do. If you could make one statement to remind yourself why exercise is important, what would it be? Write it here.

_____

_____

Applying this treasure at home: What commitment can you make to yourself and your foodie friend to make exercise an important part of your daily life? Record this on your Action Plan and share it with your foodie friend.

Day Three—Keeping the Treasure in Your Heart

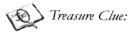 *Treasure Clue:*

I have hidden your word in my heart that I might not sin against you.

—Ps. 119:11 NIV

One of the best companions to an exercise program is the discipline of Scripture memory. Reciting verses as you walk, jog, or bike is a way to incorporate both disciplines into your daily schedule.

A small boy forgot his lines in the Sunday school presentation. His mother sat on the front row and tried to prompt him by gesturing and silently forming the words with her lips. It was no use. The boy's memory was blank.

Finally she leaned forward and whispered his cue: "I am the light of the world."

With a broad smile and beaming confidence the child said in a loud clean voice, "My mother is the light of the world."[209]

How's your memory? Have you ever been in a conversation and knew a certain verse would give definition to your topic, but you couldn't recall it? You might know bits and pieces, but the remainder escapes you. Or have you been under the teaching of someone who dared anyone to defend the Bible? Reciting Scripture would have given you a defense, but you couldn't quite remember anything that would be useful in the situation. It is common for us to memorize Scripture for comfort and discernment but we need to be ready in all situations. Scripture memory will prepare us for anything.

Write out one of your favorite verses from memory. Don't worry if it isn't word perfect.

_____

_____

_____

_____

Why do you like this verse? How does God use it in your life?

_____

_____

_____

Are you ready to have more treasures in your heart? If the thought of memorizing Scripture intimidates you, you are not alone. Most of us fall back from the topic of Scripture memory because of fears—fear of not being able to succeed, letting God down, not being seen as a "spiritual Christian" unless this is accomplished, memory difficulties, and so on. Don't let these fears keep you from trying. The Holy Spirit will be your guide. Remember, He has been guiding us all along this expedition, and He will not leave you now. We need to keep God's Word in our hearts and minds in order to keep our guard on our treasure and not let Satan steal it.

Write out a prayer to God and tell Him your concerns about Scripture memory.

_____

_____

_____

_____

Scripture memory is taught all throughout the life of most Christians. Since I am a competitive person, whenever a reward was dangled in front of me I would challenge myself to meet it. During my growing-up years, those rewards included candy, badges, certificates, beating the boys in Bible drills, or just hearing a gratifying "well done" from a favorite teacher. But then adulthood set in and life became busy. Scripture memory was no longer on the top of my to-do list, and the rewards slipped from my focus. Thankfully God sent a mentor into my life, Bette, who encouraged me to join an *Experiencing God* class. The class had two requirements: no absences or tardies were allowed for twelve weeks and lessons and memorization had to be completed on time!

Have you ever taken a class or Bible study, knowing you might not do all the lessons on time? How would your attitude and expectation level change if these disciplines were put in place?

My life as a working mother and wife was busy. There were many times I took Bible study classes to just get the main points and hope it would penetrate and make an impact. This is possible, but a life-changing impact happens when we give God everything we have to offer. That meant coming prepared, on time, and ready to go. I decided to take my friend up on this challenge—all scriptures memorized, all lessons completed on time with no absences. I took this challenge to give God my all, expecting God to show Himself to me.

Bette encouraged me through the challenge. Her life was an example that resonated with God at work in such a way that He continually revealed Himself to her and she could identify each step He made in her life. That model transformed my view of a Christian life. I went from using God for my benefit to seeking Him first. That is a continual challenge and experience each day I live.

Going through *Experiencing God* with total dedication transformed my spiritual life. The twelve weeks of class unfolded and as I spent hours memorizing, reading, and praying, my senses began to awaken to the Holy Spirit. You see, it was not the Holy Spirit that moved or changed, it was I who had previously been unable to see, hear, feel, or experience Him due to the life that I was living. It was full of "other" things. I was so blessed. I began to see why treasuring God's Word in my heart could help me sense when He was prompting me to join Him in His plan.

My life is still full of continuous ups and downs, but when I am down I know how to get up. It is easier to get up the less time you are down. Don't let any step we have learned through this study stay off your daily goals for too long. Encourage your foodie friend if he or she is down; lift up your family members. Life is more enjoyable when we are up. The Scripture we memorize will give us that lift.

Let me encourage you to take this challenge that has great rewards. Make Scripture memory and prayer an important part of your daily walk.

Scriptures will help you in five areas:

- Handling difficult situations—"I can do all things through Christ" (Phil. 4:13 KJV).
- Overcoming temptation—Knowledge of Scripture and the strength that comes with the ability to use it are an important part of putting on the full armor of God in preparation for spiritual warfare. "No temptation has overtaken you but such as is common to man; and God is faithful, who will not allow you to be tempted beyond what you are able, but with the temptation will provide a way of escape also, so that you will be able to bear it" (1 Cor. 10:13 NASB).
- Finding direction—"Your word is a lamp to my feet and a light to my path" (Ps. 119:105 NKJV).
- Gaining wisdom—"Always be prepared to give an answer to everyone who asks you to give a reason for the hope that you have" (1 Peter 3:15 NIV).
- Making us more powerful and effective evangelists—It transforms our entire world-view from the secular to the heavenly. "Do not be conformed any longer to the pattern of this world, but be transformed by the renewing of your mind. Then you will able to test and approve what God's will is—his good, pleasing, and perfect will" (Rom. 12:2 NIV).

Treasure Clues

Each week in this course began with a Treasure Clue. If you have been memorizing these weekly, you already have a treasure chest full of God's Word. Let's look back on some of the verses in our treasure hunt:

Week 1—"My son, if you will receive my words and treasure my commandments within you…then you will…discover the knowledge of God" (Prov. 2:1, 5 NIV).

Week 2—"My son, give attention to my words; incline your ear to my sayings. Do not let them depart from your sight; keep them in the midst of your heart. For they are life to those who find them and health to all their body" (Prov. 4:20-22 NASB).

Week 3—"I tell you the truth, he who believes has everlasting life" (John 6:47 NIV).

Week 4—"Sow the fields, and plant vineyards, which may yield fruits of increase" (Ps. 107:37 KJV).

Week 5—"To everything there is a season, and a time to every purpose under the heaven: A time to be born, and a time to die; a time to plant, and a time to pluck up that which is planted" (Ecc. 3:1-2 KJV).

Week 6—"Open my eyes, that I may behold wonderful things from Your law" (Ps. 119:18 NASB).

Part II—"'For I know the plans that I have for you,' declares the Lord, 'plans for welfare and not for calamity to give you a future and a hope'" (Jer. 29:11 NASB).

Week 7—"But this kind does not go out except by prayer and fasting" (Matt. 17:21 NASB).

Week 8—"Pleasant words are as a honeycomb, sweet to the soul, and health to the bones" (Prov. 16:24 KJV).

Week 9—"We will stand before this house and before You (for Your name is in this house) and cry to You in our distress, and You will hear and deliver us" (2 Chron. 20:9 NASB).

Week 10—"He gives strength to the weary, and to him who lacks might He increases power. Though youths grow weary and tired, and vigorous young men stumble badly, Yet those who wait for the Lord will gain new strength; They will mount up with wings like eagles, They will run and not get tired, They will walk and not become weary" (Isa. 40:29-31 NASB).

Week 11—"I will praise You, for I am fearfully and wonderfully made; Marvelous are Your works, and that my soul knows very well" (Ps. 139:14 NKJV).

Week 12—"Whatever you do in word or deed, do all in the name of the Lord Jesus, giving thanks through Him to God the Father" (Col. 3:17 NASB).

The following are some other key verses from our study that are part of your complete health.

Fullness—"I have come that they may have life, and have it to the full" (John 10:10 NIV).

Personal relationship—"For God so loved the world, that He gave His only begotten Son, that whoever believes in Him shall not perish, but have eternal life" (John 3:16 NASB).

Commitment—"We urge you, brethren, to excel still more" (1 Thess. 4:10 NASB).

Discipline—"Be self-controlled and alert. Your enemy the devil prowls around like a roaring lion looking for someone to devour" (1 Peter 5:8 NIV).

Trust—"Those who know your name will trust in you, for you, Lord, have never forsaken those who seek you" (Ps. 9:10 NIV).

Purity—"Finally, brothers, whatever is true, whatever is noble, whatever is right, whatever is pure, whatever is lovely, whatever is admirable—if anything is excellent or praiseworthy—think about such things" (Phil. 4:8 NIV).

Contentment—"I have learned the secret of being content in any and every situation, whether well fed or hungry, whether living in plenty or in want. I can do everything through him who gives me strength" (Phil. 4:12-13 NIV).

Perseverance—"Let us not become weary in doing good, for at the proper time we will reap a harvest if we do not give up" (Gal. 6:9 NIV).

Taking this treasure to heart: From the verses you just read, which one(s) would be good to memorize?

_____

_____

Applying this treasure at home: A friend of mine used to write songs with the words of the verse she was learning. It made the memorizing easier. How can you encourage your family to memorize Scripture?

_____

_____

Day Four—A Bible Challenge—Memorizing Verses

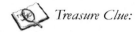 *Treasure Clue:*

Jesus said…"Man does not live on bread alone, but on every word that comes from the mouth of God."

—Matt. 4:4 NIV

If you could make a plan, would you like to memorize one verse per week? If so, it would give you fifty-two new verses a year to treasure in your heart and mind. If you could do one verse per month, it would give you twelve verses a year in your heart and mind.

Do you want it to be simple? Follow these five simple steps: read, visualize, write, say, and memorize.

Find a Treasure Clue that makes an impact on your life today. Write it down on a card that can be placed in your purse or on a mirror where you will see it often. Some people prefer to buy blank three-by-five spiral note cards. This is a handy way to flip through the verses as you learn them.

Daily Guide for Single Verse Memory

Study the following guide for Scripture memory. Repeat the process each week, adding new verses as you go.

- Day One—Read the verse out loud ten times. Always memorize the verse address (or reference) along with it. Read the verses surrounding it to get a full picture of the scene that is taking place. As you visualize it and hear the verse spoken out loud, the memory will become more natural.
- Day Two—Read the verse and address again. Recite it ten times. Continue for one week.
- Days Four-Six—Review the new verse along with last four verses learned.
- Day Seven—Recite all the verses you have learned.

What is the first verse you want to memorize? Write it here.

_____

_____

_____

Paul said, "All Scripture is God-breathed and is useful for teaching, rebuking, correcting, and training in righteousness" (2 Tim. 3:16 NIV).

A Treasure Challenge

Dr. Andrew Davis, senior pastor at First Baptist Church in Durham, North Carolina, gives us a charge to take our treasure a step further and consider memorizing whole chapters and books of the Bible. His theory is that when we memorize individual verses we tend to miss intervening verses that we do not feel are as momentous. Furthermore, most of Scripture is written to make a case, there is a flow of argumentation that is missed if *just* individual verses are memorized. In addition, there is also a greater likelihood of taking verses out of context by focusing on individual verses.

The first step to memorizing books is to memorize chapters. This requires a commitment. Go to the Lord in prayer and ask Him if He wants you to invest time in Scripture memorization. Listen to Him. Write out your prayer, concern, and conviction here.

_____

_____

_____

_____

This prayer is more than just leaving a message on voice mail. When you seek His guidance on this issue, do it with a sincere inquisition. Once He has confirmed it in your heart and mind, humbly ask the Holy Spirit for help. Ask Him to protect you from spiritual pride. Knowledge of the Bible is necessary for spiritual maturity and for increasing the yield of our treasure chest, but biblical knowledge without love for God and neighbor "puffs up" a person and makes him or her useless to God and actually harmful to the church. We don't want to use Scripture memory for our own glory.[210]

A Moderate Challenge—Memorizing Chapters

Memorizing chapters takes memorizing verses to a new level. This challenge includes similar steps as memorizing verses.

Choose the chapter that is tugging at your heart. In prayer, ask God if this is a chapter you should focus on. Read the whole book of the Bible to get the picture of what is taking place. In the case of Psalms and Proverbs, this is not necessary; just read the chapters before and after.

In Psalms, make note of the author and understand the background. Write down the chapter. Read it aloud. Then divide it into sections of how many verses you want to learn each day, and follow this guide:

- Day One—Read the first verse (or section) out loud ten times, looking at each word as if photographing it with your eyes. Always include the verse number. Then cover the page and recite it ten times. You're done for the day.
- Day Two—Recite yesterday's verses ten times, being sure to include the verse numbers. Look in the Bible if you need to, just to refresh your memory. Then follow the Day One plan for the next set of verses.
- Day Three—Recite yesterday's verses ten times. Check your Bible if you need help. Then recite all the previously learned verses together ten times out loud. Next, add the new verses for the day. Continue to follow this plan until the chapter is memorized. Check back to the Bible to make sure you are not leaving out words or changing the sequence. Always recite the verse numbers.

When the chapter is completed, recite it completely *each* day for one hundred days. By then the chapter will be a treasure for you to recall when needed. Recite these verses while driving or waiting in line.

The reason Scripture memory is in the same week as exercise is because together they make for a great experience. If you enjoy using a treadmill or stationary bike, it is easy to recite verses out loud while you are trudging along. When I walk outside, I carry my spiral note cards and flip through the verses. If you are a hiker, the verses are easy to carry in your backpack for easy review and reflection. Biking, jogging, running, and other activities are good times to recite verses out loud. All of these activities keep your mind occupied, and time flies by quickly.

The Ultimate Challenge—Memorizing Whole Books of the Bible

This may be a challenge, but it is one not to be avoided. The same pattern used to memorize chapters can be applied to memorizing books. Choose your first book. You might want to choose a short one, lest you get discouraged and give up. The greatest obstacle to lasting achievement in this arena is a lack of perseverance—just giving up. Follow the simple plan outlined above.

For a more detailed guide on memorizing Scripture download the free e-book *An Approach to Extended Memorization of Scripture* by Dr. Andrew Davis on the Designed Healthy Living website.

Which challenge are you ready for: verses, chapters, or books? _____

Where are you going to start? _____

What is the time frame you are going to use to memorize your selection?

_____

Share this with your foodie friend for accountability.

Taking this treasure to heart: What truth did you learn this week that you want to apply to your life?

_____

_____

_____

Applying this treasure at home: What steps or actions will you apply in your life or encourage in your family's life from what you learned this week? Record this on your Action Plan and share it with your foodie friend.

FABULOUS FOODIE FRIDAY

Foodie Time

Let's bring some creative fun into our foodie night this week. This event will liven up any party. After you read the directions be creative to fit the occasion or group of friends. This will require planning ahead of time.

Plan a menu with foods everyone will enjoy. Make sure some of the foods require utensils for eating and some are finger foods. Then make a list that includes: each food, each drink, each condiment needed, each utensil guests will need, and napkins. Do not put them in any kind of order; just mix them up.

Then assign a character name (like Disney characters), a word (such as various baseball terms), a letter, or a number to each listed item. For our purposes in this explanation, we'll use baseball terms. For example:

Ice cream – shortstop
Buckwheat corn muffins – first base
Butter – home plate
Chinese green beans – home run
Fork – second base
Glass of tea – umpire
Glass of water – catcher
Jelly – out
Black bean soup – error
Strawberry rhubarb pie – strike
Napkin – Cardinals
Knife – Fred bird
Poppy seed dressing – outfield
Spoon – Busch Stadium
Strawberry spinach salad – pitcher
Stuffed mushrooms – base hit
Vegetable lasagna – coach

Then make a list of just the baseball terms and make a copy for each guest. When guests arrive, explain that you will be having a three-course meal and they will need to choose which items they would like for each course. The trick is that they don't know what the actual menu items are—they pick from the list of baseball terms. They should write a "1" by the items they would like for their first course, a "2" by the items they would like for their second course, and a "3" by the items for the third course.

Their menus would look like something like this:
Base hit – 1
Busch Stadium – 2
Cardinals – 3
Catcher – 1
Coach – 2

Error – 3
First base – 1
Fred bird – 2
Home plate – 3
Home run – 3
Out – 1
Out field – 2
Pitcher – 1
Second base – 1
Shortstop – 2
Strike – 2
Umpire – 3

When guests are finished filling out these papers, have them write their names at the top and turn them in. Then it's up to you to serve each person the right items for each course of the meal, matching their choices to your original list. For example, the person who filled out the menu above would get the following items for the first course:

Base hit – stuffed mushrooms
Catcher – glass of water
First base – buckwheat muffins
Out – jelly
Pitcher – strawberry spinach salad
Second base – fork

This person did really well with her choices. However, notice that she didn't get the dressing for her salad. She'll get that later with her other food.

This may sound confusing, but it's a lot of fun, especially when people choose items that don't go well together, or they get soup without a spoon! Make sure to serve the meal a course at a time and do not give in and let them have the items they did not select for a particular course. This just adds to the fun.

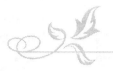

The Fullness of Christ and Health

DAY ONE—ULTIMATE JOY

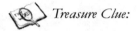 *Treasure Clue:*

Whatever you do in word or deed, do all in the name of the Lord Jesus, giving thanks through Him to God the Father.

—Col. 3:17 NASB

Last week I took my children to a restaurant. My six-year-old son asked if he could say grace. As we bowed our heads he said, "God is good, God is great. Thank You for the food, and I would even thank You more if Mom gets us ice cream for dessert. And liberty and justice for all! Amen!"

Along with the laughter from the other customers nearby, I heard a woman remark, "That's what's wrong with this country. Kids today don't even know how to pray. Asking God for ice cream! Why, I never!"

Hearing this, my son burst into tears and asked me, "Did I do it wrong? Is God mad at me?" As I held him and assured him that he had done a terrific job and God was certainly not mad at him, an elderly gentleman approached the table.

He winked at my son and said, "I happen to know that God thought that was a great prayer."

"Really?" my son asked.

"Cross my heart," the man replied.

Then in a theatrical whisper he added (indicating the woman whose remark had started this whole thing), "Too bad she never asks God for ice cream. A little ice cream is good for the soul sometimes."

Naturally, I bought my kids ice cream at the end of the meal. My son stared at his for a moment and then did something I will remember the rest of my life.

He picked up his sundae and without a word, walked over and placed it in front of the woman. With a big smile he told her, "Here, this is for you. Ice cream is good for the soul sometimes; and my soul is good already."[211]

This final week and Treasure Clue bring the final turn on the map—our relationship with the Lord and how joy and gratitude overflow from that relationship.

Anyone can apply the teachings and experience the benefits of the treasures God has given us. Health will improve; ability to handle stress and family relationships will improve. But doing all these things will not give a person the true balance in life for ultimate healing until we make sure the spiritual side is in complete alignment with the plan Jesus has for our life. Jesus is "ice cream" to our soul.

Thankful for the Treasure

"Whatever!" Have you heard that term lately? Talking to a disgruntled teen can sometimes bring about a "whatever" response. What does that mean? Does it mean, "Yes, I will do whatever you ask," or does it mean "Whatever. Will you stop telling me what to do?" In order to find the meaning, I looked it up in the dictionary. Yes it was there. Whatever—A term used to dismiss a previous statement and express indifference. It is used as a *powerful conversational blocking tool.*[212]

Read the Treasure Clue again. Do you think this is what Paul meant when he wrote the word *whatever* to the Colossians?

Have you ever said "whatever" to God, meaning a "powerful communication blocking tool"? Will that mindset contribute to your health? _____

In my New American Standard Bible, the heading of this chapter in Colossians is titled "Put on a New Self." Read the Treasure Clue again. How would you define the biblical meaning of *whatever*?

_____

_____

_____

If we wanted to put on a new self, would we refer to the biblical meaning of *whatever* or the new slang meaning? _____

How does your new design for health fit into this verse?

_____

_____

_____

_____

Giving thanks includes not only avocadoes, tomatillos, forgiveness, and relationships, but it also means every part of our life. "Whatever you do" means everything you do. In *all* things give thanks.

What are you most thankful for from this study? List the top four things. It could be a deeper relationship to God now that you see Him as your all-provider. It could be a new food or a deeper friendship with your foodie friend. The list is endless.

1. _____
2. _____
3. _____
4. _____

In your life and circumstances, what are you most thankful for today?

_____

_____

_____

Motivations for Thankfulness

What or who motivates us to be thankful? _____
There are many things that motivate us. I will talk about a few of them in detail below.

PARENTS OR PARENTAL AUTHORITY

For some people, the motivation to be thankful comes from our mothers. This reminds me of a story told about a four-year-old girl and her mother who were strolling through an open-air market. As the little girl stared at a large pile of oranges, a generous vendor took one from the pile and handed it to the little girl. "What do you say to the nice man?" the mother asked her daughter. The little girl looked at the orange, then thrust it toward the man and said, "Peel it!"

Being a mother, I can relate to how this mother felt at this ungrateful response. When our kids were young we tried hard to teach them how to be thankful when given a gift or when an act of service or love was rendered to them. How warmed our hearts were when we heard the words "thank you" without prompting. How it must warm the heart of our heavenly Father when we give thanks without any prompting! The more thankful we are without prompting, the more willing we will be to say "whatever" to God.

SCRIPTURES

Motivation can also come from scriptures. There are numerous scriptures that give us reason to be thankful. One of those verses is Psalm 118:1. Look up this verse and write it here.

_____

_____

_____

If this verse only stated "Give thanks to the Lord," that would be enough reason to make giving thanks important in our lives. But the verse continues with, ". . . for He is good; for His loving kindness is everlasting" (NASB). Not only are we motivated to give thanks because the Scripture asks us to, but also because it is followed with a blessing: "His loving kindness is everlasting." God continues to give more than we could ever conceive, so let us be grateful and continually rejoice.

PEOPLE

People may motivate us to be thankful. I remember when my children would bring me a gift. This gift could be flowers, a drawing, a good report from a teacher, help in the kitchen, a clean room, a kiss goodnight, or just a hug for being Mom. All of these reasons plus many more are good motivations to be thankful. With your spouse it could be roses, a favorite cooked meal, a diamond ring, a car with gas in it, clean clothes put away, or, once again, a hug for being you.

Your co-workers might also motivate you to be thankful. This might include someone who gives you encouragement, compliments, needy advice, or a pay raise.

We have lots of motivation to be thankful in our lives, and our days will go better if we make sure to be thankful for everything around us.

The Impact of Thankfulness

What is the impact on our health for being thankful? There have been several recent studies that examine what impact being thankful can have on our health and well-being. Jeffrey Froh, assistant professor of psychology at Hofstra University in Long Island, New York, focused his research on being grateful as a continuing behavior. "The one particular study that we did was we had students count blessings, which is essentially focusing on the things they were thankful or grateful for, and we had them journal daily for two weeks." [213]

The results of the study that Froh completed showed that students reported feeling more optimistic and more satisfied with their lives, they had fewer physical complaints and were more likely to exercise, and they were more likely to report better sleep. After the study ended they found that the effects of being thankful not only occurred immediately, but actually lasted up to three weeks later. A study from the University of Kentucky found that people who focus on being positive (thankful) not only live longer, but have more resistance to colds, have reduced coronary artery disease, and get sick less than others. [214] This study went on to say negative thinking (unthankfulness, unforgiveness, and stress) can actually weaken a healthy immune system.

Not only can being thankful help us maintain a healthy body, but our thankfulness will overflow to everyone. Showing thanks and appreciation to our family will teach and encourage them to do the same to friends, coworkers, and peers. Being thankful to a cashier may make the difference between her having a good day or a bad day. Being thankful to a coworker may be transferred to his home life or marriage. Being thankful to those around you will not only bless others and improve your health, but also will make an impact on more people than you can ever imagine.

Difficult times can be easier to handle with an attitude of gratitude. It will also make us a stronger witness. Joy and contentment will fill our lives instead of fear and anxiety. Attitudes toward others will be transformed. It will motivate us to look for God's purpose in our circumstances. The impact of all this will show us God is at work in and around us.

Steps Toward Being Thankful

If you find being thankful to be difficult, start by taking just a few steps. Try doing one or more of the things below to discover the treasure of thankfulness.

PRAYER

Look up Colossians 4:2 and write it here.

_____

_____

Let's face it, everyday life is not easy. People around us are dealing with cancer, job loss, loss of home, and difficult relationships. Life is hard. Sometimes taking the first step toward change is the hardest. In this case, the first step toward being thankful is praying. There have been times when I was dealing with trials in my life and prayer did not come quickly. Just saying the words, "God, thank You," is a simple start. Sometimes I would read a prayer out of a book because I did not know the words to speak. Books I suggest reading for this are Stormie Omartian's prayer books[215] or Beth Moore's *Praying God's Word*. Sometimes all we can pray is, "Lord, help me to have an attitude of thanksgiving." Each time we have a destructive thought or comment, we need to pray, "Help me to have an attitude of thanksgiving." Even though negative thoughts come to mind more quickly than thankful thoughts, the more time we spend retraining our mind to focus on being thankful in all situations, the easier it will be to have an attitude of thanksgiving.

JOURNAL

Keep a journal of things you're thankful for. Each day, write down everything for which you can give thanks. Continue to add to this list as God brings more things to mind. Here is a list to help jog your memory:

Necessities—food, shelter, water, clothing
People—family, friends
Possessions—home, job, car
Yourself—talents, accomplishments
Health—even in sickness we can be thankful

In your list, you can also learn to turn negative thoughts into positive ones. Here are some ideas.

The mess to clean up after a party means I have been surrounded by friends.
The taxes I pay mean that I'm employed.
The clothes that fit a little too snug mean I have enough to eat.
A lawn that needs mowing, windows that need cleaning, and gutters that need fixing mean I have a home.
The space I find at the far end of the parking lot means that I am capable of walking.
My huge heating bill means that I am warm.
The lady behind me in church who sings off key means that I can hear.
The piles of laundry and ironing mean I have clothes to wear.
The alarm that goes off in the early morning hours means that I'm alive.

Pick one of the above statements with which you can connect and write a statement of affirmation, making it personal in your life.

_____

_____

BLESSING AT MEAL TIMES

Give thanks before each meal. John 6:11 says, "Jesus then took the loaves, and when he had given thanks, he distributed them to those who were seated" (ESV). Meals will take a little more thought and preparation to bring the healthy changes we have learned. It makes us even more grateful that God has given us food for good health.

Little Jenny sat down to eat dinner with her family. She looked at the leftovers and said, "Hey, wait a minute. We thanked God for this *last* night!" We laugh at this, but how often do we have the wrong attitude about thankfulness?

The purpose of saying a blessing at mealtime is a thanksgiving for gifts that God has given us. Thanking God for all His provision can make a huge impact on the full value of our treasure chests. We have sought to learn how God designed our bodies, the foods that bring it optimal health, and the joy that comes from that knowledge. How can we then sit down to dinner and not feel an attitude of gratitude for all He has done? If we do not feel grateful to God for the meal but still say a prayer of grace, are we just thanking ourselves? Did we earn a right to be at the table and pay for the food we are eating? May it never be! In fact, we have not earned or even deserved what we receive. Giving thanks is an opportunity to share our gratefulness to our Father in heaven with those seated at the dinner table. Our relationship with God is evident to everyone around us. Our prayers at mealtimes are evidence of our gratitude to Him for His provisions.

NOTES

Write notes to family members, telling them how thankful you are for each of them. Author Linda Gilden has written a book, *Love Notes on His Pillow*. Love notes are another way of telling people you are thankful for them and that they are important to you. In this book, the author explains how love notes can be the fuel that ignites the fire of romance or the nuggets of encouragement that make your spouse feel more secure. She has also written *Love Notes in Lunchboxes* to help you communicate with your children.

SPEAK THE WORDS "THANK YOU"

Do you know how to help someone have a good day? Words and actions can warm almost any heart. We never know when someone is having a bad day or is near depression. Words or actions of thankfulness can be a turning point in someone's life. It is a chance for you to "be Jesus" to a stranger.

A few years ago a group of salesmen went to a regional sales convention in Chicago. They had assured their wives that they would be home in plenty of time for Friday night's dinner.
In their rush, with tickets and briefcases, one of these salesmen inadvertently kicked over a table which held a display of baskets of apples. Apples flew everywhere. Without stopping or looking back, they all managed to reach the plane in time for their nearly missed boarding.

All but one. He paused, took a deep breath, got in touch with his feelings, and experienced a twinge of compassion for the girl whose apple stand had been overturned.

He told his buddies to go on without him, waved goodbye, told one of them to call his wife when they arrived at their home destination and explain his taking a later flight. Then he returned to the terminal where the apples were all over the terminal floor.

He was glad he did.

The sixteen-year-old girl was totally blind! She was softly crying, tears running down her cheeks in frustration, and at the same time helplessly groping for her spilled produce as the crowd swirled about her, no one stopping, and no one to care for her plight.

The salesman knelt on the floor with her, gathered up the apples, put them into the baskets, and helped set the display up once more. As he did this, he noticed that many of them had become battered and bruised; these he set aside in another basket.

When he had finished, he pulled out his wallet and said to the girl, "Here, please take this twenty dollars for the damage we did. Are you OK?"

She nodded through her tears. He continued on with, "I hope we didn't spoil your day too badly."

As the salesman started to walk away, the bewildered blind girl called out to him, "Mister..." He paused and turned to look back into those blind eyes.

She continued, "Are you Jesus?"

He stopped in mid-stride, and he wondered. Then slowly he made his way to catch the later flight with that question burning and bouncing about in his soul: "Are you Jesus?"[216]

The treasures that we have been reading and studying during these past eleven weeks have shown us how God has a design for each of us. He is the one who wrote the owner's manual. But there is a lot more that He wants you to understand. God pursues a continuing love relationship with you that is real and personal. He has a plan for your life that will lead you to more wonderful experiences than you can imagine. All He asks of you is to follow His lead. Learning to handle stress, forgive others, and be thankful will allow Him to do mighty things in your life. The added health to enjoy these experiences is icing on the cake (a healthy version, not Betty Crocker). I pray that God has shown you new ways to be thankful for the treasures He has given you.

Taking this treasure to heart: Take a moment to write out what God has taught you in this lesson. Make a list of people that you need to thank either face to face, with a written note, or in a quick email.

_____

_____

_____

_____

Applying this treasure at home: What are two or three practical ways you can teach your family how to be more thankful?

_____

_____

Day Two—Laugh and Live Longer

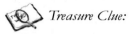 *Treasure Clue:*

A merry heart doeth good like a medicine.

—Prov. 17:22 KJV

A tourist was standing in line to buy an ice cream cone at a Thrifty Drug Store in Beverly Hills. To her utter shock and amazement, who should walk in and stand right behind her but George Clooney! Well, the lady, even though she was rattled, determined to maintain her composure. She purchased her ice cream cone and turned confidently and exited the store.

However, to her horror, she realized that she had left the counter without her ice cream cone! She waited a few minutes till she felt all was clear, and then went back into the store to claim her cone. As she approached the counter, the cone was not in the little circular receptacle, and for a moment she stood there pondering what might have happened to it. Then she felt a polite tap on her shoulder, and turning was confronted by—you guessed it—George Clooney. The famous actor then told the lady that if she was looking for her ice cream cone, she had put it into her purse![217]

There is no greater need today than for people to daily experience the warm feeling of joy and the cleansing action of contagious laughter. All around us people are tired, busy, and feel depleted. We need some wind in our sails and a rush of joy and laughter to keep us going. We should not just manage to make ends meet, but instead go forth enthusiastically. Does waking up in the morning bring joy to your heart?

Personal inventory: When was the last time you had a good belly laugh? _____
What story or situation encouraged your laughter?

_____

_____

What makes you laugh? What really turns on your funny box?

_____

_____

If your belly laugh did not take place today or yesterday, then you are in need of some medicine—medicine to make a merry heart.

Research states that we need six belly laughs a day. God must agree, since the words *happiness, joy,* and *laughter* are mentioned more than 783 times in Scripture. There are even episodes in Scripture that I am not sure were meant to be funny but my sense of humor thought they were hilarious. Check this one out.

Read 2 Kings 13:20-21. One of my favorite hobbies is people watching. It helps me get belly laughs in unusual places. Picture this scene in 2 Kings taking place, and you are a bystander watching. Yesterday (not sure exactly when) they buried Elisha—a sad day, indeed. Now today there is another death, and while they are getting ready to bury this latest victim a marauding band comes thundering down the street. The fear of the band causes them to want to ditch their friend quickly, so they toss him on the bones of Elisha.

Did you catch what happened next? The dead body—tossed in by his neglectful friends—touches the bones of Elisha and jumps to his feet. I really wish I could have seen the reaction of his friends when this newly revived man tapped them on the shoulder as they were hiding behind a rock from the marauding band. What do you think he asked them? How would they have reacted?

What are some other funny or amazing stories you recall from Scripture?

_____

_____

Make sure to share these stories with your study group or your foodie friend.

There are several stories in the Bible that I find humorous. Keep your joy glasses on when you read and you will see the humor, too.

We all need to develop our sense of humor. A good hearty laugh can transform an ordinary day into an extraordinary day in these ways:[218]

- Gives a fresh and more objective perspective on an embarrassing or difficult situation.
- Increases morale and gives a greater sense of well-being about the person and the place where the laughter occurs.
- Increases creativity and enhances problem-solving skills.
- Rejuvenates the body and mind. Think of the cleansing feeling you have after you've laughed for a few seconds.
- Gives a more positive outlook and a greater sense of hope.
- Gives a general sense of happiness and well-being for greater productivity.
- Improves learning as you relax and remember information longer.
- Can act as preventative medicine. People who are rarely ill have a healthy sense of humor and a positive outlook on life.
- Decreases and kills pain. Laughter releases powerful chemicals called endorphins, which act the same way as morphine.

- Stimulates the immune system.
- Provides an antidote for stress.
- Reduces the heart rate.

Is it any wonder we enjoy being around people who make us laugh. It makes us feel good. We feel alive. But what about those days when we can't laugh? What steals our joy?

One of the biggest stealers of our joy is discontentment. Consider these wise words the apostle Paul wrote while he was in prison: "Not that I speak from want, for I have learned to be content in whatever circumstances I am" (Phil. 4:11 NASB).

Our society constantly paints a picture that another person's life is more glamorous or rewarding than ours. We lose contentment in our present situation. Typically many people find themselves in the "if only" group. They would laugh more if only they did not have cancer, if only they had a better spouse, if only their three-year-old were potty trained, if only they had more money, if only they were more talented or more beautiful. Chuck Swindoll, in his book *Laugh Again,* challenges this idea of "if only": "Just as more money never made anyone more generous and more talent never made anyone more grateful, more of anything never made anyone more joyful."[219]

Jane Canfield has the following to say about happiness:

The happiest people are rarely the richest, or most beautiful, or even the most talented. Happy people do not depend on excitement and "fun" supplied by externals. They enjoy the fundamental, often very simple things of life. They waste no time thinking of tomorrow. They savor the moment, glad to be alive, enjoying their work, their families, the good things around them. They are adaptable; they can bend with the wind, adjust to the changes in their times, enjoy the contests of life, and feel themselves in harmony with the world. Their eyes are turned outward; they are aware, compassionate. They have the capacity to love.[220]

People who love to laugh pursue fun rather than wait for fun to come knocking on their door in the middle of the day. These contagiously joyful believers have no trouble convincing the people around them that Christianity is real and that Christ can transform a life.

Joy is the flag that flies above the castle of their hearts, announcing that the King is in residence.
—Chuck Swindoll[221]

Whom do you know who has joy every time you meet him or her?

Some other joy stealers could include: facing trials in life, having sin in our heart, placing our confidence in ourselves or in others instead of in Christ, and a lack of discipline. Let's glance at trials and sin to see how they are stealing our joy.

TRIALS IN LIFE

The purpose of trials in our life is to exercise our faith. God allows trials in order to develop perseverance in us and to teach us to focus our hope on the glory that is yet to be revealed. Trials come in many forms, such as health problems, marriage difficulties, financial crises, and criticism. Whatever form the trial takes and however severe it may be, it is intended to strengthen our character. Our faith and perseverance can grow only under the strain of trials.[222]

SIN IN OUR LIFE

David's life was one of mighty deeds for God but also showed us a man of deep failings. When he confessed his sin, he prayed, "Restore to me the joy of your salvation" (Ps. 51:12 NIV). When we are not experiencing joy, we should examine our hearts and our lives. Have we done something that is displeasing to God that we need to confess and forsake or leave behind? Or are we holding on to some sinful attitude, such as jealousy or bitterness, or a critical and unforgiving spirit? The fruit of joy cannot exist when such attitudes control our hearts. All sin, whether in attitude or action, must be dealt with if we are to display the desirable quality of joy.[223]

Searching Scripture for Joy

Read these verses and fill in the blanks. Think about what you can learn from these verses that will help you attain and maintain joy.

Philippians 3:1 (NKJV) " _____ in the Lord."

I Thessalonians 5:16-18 (NKJV) " _____ always: _____ without ceasing, in _____ give thanks; for this is the will of God in Christ Jesus for you."

Romans 14:17-18 (NKJV) "For the kingdom of God is not _____ and _____, but righteousness and _____ and _____ in the Holy Spirit."

Nehemiah 8:10 (NKJV) "The _____ of the Lord is your _____.

Hebrews 12:1-3 (NASB) "Fixing our eyes on Jesus... who for the _____ set before Him endured the cross.... And has sat down at the right hand of the throne of _____."

How can you apply the attitude of those in these verses to your own situations and experience joy?

_____

_____

Develop Your Sense of Humor

In the book *Ten Steps To Revolutionize Your Life*, author Renee C. Cobb teaches the ease of developing your sense of humor.[224] Actually raising your awareness of how often you laugh—particularly at yourself—is a great place to begin. This will awaken your awareness to life around you. Here are some things that will help.

- Laugh at yourself. If you take yourself too seriously, you'll be the only one who does. Laughing will raise your sense of self, because it allows you to be more objective and allows other people to laugh with you.
- Help your family find and develop their sense of humor. Keep a family funny book. Everyone will enjoy life more, and you will record wonderful memories to last forever. Your family will remember home as a fun place.
- Think funny. See the funny or flipside of every situation. Think about what makes something funny and look for similar factors to apply in other situations.
- See the potential humor of a problem. Try to see a problem from a different or unusual point of view. If you have children, use this technique with them to help each of them with problem solving. This will be one of the most significant skills they will ever learn!
- Adopt the perspective of a child. This does not mean you have to act silly, but to approach situations with an open mind or even outrageous thoughts. Let your inner child play occasionally.
- Share your humor. By sharing your sense of humor and doing and saying funny things, you will not only provide laughter and happiness for others, but you'll help others gain a new perspective.
- Add humor to your daily activities. This will be your greatest source of humor. Nothing is funnier than real life. Listen to the everyday things comedians talk about. You have experiences that are abundant with humor. Start looking for them and then write them in your journal or family fun book.
- Read humor. Buy joke books, funny stories, comic strips, etc. Share your favorites with someone who needs them.

- Watch old funny movies. Old movies are typically better than new ones since the newer ones contain disrespect, as well as negative and self-esteem-damaging humor.
- Plan a laugh lunch. This could be for a friend who is going through a difficult time. Invite several friends. A condition of their attendance is to come ready to tell the funniest things they know. You might also ask each one to bring a gag gift that will make your sad friend laugh. Be sure everyone knows the agenda ahead of time.
- Celebrate with someone. Find excuses to create celebrations—to recognize a friend or family member for a success. It could be to celebrate improved behaviors, attitudes, grades, a project finished successfully, farewells, the first day of spring, or…just because.

Be careful about situations where laughter is not appropriate. There are times you will need to hold back and not let others see you laughing, as these ladies experienced.

Four friends went everywhere together and shared all their spare time. One day one of them passed away. The remaining friends went together to the funeral home for the viewing. They waited their turn patiently to view the body. They were, of course, grieved, and the emotion mounted. They didn't recognize any of their friend's relatives in the room since they were all from out of town. Finally, it came their turn to approach the casket. As they looked down, it was a MAN! One of the friends punched the other friends and whispered, "THAT ain't Gladys!" Suddenly, the three of them lost control.

Not wanting to be disrespectful, they covered their faces as if they were crying. Shoulders shaking from laughter, they stood over "Fred" while his family surrounded them. Thinking they were crying over their dearly departed, the three women were hugged and patted, and told, "It's OK. It's all right. He's in a better place than we are." This, of course, made matters worse. They finally tore themselves away in what then appeared to be grief-stricken hysteria and retreated to the hallway.

Several minutes later when they finally gained their composure, they set about to find where in the world they had put Gladys. What a great release from the pain, tension, and grief of the moment![225]

Days will come along when laughter is absent, but it is up to us to not let this happen too often, and especially not for long periods of time. Joy comes from the heart, and we can have joy in the midst of trials and hard times. It is a choice. Do you choose to let sickness, problems, sin, and conflict steal your joy? Even in tough times we can be joyful. We can praise the Lord at all times, no matter what.

Taking this treasure to heart: Open your Bible and find a verse about having joy or praising God in all things. Write it on the next page and share it with your class or your foodie friend. If you are not sure how to find a verse like this, go to the end of the Bible and find the concordance. Look up the words *joy, rejoice, happy,* and *praise.* There will be a list of verses to look up. See which one fits what we are talking about. If you still cannot find one, read Psalms and Proverbs to find several pertinent verses.

_____

_____

_____

Applying this treasure at home: What ways can you add joy to your home? From what you learned this week, write out one step you are going to make to bring fun into your home.

_____

DAY THREE—MAKING THE TREASURE PERSONAL

Treasure Clue:

For God so loved the world, that He gave His only begotten Son, that whoever believes in Him shall not perish, but have eternal life.

—John 3:16 NASB

Let's personalize this verse again. Write your name in the blanks:

For God so loved _____ that He gave His only begotten Son, that if _____ believes in Him _____ shall not perish, but _____ will have eternal life.

Read this verse out loud. Now read it again out loud until you really believe it and want everyone to know it. If you don't believe it, then continue reading and let's see if that changes.

John 3:16 is the beginning of a personal love relationship between you and God. This is also the final revelation in the treasure chest of life that will make the biggest transformation in your health, your outlook in life, and your relationships with others.

Jesus said, "This is eternal life; that they may know you, the only true God, and Jesus Christ, whom you have sent" (John 17:3 NIV). The heart of eternal life and the heart of this treasure hunt we have been pursuing are the same—knowing Jesus Christ in a relationship that is real and personal to you. Knowing God does not come through a method, a church, a baptism, a religion, or a program. It is a relationship with a Person. It is an intimate love relationship with God. Through this relationship, God reveals His will and invites you to join Him where He is already at work. When you obey, God accomplishes through you something only He can do. Then you come to know God in a more intimate way by experiencing Him as He works through you.[226]

Revealing the Secret to the Ultimate Treasure

Our journey has been fun and rewarding. But if we end too early, we will miss the grand finale. The grand finale is the secret to everything we have learned. Throughout the weeks we have filled this virtual treasure chest. All along we have taken for granted the actual box that holds the treasure. Did you ever wonder what the chest or box that holds our treasure and keeps it safe actually is? What do we have to do to protect it? The answer to our secret is our relationship with God. That is "the box" that holds everything together neatly in one location. Without this box, our treasures will spill over the ground and roll away. The chest itself is built of strong wood with the aroma of fresh cut pine but the softness of oak. Our relationship with God always comes with a pleasant aroma, firm enough to hold us together and soft enough to have compassion in our darkest moments. Everything we have accomplished up to this point on our hunt will be null and void without the relationship with God through which we will truly experience eternal life. This is the greatest treasure. Jesus said, "I have come that they may have life, and have it to the full" (John 10:10 NIV). Are you ready to see your treasure chest overflowing? This is a gift that you may have if you are willing to respond to God's invitation for an intimate love relationship with Him.

There is an old hymn, "In the Garden," that describes a personal relationship with God. Does this describe your relationship with the One who loves you best?

> And He walks with me and He talks with me
> And He tells me I am His own,
> And the joy we share as we tarry there,
> None other has ever known.[227]

If these words do not describe your relationship, there is work to be done. Many of you have already accepted Christ as your Savior and you recognize Him as Lord of your life. If you have not done this, you can still apply the teachings in this Bible study and you will receive the promised health benefits, because the Lord God made everything and it is all good. However, without Christ in your life you will not have life to the fullest as described in the song on the last page, "He walks with me and He talks with me." Total health involves the body, the soul, and the spirit. Without the spiritual side you will be out of balance. "The man without the spirit does not accept the things that come from the Spirit of God, for they are foolishness to him, and he cannot understand them, because they are spiritually discerned" (1 Cor. 2:14 NIV). If you sense a need to accept Jesus as your Savior and Lord, now is the time to settle this matter.

Wordless Book—Full of Colors

Fruits and vegetables come in all varieties of colors. Each color represents a bounty of nutrients bringing us a rich life of vitality. Colors can also bring us vitality in our spiritual life as well.

On a mission trip to Wisconsin, I was leading a group of sixty teenagers. Our trip consisted of a youth musical that was performed in community parks and neighborhoods. The music had a message: God loves you. A portion of the youth were to go throughout the crowd and see if anyone had questions about the songs and if they knew the Jesus the kids were singing about. As one of the youth leaders, I spent most of my time watching out for the safety of our youth, so speaking to those in the crowd was not high on my list. That is, until one evening toward the end of the week. Two ladies sitting under a tree were very intently watching and listening. After I made sure all the youth were in place and accounted for, I made my way to these ladies. Our conversation was very polite, and then I asked them if they understood the songs. "We would like to learn what they are singing about," was their response. I opened my Wordless Book[228] and shared with them the colors of God's love. Now I would like to share with you the colors of God's love.

GOLD

What does gold remind you of? Are you thinking of jewelry or money? Those are definitely gold, but the gold I am referring to is in heaven. Heaven is a special place where God lives. The Bible tells us that in heaven the street of the city is pure, clear gold—like glass. God tells us many other things about His home. No one is ever sick there. Every person in heaven will be perfectly happy—always. The most wonderful thing about heaven is that God the Father and His Son, Jesus, are there. God is the one who made everything: the stars, the flowers, the ocean—everything in the universe. He made you and loves you very much.

Because God made you and loves you, He wants you to be a part of His family and be with Him in heaven someday. What a special place that will be! It is perfect. God is also perfect and holy. But there is one thing God will not allow in heaven and that is sin.

Darkness

The darkness—or black color—represents the sin in our life. Sin is anything we think, say, or do that displeases God. Sin has caused sorrow and sadness in our world. Can you think of some things you do that are sin? _____ Stealing, lying, disobeying, saying harmful words—all of these are examples of sin.

But the Bible says, "For all have sinned" (Rom. 3:23 NKJV). Read and mark this verse in your own Bible. "All" means every one of us. No one has ever lived and not sinned, except Jesus. We sin because we were born with a "want to" to do wrong things. God has said sin must be punished. The punishment for sin is death—which means separation from God forever.

He knew we could not be good enough to please Him. So He made a way for our sin to be forgiven. God has a wonderful plan so you and I don't have to be punished for our sins.

Red

The red represents the color of the blood Jesus shed on the cross. God loves us so much He sent His only Son, the Lord Jesus Christ, to this world. One day Jesus was wrongly accused and was nailed on the cross to die. The nails in His hands and feet caused Him to bleed. The red color represents this blood Jesus shed for us to cover our sins now and forever. Remember Romans 3:23 stated that we have all sinned, but in Romans 6:23 we see that God gave us a gift. "For the wages of sin is death, but the gift of God is eternal life in Christ Jesus our Lord" (NKJV).

God is offering you a gift. Have you ever considered it a gift before? _____

Hebrews 9:22 says, "Without the shedding of blood there is no forgiveness of sins" (ESV). This means His blood became the forgiveness of our sins. Jesus took the punishment for our sins. All our lies, meanness, bad temper—all of it. The Lord Jesus died and was buried.

1 Corinthians 15:3-4 says, "That Christ died for our sins according to the Scriptures, and that He was buried, and that He rose again the third day according to the Scriptures" (NKJV). This was the work the Lord Jesus had come to do—to be able to save us from our sins. But after three days in the tomb, the most wonderful thing happened. God gave Jesus life again. God raised Him up from the dead! The Lord Jesus came back to life! He walked on this earth

and many people saw him. Then the Lord Jesus went back to heaven and is there right now with His Father, God.

This means because of what He did for you, you can have your sins forgiven.

WHITE

The white represents cleanness or purity. God wants to forgive Your sins, take them away, and make you His child.

John 1:12 says, "As many as received Him, to them He gave the right to become children of God, to those who believe in His name" (NKJV). Let's take that verse apart. "Received Him… to those who believe in His name." Receiving Him means you believe with all your heart that Jesus died on the cross for your sins and rose again. You need to be willing to turn from your sin and believe that only the Lord Jesus can forgive you. Then you will become a child of God. That's what the rest of the verse means when it says, "to them He gave the right to become children of God, to those who believe in His name." You can tell the Lord Jesus right now that you have sinned and you believe He died for you. Would you like to do that right now?

Tell Jesus in your own words that you have sinned and done wrong things. Tell him you believe He died for you. Right now, ask Him to forgive your sins and become your Father. Thank Him for answering you and forgiving you right now.

After you have completed this, answer these questions.

Whose child are you now? _____

The answer is God's child. Yippee! That's a definite praise tickle!

How do you know? _____

Go back and refer to John 1:12 if you are not sure of the answer. When you believe on the Lord Jesus Christ and receive Him, you become a child of God. Isn't that wonderful?

Remember these promises:

Hebrews 13:5 (NKJV)—"I will never leave you." You can place your name in this verse: "God will never leave _____."

Hebrews 13:6 (NKJV)—"The Lord is my helper." "The Lord is _____'s helper."

When you become God's child, He wants you to get to know Him better.

GREEN

The green color reminds me of all the growing plants and foods we have studied in this treasure hunt. It reminds me of new life—everlasting life. When you receive the Lord Jesus as your Savior from sin, you are like a newborn baby in God's family. God wants you to grow by learning more about Him. As you learn more about the Lord Jesus, you will learn how to please Him. You have His power and strength to do what is right. But when you do something that is sin, what can you do? Open your Bible to 1 John 1:9. Write it out here:

_____

_____

_____

God knows when you sin, but He wants you to confess your sin. To confess means to tell on yourself to God or to admit the wrong you have done. As soon as you realize you have done something wrong, tell the Lord right away. He will forgive you from that sin because that is what He promised to do. Ask Him to help you to not do it again.

Remember, because you are God's child now, you can ask Him to give you the power and strength to obey Him and do what is right. Isn't He a wonderful Savior and friend?

If this decision is new for you today, record it here and in your Bible.

_____ has accepted Jesus Christ as his or her (circle one) Personal Savior, Friend, Father, Provider, Caretaker, Comforter on this date: _____.

Scripture tells us no one can take you away from Jesus. No one can come between you and your relationship with the Father. Are you excited? I am for you. Please send the Designed Healthy Living staff an email so we can rejoice in your decision. We will be praying for you.

After making this decision either many years ago or just recently, we need to think in terms of growing as a Christian. As we look at nature, green represents growth and our lives need to be continually growing. The more time we spend with our friends, the more we get to know them. Spending time with our Lord will accomplish the same thing.

If you need help with any of these principles or colors, talk to the leader in your class, the pastor of the church, or a Christian friend. If you have just made this very important decision, call someone and share it with him or her.

Life will not always be easy, but you now have someone to lead you through without getting tangled up in the "briar patches."

Applying this treasure at home: If this is the first day of your new life in Christ, record the date on your Action Plan. If you have recommitted your life to Christ and desire Him to be a bigger part of your life, also record this date on the Action Plan. These dates are a record of the life-changing event that has taken place. It is a time of celebration. The angels are rejoicing, and so should you!

Congratulations! This decision allows God's treasures to continually fill you up daily. There is no one between you and God. He is there for you *all* the time.

Day Four—Reflecting on Your Action Plan

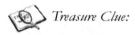 *Treasure Clue:*

Finally then, brethren, we request and exhort you in the Lord Jesus, that as you received from us instruction as to how you ought to walk and please God (just as you actually do walk), that you excel still more.

—1 Thess. 4:1 NASB

". . . excel still more." To get the full meaning of what this verse is saying, read 1 Thessalonians 4:1-12.

We have completed our very in-depth study of health. Where do we go from here? These verses in 1 Thessalonians give us the answer.

Verse 1 says we are "to walk and please God that you may excel still more." Verse 10 again says "to excel still more" and verse 12 to "not be in any need" (NASB).

This chapter is full of sanctification, which means continually working to be holy in everything we do. It is filled with words on sanctification, love, and how we should conduct ourselves.

The words "excel still more" really jumped out at me. I have been working to follow a healthy eating plan for many years now, and the benefits have been wonderful. The best part has been how God reveals all the different ways He can work in my life, and still there is so much more! I must admit that I do struggle many times. Over the holidays I tend to drop my guard like we have studied in these last weeks, and this will cause a weight gain. But getting back on track after only five pounds gained is easier than waiting until it is twenty or thirty or more.

Discipline is a daily activity and we know it is worth it. But these verses take it a step further—excel still more.

What do you think the definition of *excel* is?

It means to be very good, to be outstanding, to do better than a given standard or than a previous achievement.

When I realize that my goal is sanctification—to be made holy—then God is telling me that I need to continue to excel. Excel means to do better than previous personal achievement. It does not mean that I will have arrived, but that I can continue to excel each day and year.

This also means that for those of you who are just starting to make changes in your health and food choices, you can begin to excel today. 1 Thessalonians 4:12 ends with "not be in any need." What a blessing that verse is!

Reflecting on Your Action Plan

Your Action Plan has twelve weeks of steps to personally help you bring about the ultimate treasure of health to its fullest. Our journey has taken us to the depths of many pitfalls and to the mountains of great rewards. Look at your sheet. How many goals have you reached?

_____

How do you feel? Rate each category on a scale of one to ten, with one being few changes and ten meaning you've made many changes.

Mentally—less stress, able to forgive, joy, enjoying life to the fullest

_____

_____

Physically—noticing changes in weight, attitude, enjoying new foods, enjoying life to the fullest

_____

_____

Spiritually—deeper awareness of God in all you do: eating, working, playing, worshipping, and enjoying life to the fullest

_____

_____

Are you surprised with the changes in your life? _____

What changes surprised you most?

_____

Which change was the most difficult?

_____

Record the praise tickles shared in class.

_____

_____

_____

_____

Go to the Assessment Form in the Appendix and record your health today. If you have been seriously making changes, there should be many praise tickles revealed on this form. Share these with the class this week and with your foodie friend. We encourage you to email your results to the Designed Healthy Living staff so we can rejoice with you.

Results from Your Hunt

Feelings of success come from being able to see a list of accomplishments. In the Appendix of this book you will find **Results from Your Hunt**. These pages let you check off the particular items you have accomplished from this journey. Many times people take this course and feel like it was so much information to absorb that they did not make many noticeable changes. After checking off the changes they did make it is reassuring to know that small changes to a lifestyle can add up to a big difference.

Now you are ready to move forward. From here on out, follow these steps:

- Continue to fill, enjoy, and protect the treasure you have discovered.
- Share the Treasures of Healthy Living with others who are looking for God's design for their health.
- Continue to meet with your foodie friend and enjoy food and fellowship together.
- Become a member of the Fabulous Foodie Friday club. Go to www.designedhealthyliving.com and sign up. It's free, and you can share your Fabulous Foodie Friday ideas and comments. Play with your food and share the fun. Share recipes, ideas, and pictures of your foodie events.

- Excel still more!

Congratulations; you made it! You have completed twelve weeks of a life-changing adventure!

FINAL FABULOUS FOODIE FRIDAY

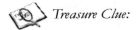 *Treasure Clue:*

The LORD your God will bless you in all your harvest and in all the
work of your hands, and your joy will be complete.

—Deut. 16:15 NIV

Out with the bad and in with the good. The work of your hands has included clearing out the cabinets in the kitchen, the pantry, and the refrigerator. You have learned the value of eating for the length of your days. You can bank on this knowledge for the rest of your radical life. My prayer is God's blessing as you continue this journey. Make plans now with your foodie friends to continue your Foodie Fridays. Send us your favorite foodie ideas so we can share them with everyone else. True foodies are always looking for good food, good recipes, and good friends. You can never have enough foodie friends.

Foodie Time

It's harvest time. You have worked hard; now it is time to reap the harvest of your knowledge. Enjoy a feast of celebration with your foodie friends. Invite others to come and join you. Make sure everyone brings a new food never shared before and brings the recipes for you to add to your recipe scrapbook.

Celebrate your feast by making it BYOP—bring your own plate. The plate might be a special heirloom or one designed by little hands that you treasure. The idea of sharing your favorite plate is also a way to save money on purchasing paper plates. Let everyone share what makes his or her plate so special. Listening to the stories makes it very interesting. This idea could be transferred to the cup or mug as well. Fun memorable stories abound all around us, and foodie friends are the ones who care enough to listen.

Fabulous Foodie Friends Forever

APPENDIX

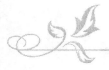

Action Plan

LET'S MAKE IT PERSONAL!

List the simple steps you are willing to take from your lesson each week. Use this sheet to check off the items when completed and watch the progress gained toward a healthier life.

Week One—Treasure of Health ☐

What changes am I willing to implement into my lifestyle from my studies this week?

_____

_____

_____

Week Two—Beverages ☐

What changes am I willing to implement into my lifestyle from my studies this week?

_____

_____

_____

Week Three—Grains ☐

What changes am I willing to implement into my lifestyle from my studies this week?

_____

_____

_____

Week Four—Vegetables and Fruits □

What changes am I willing to implement into my lifestyle from my studies this week?

_____

_____

_____

Week Five—Herbs, Spices, Oil, and Vinegar □

What changes am I willing to implement into my lifestyle from my studies this week?

_____

_____

_____

Week Six—Protein and Meat □

What changes am I willing to implement into my lifestyle from my studies this week?

_____

_____

_____

Week Seven—Fasting and Self-Discipline □

What changes am I willing to implement into my lifestyle from my studies this week?

_____

_____

_____

Week Eight—Sweets ☐

What changes am I willing to implement into my lifestyle from my studies this week?

_____

_____

_____

Week Nine—Environment and Toxins ☐

What changes am I willing to implement into my home and environment from my studies this week?

_____

_____

_____

Week Ten—Stress and Forgiveness ☐

What changes am I willing to implement into my lifestyle from my studies this week?

_____

_____

_____

Week Eleven—Exercise ☐

What changes am I willing to implement into my lifestyle from my studies this week?

_____

_____

_____

Week Twelve—The Fullness of Christ and health ☐

What changes am I willing to implement into my lifestyle from my studies this week?

_____

_____

_____

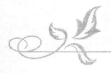

Daniel Fast Journal

In those days I, Daniel, was mourning three full weeks. I ate no pleasant food, no meat or wine came into my mouth, nor did I anoint myself at all, till three whole weeks were fulfilled.

—Dan. 10:2-3 NKJV

Get ready to experience God in His fullness and acquire the most in your health! The Daniel Fast is a great way to set yourself aside and enjoy the richness of the blessings that God has stored up for you!

Dates for this fast: _____ through _____

Week 1—Write down how the Daniel Fast impacts your everyday life.

Day 1

_____

_____

_____

Day 2

_____

_____

_____

Day 3

_____

_____

_____

Day 4

_____

_____

_____

Day 5

_____

_____

_____

Day 6

_____

_____

_____

Day 7

_____

_____

_____

Week 2—Continue to journal your experience. What improvements have you noticed physically, mentally, and/or spiritually? What changes would you like to make this week?

_____

_____

Daniel Fast Journal

Day 1

_____

_____

_____

Day 2

_____

_____

_____

Day 3

_____

_____

_____

Day 4

_____

_____

_____

Day 5

_____

_____

_____

Day 6

_____

_____

_____

Day 7

_____

_____

_____

Week 3—As the Daniel Fast comes to the final week, congratulate yourself for making it this far. This last week will be easy – don't give up. What obstacles have you experienced that you want to remove this final week? What challenges are you experiencing?

_____

_____

Day 1

_____

_____

_____

Day 2

_____

_____

_____

Daniel Fast Journal

Day 3

_____

_____

Day 4

_____

_____

Day 5

_____

_____

Day 6

_____

_____

Day 7

_____

_____

_____

As you look back over your Daniel Fast Journal, what are the top three experiences or improvements to your health?

1. _____

2. _____

3. _____

Write a prayer of your thoughts and overall expression to God for bringing you through this experience. If it was hard but rewarding, include that in your prayer. How did you see God in a new way through this experience?

_____

_____

_____

_____

_____

_____

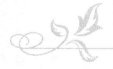

Health Assessment

How Are You Feeling Today?

Fill in the boxes or check any symptoms that apply to you.
Begin Date: _____

Date	Begin date	4 weeks	8 weeks	12 weeks
Help, I'm tired all the time!				
Blood Pressure				
Cholesterol				
Weight				
Triglycerides				
Exercise - # of times per week				
Acne				
Allergies				
Anxiety attacks				
Attention problems				
Bad breath				
Belching				
Bladder infections				
Blood clots				
Body odor				
Cold hands or feet				
Constipation				
Cravings for sweets or carbs				
Dandruff				
Depression				

Difficulty concentrating				
Dry, scaly skin				
Eczema, psoriasis				
Exhaustion				
Fatigue				
Fertility problems				
Fibromyalgia symptoms				
Food sensitivities				
Frequent illness				
Gas / bloating				
Have bitterness / lacking joy				
Headaches				
High stress level				
Indigestion				
Insomnia				
Joint Pain				
Less than three veggies daily				
Low sex drive				
Low fiber intake				
Medications (Rx or OTC)				
Mood swings				
Muscle cramps				
Nausea				
Number of laughs a day				
PMS				
Poor concentration				
Shortness of breath				
Smelly feet				
Use of alcohol or drugs				
Vegetables-how many do you eat per day?				
Yeast infections				

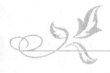

Results of My Hunt

- ☐ I have added a healthy yogurt to my weekly diet.
- ☐ I have started making yogurt smoothies for my family.
- ☐ I added a good calcium magnesium supplement.
- ☐ I substituted yogurt in a recipe and tried a new dish using yogurt.
- ☐ I added more calcium-rich foods to my family's daily routine.
- ☐ My family is doing a better job of washing their hands throughout the day with pH balanced soap.
- ☐ I included grapes as a lunch item or snack for my family and myself.
- ☐ I added these cancer- and heart-protective foods to our meals: carrots, onions, broccoli, and tomatoes
- ☐ I increased our vegetables to three to five a day.
- ☐ I increased our fruits to two to four a day.
- ☐ I added a good vitamin E supplement.
- ☐ I began a daily exercise routine.
- ☐ I started using a natural sun block.
- ☐ I started drinking at least eight 8-oz. glasses of water a day, thirty minutes before a meal and two hours or more after a meal.
- ☐ I started my morning with water alone.
- ☐ I did the Nutritional Deficiency questionnaire from the website.
- ☐ I purchased Ezekiel Bread this week.
- ☐ I purchased a grain mill and started making my own whole grain foods.
- ☐ I substituted whole grain pasta for white refined pasta.
- ☐ I switched to Rumford baking powder without aluminum.
- ☐ I began a B-Complex supplement.
- ☐ I purchased olive oil – extra virgin or cold pressed.
- ☐ I substituted olive oil in a recipe.
- ☐ I made my own salad dressing using healthy oil.
- ☐ I made yo-cheese using my yogurt funnel and used this in a recipe.
- ☐ I switched back to butter.
- ☐ I purchased some mozzarella soy cheese and tried it with my family.

- ☐ I purchased some raw nuts and served them with breakfast, lunch, or a snack.
- ☐ I tried a tofu product or used it in a recipe.
- ☐ I made homemade french fries in the oven instead of frying them.
- ☐ I switched to healthy chips.
- ☐ I used flax seeds in a recipe – freshly milled.
- ☐ I purchased a healthier choice deli meat with no preservatives.
- ☐ I was able to pass up a scavenger dish.
- ☐ I tried substituting honey in a recipe.
- ☐ I purchased some sucanat and used it in a recipe.
- ☐ I shared the facts about Aspartame with someone.
- ☐ I purchased a healthier breakfast cereal that includes a quality sweetener.
- ☐ I was able to pass up a soda.
- ☐ I added a good quality protein to my smoothie.
- ☐ I switched to sea salt.
- ☐ I switched to real vanilla.
- ☐ I used fresh garlic in a food dish.
- ☐ I added a good vitamin C supplement.
- ☐ I prepared steamed vegetables.
- ☐ I started washing my fruits and vegetables.
- ☐ I baked sweet potatoes instead of white potatoes.
- ☐ I used fresh herbs in a food dish instead of dried.
- ☐ I switched to non-fluoride toothpaste.
- ☐ I purchased unsweetened juice.
- ☐ I tried a milk alternative such as soy, rice, and almond.
- ☐ I made lemonade using stevia or honey.
- ☐ I made popsicles for my children using fruit, juice, yogurt, etc.
- ☐ I switched to at least eight of the name brands or similar type healthier items listed on the shopping guide from the manual.
- ☐ I made it through the entire class.
- ☐ I have encouraged someone to take the next Designed Healthy Living Class.
- ☐ I converted one of my family's recipe with healthier ingredients.
- ☐ I threw away the bleach.

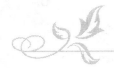

Endnotes

1. Dan and Nancy Dick, *Daily Wisdom from the Bible* (Uhrichsville, OH: Barbour Press, 2004), 18.
2. http://www.bcma.org/files/Eat_Together.pdf.
3. Beth Moore, *Praying God's Word*, (Nashville: B&H, 2000), 149.
4. Ibid., 150.
5. Steve Reynolds, pastor and author *of Bod4God,* (Ventura, CA: Regal) 2009, written with permission.
6. Alan Crippen II, "Sensible, well, informed," *Citizen Magazine*, February 2009, 8-9.
7. Debbie Grice, RN, used with permission.
8. S.I. McMillen and David Stern, *None of These Diseases* (Grand Rapids: Revell, 2000), 18.
9. Reginald Cherry, *The Bible Cure*, (Harlan, IA: Guideposts, 1998), 27.
10. Hope Egan and Amy Cataldo, *What the Bible Says about Healthy Living Cookbook* (Shelbyville, TN: Heart of Wisdom Publishing, 2009),v.
11. Rex Russell, M.D., *What the Bible Says about Healthy Living* (Ventura, CA: Regal, 2006), 29.
12. *The New York Times,* March 17, 2005, http://www.nytimes.com (Accessed January 25, 2009).
13. The Mayo Clinic Staff, "Mediterranean diet: Choose this heart-healthy diet option," Mayo Clinic Online, http://www.mayoclinic.com/health/mediterranean-diet/CL00011 (Accessed October 2009).
14. Steve Parker, *The Advanced Mediterranean Diet: Lose Weight, Feel Better, Live Longer* (Gilbert, Arizona: Vanguard Press, 2007), 130.
15. To read the documented research, visit: http://www.oldwayspt.org/med_studies (accessed September 2009).
16 This song was taught to me by Dan and Joan Terry, CEF missionaries. The original author is unknown.
17. Charles and Frances Hunter, *Laugh Yourself Healthy* (Lake Mary, FL: Christian Life, 2008), 85-86.
18. B. Batmanghelidj, *Your Body's Many Cries for Water.* www.watercure.com. Accessed June 2009.
19. Sloan Barnett, *Green Goes with Everything* (New York: Atria Books, 2008), 172.

20. Russell, *What the Bible Says about Healthy Living*, 219.

21. The Nourisher, "Vonderplanitz and Campbell Douglass's testimony on Raw Milk," *Nourished Magazine* Online, December 2008, http://editor.nourishedmagazine.com.au. Also see: http://www.realmilk.com/milkcure.html (accessed September 2009).

22. J. Crewe, "Raw milk cures many diseases," *Certified Milk Magazine*, January 1929, 3-6.

23. Silas Weir Mitchell, Fat and Blood: An Essay on the Treatment of Certain Forms of Neurasthenia and Hysteria (Charleston, SC: BiblioBazaar, 2007) 119-154. Bernard MacFadden, *The Miracle of Milk: How to Use the Milk Diet Scientifically at Home* (Pierides Press, 2008), 55.

24. E. Mattick and J. Golding, "Relative value of raw and heated milk in nutrition," *The Lancet*, March 21, 1931, 703-6.

25. "Functional Domain of Bovine Milk," PubMed, June 2002, http://www.pubmedcentral. nih.gov/articlerender.fcgi?artid=128229.

26. Pat Hagan, "Untreated Milk Cuts Children's Allergies," Daily Mail, August 2006, http://www.dailymail.co.uk/health/article-399520/Untreated-milk-cuts-childrens-allergies.html.

27. http://journals.cambridge.org/action/display Abstract from Page=online&aid=887004, Accessed January 2009.

28. "Dairy Chemistry and Physics," University of Guelph, http://www.foodsci.uoguelph.ca/dairyedu/chem.html#vitamin.

29. M.L. Power et al., "The role of calcium in health and disease" *American Journal of Obstetricians & Gynecology*, 181:1560-9.

30. http://content.nejm.org/cgi/content/abstract/328/12/833 (kidney stones). M. Nishida et al., "Calcium and the risk for periodontal disease," *Journal of Periodontology* 71(7):1057-66.

31. K. Shahani, "Enzymes in Bovine Milk," Journal of Dairy Science, http://jds.fass.org/cgi/reprint/56/5/531.

32. T. Olivecrona et al., "Lipases in Milk," in *Advanced Dairy Chemistry: Vol. 1: Proteins*, 3rd ed., Patrick F. Fox and Paul McSweeney, eds. (New York: Springer, 1998), 473-488. Shakel-Ur-Rehman et al, "Indigenous Phosphatases in Milk" in *Advanced Dairy Chemistry: Vol. 1: Proteins*, 3rd ed., 523-533). K. Pruitt, "Lactoperoxidase" in *Advanced Dairy Chemistry: Vol. 1: Proteins*, 3rd ed., 563-568.

33. Chantal Matar, "The Effect of Milk Fermentation," *Journal of Dairy Science*, 1996, http://jds.fass.org/cgi/reprint/79/6/971 (accessed September 2009).

34. Russell, *What the Bible Says about Healthy Living*, 215.

35. J. M. Farberm, "Thermal Resistance of Listeria Monocytogenes in Inoculated and Naturally contaminated Raw Milk," *International Journal of Food Microbiology*, 7:4 (Dec. 1988): 277-286.

36. Russell, *What the Bible Says About Healthy Living*, 218.

37. Marie-Caroline Michalski and Caroline Januel, "Does homogenization affect the human health properties of cow's milk?" *Trends in Food Science & Technology,* 17:8 (August 2006): 423-37.
38. The George Mateljan Foundation, "Pasteurization," The World's Healthiest Foods Web site, http://whfoods.org/genpage.php?tname=george&dbid=149#answer (accessed June 2009).
39. Ibid., 219.
40. Russell, *What the Bible Says about Healthy Living,* 29.
41. Doris Rapp, *Is This Your Child's World* (New York: Quill, 1991) 59-60.
42. James Riddle, *The Complete Personalized Promise Bible* (Tulsa, Oklahoma: Harrison House, 2004),419.
43. Patrick J. Bird, Ph.D., "*Grape Juice and Heart Attacks,*" University of Florida College of Health and Human Performance web site: http://www.hhp.ufl.edu/keepingfit.
44. American Heart Association, "*The Heart-Healthy Cup Runneth Over—Grape Juice,*" Meeting Report, http://www.scienceblog.com/community/older/1998/A/199800317.html.
45. Joseph Maroon, *The Longevity Factor* (New York: Atria Books, 2009), 193.
46. Dr. Steve Chaney, interview by Annette Reeder.
47. "Organic Grape Juice," Organic Food Corner, http://www.organicfoodcorner.com/fruits/grape-juice.php (accessed September 2009).
48. Encarta Encyclopedia: English (North America) Microsoft Office Outlook 2003.
49. All data regarding the effects of alcohol are from the following: Sharon Rady Rolfes, Kathryn Pinna, and Ellie Whitney, *Understanding Normal and Clinical Nutrition,* 7th ed. (Belmont, CA: Wadsworth, 2007), 240-9.
50. Joyce Rogers, *The Bible's Seven Secrets to Healthy Eating* (Wheaton, IL: Crossway, 2001), 63.
51. James Riddle, *The Complete Personalized Promise Bible,* 491.
52. Rolfes, Pinna, and Whitney, *Understanding Normal and Clinical Nutrition,* 7th ed., 240-9.
53. L. Erickson, "Rooibos Tea: Research into antioxidant and antimutagenic properties," American Botanical Council's *Herbal Gram* 59 (2003): 34–45.
54. A. Rietveld and S. Wiseman, "Antioxidant effects of tea: evidence from human clinical trials," *Journal of Nutrition,* 133(10):3285S–3292S.
55. Brian Wansink, Ph.D., *Mindless Eating* (New York: Bantam Books, 2006), 189.
56. Miriam Feinberg Vamosh, *Food at the Time of the Bible,* (Nashville: Abingdon, 2004), 25.
57. Joyce Rogers, *The Bible's Seven Secrets to Healthy Eating* (Wheaton, IL: Crossway, 2001),
58. Russell, *What the Bible Says about Healthy Living,* 105-6.
59. Whole Grains Council, www.wholegrainscouncil.org (accessed May 20, 2009).
60. Phyllis Balch, Dietary Wellness, (Penguin Group, New York, 2003, 108.

61. J.G. Brook et al., "Dietary Soy Lecithin Decreases Plasma Triglyceride Levels and Inhibits Collagen and ADP Platelet Aggregation," *Biochem Med Metabol Biol* 35(1986): 31-9.

62. http://www.breadbeckers.com/phytic_acid_friend_or_foe.htm, Accessed October 2009. This article can also be found on the Designed Healthy Living website; www.designed-healthyliving.com.

63. Vamosh, *Food at the Time of the Bible*, 54-56.

64. Lendon Smith, *Feed Your Kids Right* (New York: Dell, 1081), 85.

65. www.wholegrainscouncil.org (accessed May 20, 2009).

66. Rolfes, Pinna, and Whitney, *Understanding Normal and Clinical Nutrition*, 7th ed., 52-53.

67. www.wholegrainscouncil.org (accessed June 2009).

68. www.wholegrainscouncil.org (accessed May 20, 2009). William Sears, *The Family Nutrition Book* (Little Brown and Company: New York, 1999). Sue Gregg, *A Busy Woman's Guide to Healthy Eating* (Eugene, OR: Harvest House, 2001). Donna Spann, *Grains of Truth* (Lorton, VA: Today's Family Matters, 2005). Marion Nestle, *What to Eat* (New York: North Point Press, 2004). Phyllis A. Balch, CNC, *Dietary Wellness* (New York: Avery, 2003).

69. EZ-Gest® is an enzyme product that supplies all the necessary enzymes to digest all food categories. It can be found at www.shaklee.com or www.mytreasures.myshaklee.com.

70. Carolyn Wyman, *Better Than Homemade* (Philadelphia, A: Quirk Books, 2004), as referenced in Wansink, *Mindless Eating*, 202.

71. Anonymous, "Position of the American Dietetic Association: Phytochemicals and Functional Foods," *Journal of American Dietetics Association* (April 1995): 493-6.

72. Russell, *What the Bible Says about Healthy Living*, 188.

73. Walter C. Willett, *Eat, Drink, and Be Healthy: The Harvard Medical School Guide to Eating Healthy* (New York: Simon & Schuster, 2001), 115.

74. American Cancer Society, "Cancer Facts & Figures 2008" citation (Atlanta: American Cancer Society, 2008).

75. K.J. Joshipura et al., "Fruits and Vegetable Intake in Relation to Risk of Ischemic Stroke," *Journal of the American Medical Association* 282 (1999): 1233-39.

76. Ibid., 120.

77. Ibid., 122.

78. Anonymous, "Mini Snack Portions Back," Tuft's Healthy Newsletter, September 2008, http://www.tuftshealthletter.com/ShowArticle.aspx?RowID=589 (accessed March 2009).

79. CDC, "Can Eating Fruits and Vegetables Help People Manage Their Weight," 2007, http://www.cdc.gov/nccdphp/dnpa/nutrition/pdf/rtp_practitioner_10_07.pdf (accessed March 2009).

80. Center for Nutrition Policy and Promotion, "Improving the nutrition and wellbeing of Americans," www.usda.gov/cnpp (accessed March 2009).

81. Ian Sample, "Organic Food Is Healthier," *The Guardian*, 2007, http://www.guardian.co.uk/science/2007/oct/29/organics.sciencenews (accessed August 2009).

82. EWG specializes in providing useful resources to consumers while simultaneously pushing for national policy change. Resources include Skin Deep (http://www.cosmeticsdatabase.com) and the Shoppers' Guide to Pesticides in Produce (http://www.foodnews.org/walletguide.php).

83. Environmental Working Group, "Shopper's Guide to Pesticides," 2009, http://www.foodnews.org/methodology.php (accessed May 2009).

84. Richard Brouse, M.D., "Jeopardizing the Future, Genetic Engineering, Food and the Environment," 2004.

85. Nestle, *What to Eat*, 56.

86. Caroline M. Apovian, M.D., FACN, Nutrition and Weight Management Center, "Foods-Fresh vs. Frozen or Canned," Medical Encyclopedia, 2007, http://www.drugs.com/search.php?searchterm=Caroline%20M.%20Apovian&is_main_search=1 (accessed January 16, 2009).

87. Russell, *What the Bible Says about Healthy Living*, 186

88. Ibid.

89. Wal-Mart, "Wal-Mart Commits to America's Farmers as Produce Goes Local," 2008, http://www.walmartstores.com (accessed January 29, 2009).

90. Rolfes, Pinna, and Whitney, *Understanding Normal and Clinical Nutrition*, 7th ed., 70.

91. Author unknown.

92. James A. Duke, Ph.D., *The Green Pharmacy* (Emmaus, PA: Rodale, 1997), 8.

93. Linda C. Tapsell, "Dietary Guidelines for Health—Where Do Herbs and Spices Fit?" *Nutrition Today* 43 (July/August 2008): 132-7.

94. Duke, *The Green Pharmacy*, 7.

95. Jethro Kloss, *Back to Eden* (Twin Lakes, WI: Lotus Press, 2005).

96. Elliot Essman, "Bitter is Better," Style Gourmet, 2007, http://www.stylegourmet.com/articles/020.htm. This article referenced the The Environment News Service reports. A recent review by Dr. Adam Drewnowski, at the University of Washington (UW) Nutritional Sciences Program.

97. This information was gathered from the following sources and other references listed. Wayne Little, "Discovery of Taste Receptor," National Institute Health, 2000, http://www.nih.gov/news/pr/mar2000/nidcr-16.htm (accessed June 2009). J. Kimball, "The Sense of Taste," Biology Pages Pdf, 2007, http://users.rcn.com/jkimball.ma.ultranet/BiologyPages/T/Taste.html. Elliot Essman, "Bitter is Better," Style Gourmet, 2007, http://www.stylegourmet.com/articles/020.htm.

98. Whole Foods Market, http://www.whfoods.org (accessed May 2009).

99. Rev. Tom Faggart, "On Making a Difference," Lectionary Sermons of the Week, June 2009, www.clergyresources.net (accessed June 2009).

100. Nestle, *What to Eat.*

101. Sharon Tyler Herbst and Ron Herbst, *The New Food Lovers Companion* (Hauppauge, NY: Barrons Educational Series, 2007).

102. Pamela Hoeppner, *The Breast Stays Put* (Longwood, FL: Xulon Press, 2008), 221.

103. Pamela Hoeppner, *The Breast Stays Put* (Publisher's Location: Xulon Press, 2008), 221-2.

104. Mike Adams, "Interview with Dr. Russell Blaylock on devastating health effects of MSG, aspartame and excitotoxins," NaturalNews.com, September 7, 2006, http://www.natural-news.com/020550.html (accessed June 2009).

105. Russell, *What the Bible Says About Healthy Living*, 136.

106. Udo Erasmus, *Fats that Heal, Fats that Kill: The Complete Guide to Fats, Oils, Cholesterol and Human Health* (BC Canada: Alive Books, 1993), 43.

107. Erasmus, *Fats that Heal, Fats that Kill*, 253. See also: Vamosh, *Food at the Time of the Bible*. Rolfes, Pinna, and Whitney, *Understanding Normal and Clinical Nutrition*, 7th ed. Marianne Ritchie, *Planning, Planting and Harvesting Your Herb Garden* (Richmond: Thyme to Plant, 2005). Jeffrey S. Bland et al., *Clinical Nutrition: A Functional Approach* (Washington: Institute for Functional Medicine, 2004). Sears, *The Family Nutrition Book*.

108. Erasmus, *Fats that Heal, Fats that Kill*, 438.

109. Willett, *Eat, Drink, and Be Healthy*.

110. Ibid.

111. Carol Johnston PhD, "Vinegar Helps Lower Blood Glucose," Arizona State University, 2008, http://researchstories.asu.edu/2008/01/vinegar_helps_lower_blood_gluc.html (accessed July 2009).

112. Amy Barclay de Tolly, "Edible Flowers," About.Com Home Cooking Guide, http://homecooking.about.com/library/weekly/blflowers.htm (accessed July 2009).

113. Charles Swindoll, *Laugh Again* (Dallas, TX: Word, 1992), 63.

114. John Piper, *Desiring God* (Sisters, OR: Multnomah, 1996), 26.

115. Russell, *What the Bible Says about Healthy Living*, 26.

116. Rogers, *The Bible's Seven Secrets to Healthy Eating*, 88.

117. Russell, *What the Bible Says about Healthy Living*, 28.

118. Rogers, *The Bible's Seven Secrets to Healthy Eating*, 146.

119. Bruce Miller, M.D., *Protein, A Consumer's Concern* (Dallas, TX: Bruce Miller Enterprises, 1997), 4.

120. Ibid., 12.

121. Ibid., 15.

122. Ibid., 25.
123. Erasmus, *Fats That Heal, Fats that Kill*, 43, 73.
124. Russell, *What the Bible Says about Healthy Living*, 146.
125. Bernard Ward, *Healing Foods from the Bible* (New York: Globe Communications, 1994) 69.
126. Erasmus, *Fats That Heal, Fats that Kill*, 234.
127. Won O. Song and Jean M. Kerver, "Nutritional Contribution of Eggs to American Diets," *Journal of the American College of Nutrition* 19 (90005): 556S-562S.
128. William Douglas, *The Milk of Human Kindness*, (Lakemont, GA: Copple House Books, 1985), 213.
129. Russell, *What the Bible Says about Healthy Living*, 149.
130. Russell, *What the Bible Says about Healthy Living*, 160.
131. David Meinz, *Eating by the Book* (Nashville, TN: Gilbert Press,1999).
132. D. Thomas Lancaster, *Man Alive! There's More, Holy Cow* (Marshfield, MO: Fruits of Zion), p. 55.
133. Elmer A. Josephson, *God's Key to Heath and Happiness* (New Jersey: Revell, 1962), 82.
134. Russell, *What the Bible Says About Healthy Living*, 154.
135. Jayne Hurley and Bonnie Liebman, "Lower-Fat: Hot Dogs, Bacon, & Sausage: The Best of the Worst," *Nutrition Action Health Newsletter* July/August 1998, http://www.cspinet.org/nah/7_98meat.htm (accessed September 2009).
136. Amalia Gagarina M.S. R.D., "Eating Processed Raises Stomach Cancer Risk," Armenian Medical Network, December 2007, http://www.health.am/cr/more/raises-stomach-cancer-risk.
137. Ted Broer, *Maximum Energy* (Lake Mary, FL: Siloam Press, 2006), 169.
138. Kevin Calci, "Hepatitis A Within Oysters," *Applied & Environmental Microbiology*, August 2004, http://www.pubmedcentral.nih.gov/articlerender.fcgi?artid=544230.
139. Texas Department of Health Service, "Risk of Eating Raw Oysters and Clams," http://www.dshs.state.tx.us/idcu/disease/hepatitis/hepatitis_c/overview/raw_oysters.
140. Boston News, "Tainted Canadian Clams Cause Illness," 2008, http://www.boston.com/news/local/maine/articles/2008/07/07/tainted_canadian_clams_cause_ illnesses/
141. Paula Baille Hamilton, M.D. *The Body Restoration Plan* (Pleasanton, CA: Shaklee, 2002).
142. Rogers, *The Bible's Seven Secrets to Healthy Eating*.
143. Stormie Omartian, *Greater Health God's Way* (Eugene, Oregon: Harvest House,1996), 207.
144. Ibid.
145. Elmer Towns, *Fasting for Spiritual Breakthrough* (Ventura, CA: Regal, 1996), 31.

146. Edward Rowell, 1001 Quotes, Illustrations, and Humorous Stories, (Grand Rapids, MI, Baker Books, 2008), 46.

147. Elmer Towns, Fasting for Spiritual Breakthrough, 52.

148. Michel Quoist, *The Christian Response* (Dublin: Gill and Macmillan, 1965), 4.

149. Jerry Bridges, *Pursuit of Holiness* (Colorado Springs: NavPress, 2001), 108.

150. John Kirk, *The Mother of the Wesleys* (Cincinnati: Poe and Hitchcock, 1865), 187. As quoted in Bridges, *Pursuit of Holiness*, 108.

151. Jerry Bridges, *The Fruitful Life* (Colorado Springs: NavPress, 2008), 155.

152. Ibid., 156.

153. Bridges, *Pursuit of Holiness*, 109.

154. Hunter and Hunter, *Laugh Yourself Healthy*, 83.

155. Bridges, *Pursuit of Holiness*, 110. The concept of this story comes from the teachings of Jerry Bridges.

156. Encarta Dictionary, North America, Microsoft Word Outlook 2003.

157. Bridges, *Pursuit of Holiness*, 102.

158. I highly recommend reading each of the following books for a much more in-depth study toward holiness. Jerry Bridges, *The Fruitful Life* and *Pursuit of Holiness*. Elmer Towns, *Fasting for Spiritual Breakthrough*. Stormie Omartian, *Greater Health God's Way*.

159. Penn State University, "Honey proves better option for childhood cough than OTC," LIVE, December 2007, http://live.psu.edu/story/27584 (accessed September 2009).

160. Ibid.

161. Vamosh, *Food at the Time of the Bible*, 70.

162. Medical Training Institute of America, "Honey Contributes to Strong Bones," Basic Care Bulletin.

163. Ibid.

164. Ibid.

165. Rolfes, Pinna, and Whitney, *Understanding Normal and Clinical Nutrition*, 7th ed.

166. Jacqueline Krohn, M.D., Frances Taylor, and Eria Mae Larson, *Allergy Relief & Prevention: A Doctor's Complete Guide to Treatment and Self-Care*, (Point Roberts, WA: Hartley & Marks, 2000), 126.

167. Annette Reeder, "Ingredients in Honey," in *Treasures of Health Nutrition Manual* (Washington: Pleasant Word, 2010).

168. Russell, *What the Bible Says about Healthy Living*, 174.

169. Ibid., 171.

170. Raymond Francis, M.Sc., *Never Be Sick Again* (Deerfield Beach, FL: Health Communications, 2002), 89-91.

171. Don Colbert, M.D., and Mary Colbert, *The Seven Pillars of Health*, (Lake Mary, FL, Siloam Press, 2007), 43.

172. Mary Shomon, "Adrenal Fatigue," About.com, 2003, http://thyroid.about.com/cs/endocrinology/a/adrenalfatigue_2.htm (accessed September 2009).

173. Information for "Sugar Can Harm Us" was acquired from the following sources. Rolfes, Pinna, and Whitney, *Understanding Normal and Clinical Nutrition*. Colbert and Colbert, *The Seven Pillars of Health*. Sears, *The Family Nutrition Book*. Krohn, Taylor, and Larson, *Allergy Relief & Prevention*.

174. Barbara Howard PhD., "Sugar and Cardiovascular Disease," American Heart Association, http://www.circ.ahajournals.org/cgi/content/full/106/4/523 (accessed October 2009). Colbert and Colbert, *The Seven Pillars of Health*, 81.

175. JL Farrar, PubMed "Inhibition of protein glycation by skins and seeds of the muscadine grape," Biofactors, 2007, http://www.ncbi.nlm.nih.gov/pubmed/18525113 (accessed July 2009).

176. Bland et al., *Clinical Nutrition a Functional Approach*, 247.

177. Katherine Zeratshy, R.D. , "High Fructose Corn Syrup Seems to Be a Common Ingredient in Many Foods," Mayoclinic.com, October 2008, http://www.mayoclinic.com/health/high-fructose-corn-syrup/an01588 (accessed July 2009).

178. Krohn, Taylor, and Larson, *Allergy Relief & Prevention*, 119-122.

179. Ibid.

180. Ibid.

181. These notes were compiled from my own experiences and from Sears, *The Family Nutrition Book*.

182. Encarta Dictionary, North America, Microsoft Word Outlook Express, 2003.

183. Elizabeth Lipski, M.S., C.C.N., *Leaky Gut Syndrome*, A Keats Good Health Guide (Publisher's Location: McGraw-Hill, 1998), 25.

184. H.A. Salme and S. Sarna, "Effect of silymarin on chemical, functional, and morphological alterations of the liver. A double blind controlled study." *Scandinavian Journal of Gastroenterology*, 17 (June 1982): 417-421.

185. Paula Baile-Hamilton, M.D., *Toxic Overload* (New York: Avery, 2005), 9.

186. Ibid.

187. Sloan Barnett, *Green Goes With Everything* (New York: Atria Books, 2008), 1-2.

188. Ibid.

189. U.S. Environmental Protection Agency Green Building Workgroup, "Buildings and the Environment: A Statistical Summary," December 20, 2004, http://www.epa.gov/greenbuilding/pubs/gbstats.pdf (accessed September 2009).

190. Baile-Hamilton, *Toxic Overload*, 9.

191. Edward Rowell, *1001 Quotes, Illustrations, and Humorous Stories*, 64.

192. Barnett, *Green Goes with Everything*, 84.

193. Ibid., 85.

194. The endocrine system involves the hormone system throughout the body. It is highly affected by stress.

195. A. Tzonou et al., "Hair dyes, analgesics, tranquilizers, and perineal talc application as risk factors for ovarian cancer," *International Journal of Cancer* 55(3): 408-410.

196. Krohn, Taylor, and Larson, *Allergy Relief & Prevention*, 2.

197. FDA, "Food Allergies: What you Need to Know," FDA Web Site, August 2009, http://www.fda.gov/Food/ResourcesForYou/Consumers/ucm079311.htm (accessed June 2009).

198. Recipe from: Shelly Ballestero, *Beauty By God* (Ventura, CA: Regal, 2009), 182.

199. Ibid., 136.

200. Steve Parker, M.D., "Chocolate Linked to Lower Cardiac Death Rate After First Heart Attack," Mediterranean Blog, September 2009, http://advancedmediterraneandiet.com/blog (accessed August 2009).

201. Ray Pritchard, *The Healing Power of Forgiveness* (Eugene, OR: Harvest House, 2005), 71.

202. Name withheld, used by permission.

203. Mayo Clinic Staff, "Forgiveness: How to Let Go of Bitterness and Grudges," The Mayo Clinic, Date, http://www.mayoclinic.com/health/forgiveness/MH00131 (accessed October 2009).

204. Pritchard, *The Healing Power of Forgiveness*, 49-50.

205. Organic Natural News, "Organic Chocolate," http://www.organic-nature-news.com/organic-chocolate.html (accessed August 2009).

206. Hunter and Hunter, *Laugh Yourself Healthy*, 156.

207. Personal testimony from Senior Pastor Jeff Brauer, Winn's Baptist Church, Glen Allen, Virginia. Pastor Brauer contributed greatly to the healthy living classes and also to this book. He is an encouragement to all pastors on the importance of health in the pulpit.

208. Personal testimony from Hunter Stoner, member of Richmond University cross country team and highly awarded Celtic dancer. Hunter is studying nutrition and physical fitness. She helped write this chapter, and her love for the Lord is evident in her life.

209. Rusty Wright and Linda Wright, *500 Clean Jokes and Humorous Stories* (Uhrichsville, OH: Barbour, 1998), 209.

210. Information on memorizing chapters and books comes from Dr. Andrew Davis, *An Approach to Extended Memorization of Scripture* (Durham, NC: First Baptist Church, no date). Used with permission.

211. Author unknown, "Children Saying Grace," *Inspirational Food for the Soul*, May 2006, www.inspirationalfood.com (Accessed October 2009).

212. Encarta Dictionary, North America, Microsoft Office Outlook 2003.

213. Ann Phi-Wendt, "The Health Benefits of Being Thankful," Public Radio International, 2008, http://www.pri.org/health/health-benefits-being-thankful.html (accessed July 2009).

214. Roger Dobson, *The Benefits of Being Positive*, April 2009, http://www.independent.co.uk/life-style/health-and-families/features/the-benefits-of-being-positive-1664288.html, Accessed October 2009.

215. Stormie Omartian's books include *The Power of a Praying Wife, The Power of the Praying Parent, The Power of Praying Together,* and *Praying God's Will for Your Life.* These are all excellent books to guide you in your prayer life.

216. Neil Chadwick, "Are You Jesus," Joyful Ministry, 2008, www.joyfulministry.com/apples (accessed July 2009).

217. Swindoll, *Laugh Again*, 126.

218. Normon Cousins, The Humor Foundation, "Research Findings," date unknown, http://www.humourfoundation.com.au/index.php?page=150, Accessed August 2009.

219. Swindoll, *Laugh Again*, 21.

220. Lloyd Cory, comp., "Jane Canfield," in *Quote/Unquote* (Wheaton: Victor Books, 1977), 144.

221. Swindoll, *Laugh Again*, 22.

222. Bridges, *The Fruitful Life*, 78.

223. Ibid., 77.

224. Renee C. Cobb, *Ten Steps to Revolutionize Your Life* (Richmond, VA: Make a Difference Pub, 1996), 205-206. Used with permission.

225. Ibid., 211.

226. These concepts are from the Bible study *Experiencing God* By Henry Blackaby, (Nashville, Tennessee, Lifeway Publications).

227. Charles Austin Miles, "In the Garden," 1912.

228. The training for the mission trips that I led included memorizing the Wordless Book. This presentation comes from CEF- Child Evangelism Fellowship. CEF's international head-quarters is in Warrenton, Missouri. The words in this study are going to be almost word for word from their literature since we encouraged everyone on the team to memorize the simplicity with which the salvation message can be presented. The Children's Ministry Resource Bible, CEF, Inc. Publishing 2003, has this same teaching and I recommend anyone acquire this Bible if you work with children.

Other Books by Annette and Dr. Richard Couey:

 Treasures of Health Nutrition Manual
Available soft cover and Kindle

 Healthy Treasures Cookbook
Available soft cover

 Daniel Fast
Available as download on website and Kindle

Many more to come - be watching and praying.

Designed Healthy Living
Changing lives one meal and a prayer at a time.

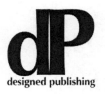
designed publishing

Designed Publishing Since 2004
Designed Healthy Living
Glen Allen, Virginia
804-798-6565
www.designedhealthyliving.com
Email: yourfriends@designedhealthyliving.com

CPSIA information can be obtained at www.ICGtesting.com
Printed in the USA
BVOW07s0458210214

345556BV00004B/47/P